AF745868

CARDIAC DEFIBRILLATION – MECHANISMS, CHALLENGES AND IMPLICATIONS

Edited by **Natalia Trayanova**

Cardiac Defibrillation – Mechanisms, Challenges and Implications
Edited by Natalia Trayanova

Published by InTech
Janeza Trdine 9, 51000 Rijeka, Croatia

Copyright © 2011 InTech
All chapters are distributed under the Creative Commons Non Commercial Share Alike Attribution 3.0 license, which permits to copy, distribute, transmit, and adapt the work in any medium, so long as the original work is properly cited. After this work has been published by InTech, authors have the right to republish it, in whole or part, in any publication of which they are the author, and to make other personal use of the work. Any republication, referencing or personal use of the work must explicitly identify the original source.

Statements and opinions expressed in the chapters are these of the individual contributors and not necessarily those of the editors or publisher. No responsibility is accepted for the accuracy of information contained in the published articles. The publisher assumes no responsibility for any damage or injury to persons or property arising out of the use of any materials, instructions, methods or ideas contained in the book.

Publishing Process Manager Romina Krebel

Technical Editor Teodora Smiljanic

Cover Designer InTech Design Team

Additional hard copies can be obtained from orders@intechopen.com

Cardiac Defibrillation – Mechanisms, Challenges and Implications,
Edited by Natalia Trayanova
p. cm.
ISBN 978-953-307-666-9

We are IntechOpen, the world's leading publisher of Open Access books

Built by scientists, for scientists

4,000+
Open access books available

116,000+
International authors and editors

120M+
Downloads

151
Countries delivered to

Our authors are among the
Top 1%
most cited scientists

12.2%
Contributors from top 500 universities

WEB OF SCIENCE™

Selection of our books indexed in the Book Citation Index in Web of Science™ Core Collection (BKCI)

Interested in publishing with us?
Contact book.department@intechopen.com

Numbers displayed above are based on latest data collected.
For more information visit www.intechopen.com

For EU product safety concerns:
IN TECH d.o.o., Prolaz Marije Krucifikse Kozulić 3, 51000 Rijeka, Croatia,
info@intechopen.com or visit our website at intechopen.com.

Meet the editor

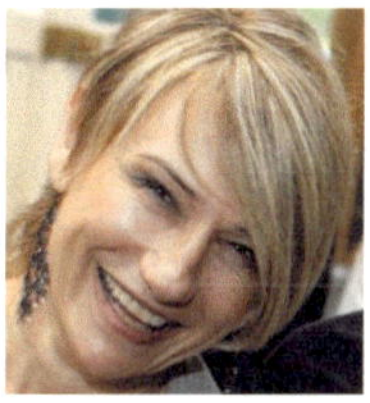

Dr. Natalia Trayanova is a Professor in the Department of Biomedical Engineering and the Institute for Computational Medicine at Johns Hopkins University, and holds an endowed professorship (William R. Brody Faculty Scholar). She is a Fellow of the Heart Rhythm Society, American Heart Association, and American Institute for Medical and Biological Engineering. She is the recipient of numerous awards, among which Excellence in Research and Scholarship Award (2005), Outstanding Researcher Award (2002), and Fulbright Distinguished Research Award (2002). She has published extensively and has presented at a large number of international meetings. Dr. Trayanova is Associate Editor of Frontiers in Computational Physiology and Medicine, served as Associate Editor of IEEE Transactions of Biomedical Engineering in the period 1997-2005, is on the Editorial Board of the journals Heart Rhythm and American Journal of Physiology (Heart and Circulatory System), and is an Area Editor of IEEE Reviews in Biomedical Engineering. Dr. Trayanova was the Vice-Chair in 2007 and the Chair in 2009 of the Gordon Research Conference on Cardiac Arrhythmia Mechanisms.

Contents

Preface

According to the American Heart Association, an overwhelming number of sudden cardiac deaths, estimated at about 400,000 per year, are thought to result from ventricular fibrillation, the most lethal of all cardiac rhythm disorders. Ventricular fibrillation is the breakdown of the organized electrical activity driving the heart's periodic pumping into disorganized self-sustained electrical activation patterns. A fibrillation episode results in the loss of cardiac outpu and, unless timely intervention takes place, death quickly ensues. Cardiac defibrillation, as achieved by the delivery of high-intensity electric shocks, is currently the only reliable treatment for ventricular fibrillation. Indeed, external defibrillators have long been used as standard therapy for ventricular fibrillation, and implantable cardioverter/defibrillators (ICDs) have been demonstrated to be an effective, lifesaving technology, superior to pharmacological therapy. Large, well-controlled prospective ICD trials have revolutionized the concept of sudden cardiac death prophylaxis. These studies have resulted in rapid growth of the patient populations for whom ICDs are indicated, with over 200,000 devices implanted every year throughout the world. In addition, over 100,000 external transthoracic defibrillators are installed in cardiac clinics, and a growing number of automatic external defibrillators are being used in public places and in households.

The increasingly large and diverse populations of patients with ICDs have exposed some of the limitations of this clinical technology. Although mean defibrillation thresholds typically range from 7 to 11J, ICDs are designed to provide up to 40J shocks. This is to accommodate the nearly 25% of patients, which have higher defibrillation thresholds, requiring programming of the ICD at near maximum output. Clinical studies have recognized the desirability of reducing shock strength, and over 200 papers have been published in the last 10 years on the topic of defibrillation thresholds. Reducing shock strength remains a major challenge to clinical defibrillation.

Although ICD therapy has proved to be efficient and reliable in preventing sudden cardiac death, defibrillation is a traumatic experience. The therapy is painful and could be detrimental to cardiac function. Furthermore, clinical data from ICD trials have suggested that 6 out of 7 shocks delivered are classified as inadequate. Issues related to inappropriate and unnecessary shocks as well as patient risk stratification and post-

ICD cardiac rehabilitation are essential to the delivery of appropriate care to ICD recipients.

Additionally, certain special populations of patients are poorly served by current ICD technology. These include children and patients of small body size. Unique difficulties surround cardiac defibrillation in the pediatric population, including high rates of lead failure, frequent inappropriate therapy, and the mismatch of device and lead size to the body.

Many of the advances in defibrillation have been accomplished through the developments in hardware and software and by experimental trial and error. Further advances in the clinical procedure of defibrillation will require increased knowledge of the basic mechanisms by which the electric fields interact with heart tissue. Therefore, research on defibrillation mechanisms, particularly aimed at developing low-voltage defibrillation strategies, remains an important basic science topic.

The objective of this book is to present contemporary views on the challenges and implications of cardiac defibrillation, and specifically, on the subjects presented above. Basic science chapters elucidate questions such as lead configurations and the reasons by which a defibrillation shock fails. The chapters devoted to the challenges in the clinical procedure of defibrillation address issues related to inappropriate and unnecessary shocks, complications associated with the implantation of ICD devices, and the application of the therapy in pediatric patients and young adults. The book also examines the implications of defibrillation therapy, such as patient risk stratification, cardiac rehabilitation, and remote monitoring of patient with implantable devices.

Natalia Trayanova, PhD
Johns Hopkins University, MD, Baltimore
USA

Part 1

Basic Mechanisms of Defibrillation

1

Mechanisms of Defibrillation Failure

Takashi Ashihara[1], Jason Constantino[2] and Natalia A. Trayanova[2]
[1]Shiga University of Medical Science,
[2]Johns Hopkins University,
[1]Japan
[2]U.S.A.

1. Introduction

Since defibrillation by high-energy electric shocks is the only effective means for termination of ventricular fibrillation, defibrillation shocks are now widely used in clinical practice for prevention of sudden cardiac death. However, the high-energy shocks could result in myocardial dysfunction and damage (Runsio et al., 1997) and in psychological trauma (Maisel, 2006). Comprehensive understanding of the ventricular response to electric shocks as well as the mechanisms of defibrillation failure is the approach most likely to succeed in reducing shock energy.

Recent experimental techniques, such as high-resolution mapping with multi-electrodes or optical recordings, have provided new characterizations of tissue responses to electric shocks. However, the mechanisms of the success and failure of defibrillation are not fully understood since the presently available experimental techniques, which provide detailed information about the myocardial surface (mostly epicardial) activity, are insufficient in resolving depth information during and after the electric shocks. Moreover, electrical or optical signal artifacts during the shock make it difficult for the researchers to get direct evidence regardig the mechanisms of electrical defibrillation.

It has been demonstrated experimentally that after the delivery of shocks of strength near the defibrillation threshold (DFT) from an implantable cardioverter-defibrillator (ICD) device, the first global activation consistently arises focally on the left ventricle (LV) (Chattipakorn et al., 2001, 2003) following an isoelectric window (a quiescent period following the shock). Understanding the origins of the isoelectric window is thus of great importance for uncovering the mechanisms of defibrillation failure. Various hypothesis have been proposed for the existence of the isoelectric window, including virtual electrode-induced propagated graded response (Trayanova et al., 2003), calcium sinkholes (Hwang et al., 2006), and activations emanating from Purkinje fibers (Dosdall et al., 2007); however, the mechanisms responsible for it remain inconclusive.

In this context, we hypothesized that submerged "tunnel propagation" of postshock activation (PA) through shock-induced intramural excitable areas underlies both fibrillation induction and failed defibrillation by shocks as well as the existence of an isoelectric window. To test this hypothesis, we analyzed the global three-dimensional activity in ventricles with the use of a recently-developed realistic computer model of stimulation/defibrillation in the rabbit heart (Trayanova et al., 2002). Simulations with this

model, termed the rabbit bidomain model of defibrillation, have proven invaluable in understanding various aspects of the response of the heart to shocks (Rodriguez et al., 2005). The bidomain model is a continuum representation of the myocardium, which takes into account both intracellular and extracellular current distributions through the myocardium.
The objectives of this book chapter are to demonstrate the use of the realistic three-dimensional bidomain rabbit ventricular model and failed defibrillation in uncovering the mechanisms of fibrillation induction and defibrillation failure.

2. Similarities between fibrillation induction and failed defibrillation

An isoelectric window (Chen et al., 1986a), the quiescent period prior to the first global PA, has been experimentally documented following strong shocks. The presence of the isoelectric window following failed defibrillation attempts (Chen et al., 1986a; Shibata et al., 1988b; Wang et al., 2001) led to the understanding that an electric shock terminates ongoing fibrillation but then reinitiates it. Hence, the mechanisms of fibrillation induction and its reinitiation (failed defibrillation) are considered to be the same. Thus, elucidating the origin of PAs resulting in fibrillation induction provides invaluable insight into the mechanisms of defibrillation failure and could contribute significantly in finding novel ways to appreciably lower the shock energy.
Indeed, striking similarities between these mechanisms have been found, particularly with regard to the propagation of the first global PA and the duration of the isoelectric window (Shibata et al., 1988a, 1988b; Wang et al., 2001). The similarity is supported by the significant correlation between the upper limit of vulnerability (ULV) and DFT (Chen et al., 1986b; Swerdlow et al., 1998). Based on these facts, we first focused on the mechanism responsible for the earliest-propagating PA in fibrillation induction by the electric shock, and then we extend the study to defibrillation failure.

3. Fibrillation induction following external shock

First, we conducted simulations of fibrillation induction following uniform-field external shocks with the use of the rabbit bidomain ventricular model, extensively validated with experimental measurements (Rodriguez et al., 2005). Biphasic shocks were delivered via plate electrodes located in the vicinity of RV and LV free walls (Figure 1A). The ventricles were immersed in the perfusing bath.
Figure 1B shows examples of arrhythmia non-induction and induction after 16- and 12-V/cm shocks, which are just above and near the ULV, respectively. Virtual electrodes (regions of positive and negative membrane polarization) induced by the shock (shock end, 0-ms panels) resulted in quick excitation of the ventricular surface (10-ms panels). Whereas no PA was induced by the 16-V/cm shock, for the 12-V/cm shock case, the earliest-propagated PA (arrows in 55-ms panel) led to the establishment of ventricular fibrillation (VF) (80-ms panel) following an isoelectric window.
The origin of the initiating PA following the 12-V/cm shock is analyzed in Figure 1C. The initiating PA originated at the boundary between a recovered area unaffected by the shock and the shock-induced depolarized area as a virtual electrode-induced propagated graded response (zigzag arrow in 10-ms panel). This occurred deep within the LV wall, and the initiating PA proceeded transmurally toward the LV epicardium (20-ms panel), where tissue had already recovered, and became the earliest-propagated PA.

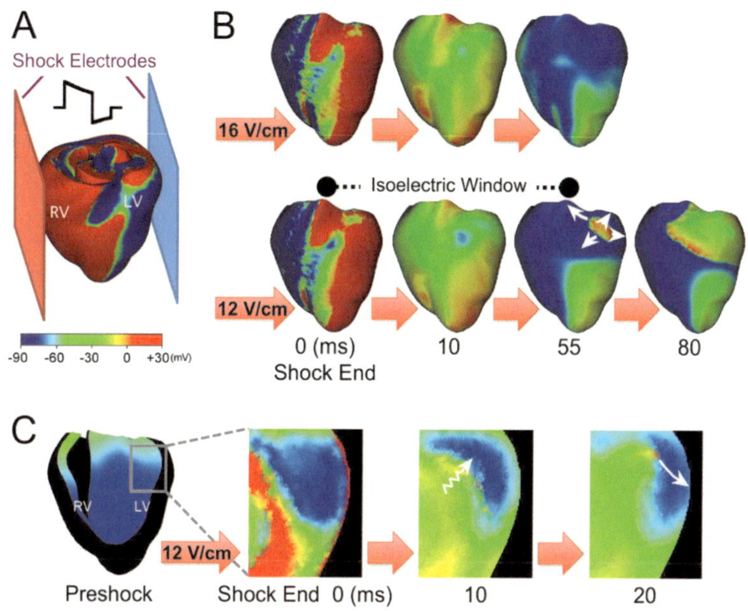

Fig. 1. Fibrillation induction following external biphasic shock.

4. Defibrillation failure following an ICD shock

We then extended the simulation study to electrical defibrillation by nonuniform-field ICD shocks. Biphasic shocks were delivered via ICD electrodes, a catheter in RV and an active can in the bath near the posterior LV (Figure 2A). For near-DFT shock episodes, we examined PA origins, and we found that around half of the earliest-propagated PAs originated from shock-induced wavefronts and the other half from pre-existing wavefronts. This means that failed defibrillation for near-DFT shocks is not always associated with termination of pre-existing wavefronts and generation of new wavefronts by the shock.

As shown in Figure 2B, the postshock excitable area in the RV after near-DFT shocks was directly depolarized by the shock and the one in the septum was immediately eradicated by break excitations elicited by the shock (black circles in 0- and 17-ms panels), whereas the main postshock excitable area was consistently located within the LV wall (red ellipsoid in 17-ms panel) since ICD electrodes generate weak virtual electrode polarization across the thick LV wall. Thus, the majority of postshock LV excitable area resulted from pre-existing excitable gaps during VF at the time of shock. This means that the larger excitable area in the LV wall allowed for postshock wavefronts of different origins to propagate unobstructed, increasing the likelihood of defibrillation failure. Thus, defibrillation shock outcome was affected by the preshock state.

As shown in Figure 2C, whereas the earliest-propagated PA arose on the epicardium immediately after the 75-V shock end (white arrows in top panel), the increase in shock strength to 100 V changed the type of the earliest-propagated PA into a delayed breakthrough after an isoelectric window (middle panel). Further increase in the shock strength to 175 V caused the prolongation of the isoelectric window from 35 to 50 ms (compare middle and bottom panels). These simulation results suggest that high strength shocks caused the entire epicardium to become refractory and created midmyocardial excitable tunnel, through which a submerged initiating PA propagated during the isoelectric window, i.e., tunnel propagation occurred. After the isoelectric window, the initiating PA became the earliest-propagated PA, often reinitiating VF.

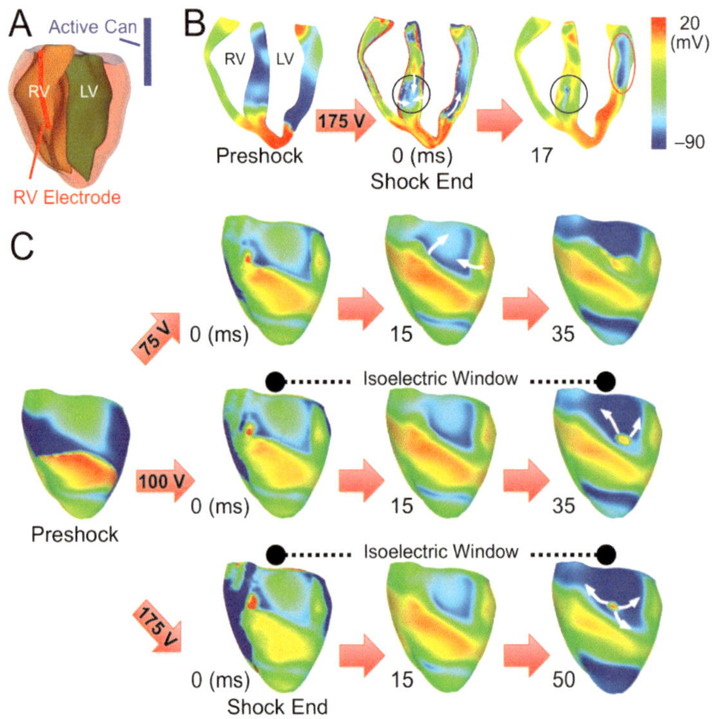

Fig. 2. Failed defibrillation following ICD shock.

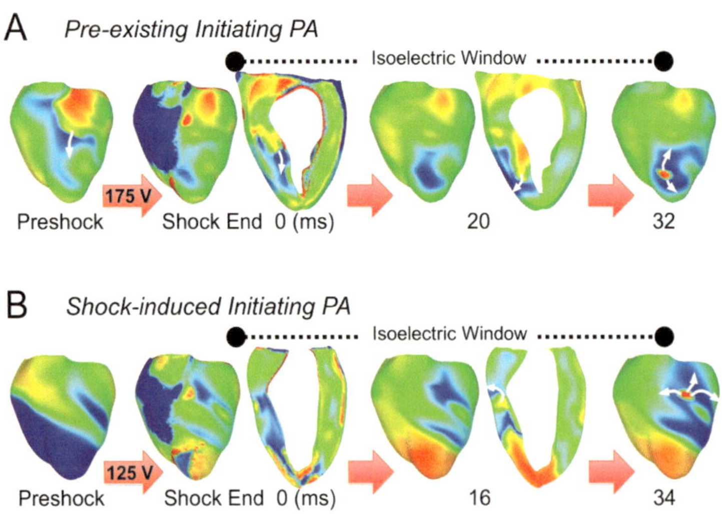

Fig. 3. Examples of initiating PA following ICD shock.

We classified the events depending on the origin of the initiating PA, which was either pre-existing fibrillatory or shock-induced wavefront.

Figure 3A shows an example of the tunnel propagation of pre-existing initiating PA after the near-DFT shock. A pre-existing fibrillatory epicardial wavefront (arrow in preshock panel) became submerged at shock end (arrow in 0-ms panel) and propagated within the midmyocardial tunnel following the 175-V shock (arrow in 20-ms panel). The tunnel formation and the submerging of the wavefront were due to the epicardium becoming refractory after this near-DFT shock (compare epicardial regions in 0- and 20-ms panels), resulting in an isoelectric window of LV epicardium. Tunnel propagation ended in a breakthrough (exit from the tunnel) on the near LV apex after the isoelectric window (32-ms panel), causing the shock to fail.

In contrast, Figure 3B shows an example of the tunnel propagation of initiating PA induced by near-DFT shock. There was no pre-existing wavefront, resulting in initiating PA at shock end (0-ms panel). After the 125-V shock, a new shock-induced wavefront propagated intramurally through the LV tunnel (arrow in 16-ms panel), emerging focally on the LV epicardium after the isoelectric window (34-ms panel), and causing the shock to fail.

5. Implications of the tunnel propagation hypothesis

The external monophasic shock study from our group (Rodriguez et al., 2005) demonstrated that shock outcome and the type of postshock arrhythmia depend on the distribution of the intramural excitable area (tunnel) formed by shock-induced deexcitation of previously refractory myocardium. We extended these findings and proposed the "tunnel propagation" hypothesis (Ashihara et al., 2008) for shock-induced arrhythmiogenesis that unifies all known aspects and findings regarding the postshock electric behavior of the heart, e.g., mechanisms of PA origin and isoelectric window after electric shocks, and the increase in isoelectric window duration for high strength shocks. Furthermore, we found that the tunnel propagation hypothesis is applicable to not only arrhythmia induction with external uniform-field shocks (Ashihara et al., 2008) but also defibrillation failure following nonuniform-field ICD shocks (Constantino et al., 2010).

As previously suggested by the ULV hypothesis (Chen et al., 1986a; Shibata et al., 1988b; Wang et al., 2001), failed defibrillation by near-DFT shock may result from the reinitiation of VF following the isoelectric window since the pre-existing VF is entirely terminated by the shock (Figure 4A). If this is the case, the shock outcome must not be affected by the preshock state of ventricles. However, both defibrillation shock outcome and the DFT have probabilistic nature (Davy et al., 1987; Yashima et al., 2003). The tunnel propagation hypothesis (Figure 4B) explains surmises that for successful defibrillation, pre-existing wavefronts may not be terminated by the strong shock but instead remain hidden in the intramural tunnel, in contrast to what was previously believed. Moreover, the tunnel propagation hypothesis can link defibrillation shock outcome to the preshock state of the ventricles. Based on the tunnel propagation hypothesis, both pre-existing and new shock-induced wavefronts propagate through the intramural excitable tunnel during the isoelectric window before the reinitiation of VF (defibrillation failure), and therefore the probability of defibrillation failure varies depending on the timing of shock delivery during VF. In fact, here we observed in the simulations that postshock propagation within the LV mid-myocardium was strongly dependent on preshock state.

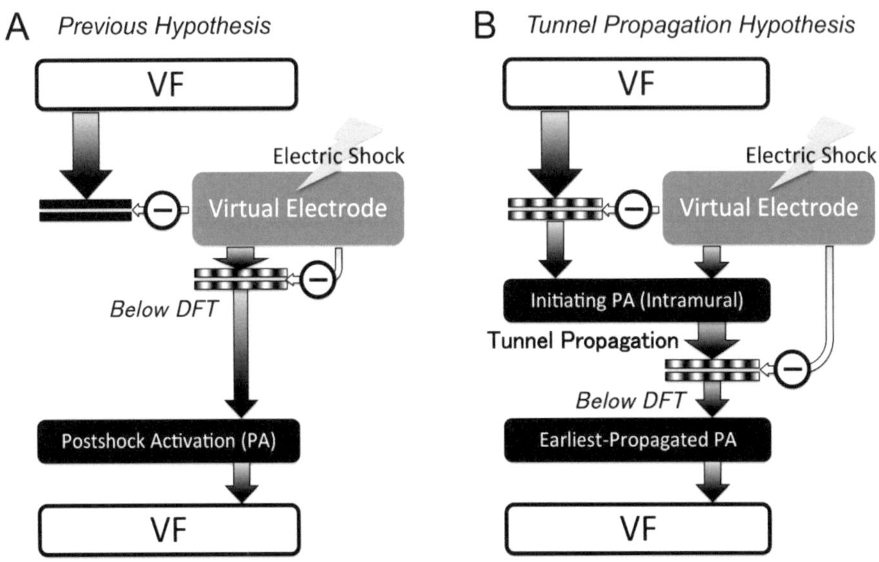

Fig. 4. Comparison between the previous hypothesis for VF reinitiation and the tunnel propagation hypothesis.

However, the concepts proposed here do not limit the origin of the initiating PAs; these might have alternative origins, such as Purkinje fibers (Dosdall et al., 2007). The tunnel hypothesis is independent of the origin of wavefronts that propagate through it.

The increase in isoelectric window after high strength shock can also be explained by the prolongation of the epicardial refractoriness (surface polarization), resulting in the longer tunnel propagation. This is because intramural virtual electrode polarization is lower magnitude than surface polarization (Entcheva et al., 1999) and thus the LV mid-myocardium, less affected by the shock, still contributes to the excitable tunnel even for higher strength shocks.

Considering the high probability of the existence of the postshock excitable tunnel even for above-DFT shocks, defibrillation success may be explained by the fact that initiating PAs, originating within the wall, cannot find an excitable exit onto the epicardium and die out in the mid-myocardium. Obtaining such insight into the mechanisms of defibrillation would have been impossible with the use of experimentation alone.

6. Conclusion

The tunnel propagation hypothesis, as part of the set of mechanisms operating during defibrillation, is expected to shed light on possible strategies for lowering DFT as well as for developing new defibrillation devices.

7. Funding sources

This work was supported by Grant-in-Aid 21790717, 22136011, and 21500420 for Scientific Research from the Ministry of Education, Culture, Sports, Science, and Technology of Japan (to T.A.), and by NIH grants R01 HL082729 and R01 HL103428 and NSF grant CBET-0933029 (to N.T.).

8. References

Ashihara, T.; Constantino, J. & Trayanova, N. A. (2008). Tunnel propagation of postshock activations as a unified hypothesis for fibrillation induction and isoelectric window. Circ Res, Vol. 102, pp. 737-745

Chattipakorn, N.; Banville, I.; Gray, R. A. & Ideker, R. E. (2001). Mechanism of ventricular defibrillation for near-defibrillation threshold shocks: a whole-heart optical mapping study in swine. Circulation, Vol. 104, pp. 1313-1319

Chattipakorn, N.; Fotuhi, P. C.; Chattipakorn, S. C. & Ideker, R. E. (2003). Three-dimensional mapping of earliest activation after near-threshold ventricular defibrillation shocks. J Cardiovasc Electrophysiol, Vol. 14, pp. 65-69

Chen, P-S.; Shibata, N.; Dixon, E. G.; Wolf, P. D.; Danieley, N. D.; Sweeney, M. B.; Smith, W. M. & Ideker, R. E. (1986). Activation during ventricular defibrillation in open-chest dogs: evidence of complete cessation and regeneration of ventricular fibrillation after successful shocks. J Clin Invest, Vol. 77, pp. 810-823

Chen, P-S.; Shibata, N.; Dixon, E. G.; Martin, R. O. & Ideker, R. E. (1986). Comparison of the defibrillation threshold and the upper limit of vulnerability. Circulation, Vol. 73, pp. 1022-1028

Constantino, J.; Long, Y.; Ashihara, T. & Trayanova, N. A. (2010). Tunnel propagation following defibrillation with ICD shocks: hidden postshock activations in the left ventricular wall underlie isoelectric window. Heart Rhythm, Vol. 7, pp. 953-961

Davy, J. M.; Fain, E. S.; Dorian, P. & Winkle, R. A. (1987). The relationship between successful defibrillation and delivered energy in open-chest dogs: reappraisal of the defibrillation threshold concept. Am Heart J, Vol. 113, pp. 77-84

Dosdall, D. J.; Cheng, K. A.; Huang, J.; Allison, J. S.; Allred, J. D.; Smith, W. M. & Ideker, R. E. (2007). Transmural and endocardial Purkinje activation in pigs before local myocardial activation after defibrillation shocks. Heart Rhythm, Vol. 4, pp. 758-765

Entcheva, E.; Trayanova, N. & Claydon, F. J. (1999). Patterns of and mechanisms for shock-induced polarization in the heart: a bidomain analysis. IEEE Trans Biomed Eng, Vol. 46, pp. 260-270

Hwang, G-S.; Hayashi, H.; Tang, L.; Ogawa, M.; Hernandez, H.; Tan, A-Y.; Li, H.; Karagueuzian, H. S.; Weiss, J. N.; Lin, S-F. & Chen, P-S. (2006). Intracellular calcium and vulnerability to fibrillation and defibrillation in Langendorff-perfused rabbit ventricles. Circulation, Vol. 114, pp. 2595-2603

Maisel, W. H. (2006). Pacemaker and ICD generator reliability; meta-analysis of device registries. JAMA, Vol. 295, pp. 1929-1934

Rodriguez, B.; Li, L.; Eason, J. C.; Efimov, I. R. & Trayanova N. A. (2005). Differences between left and right ventricular chamber geometry affect cardiac vulnerability to electric shocks. Circ Res, Vol. 97, pp.168-175

Runsio, M.; Kallner, A.; Kallner, G.; Rosenqvist, M. & Bergfeldt, L. (1997). Myocardial injury after electrical therapy for cardiac arrhythmias assessed by troponin-T release. Am J Cardiol, Vol. 79, pp. 1241-1245

Shibata, N.; Chen, P-S.; Dixon, E. G.; Wolf, P. D.; Danieley, N. D.; Smith, W. M. & Ideker, R. E. (1988). Influence of shock strength and timing on induction of ventricular arrhythmias in dogs. Am J Physiol, Vol. 255, pp. H891-H901

Shibata, N.; Chen, P-S.; Dixon, E. G.; Wolf, P. D.; Danieley, N. D.; Smith, W. M. & Ideker, R. E. (1988). Epicardial activation after unsuccessful defibrillation shocks in dogs. Am J Physiol, Vol. 255, pp. H902-H909

Swerdlow, C. D.; Kass, R. M.; O'Connor, M. E. & Chen, P-S. (1998). Effect of shock waveform on relationship between upper limit of vulnerability and defibrillation threshold. J Cardiovasc Electrophysiol, Vol. 9, pp. 339-349

Trayanova, N.; Eason, J. & Aguel, F. (2002). Computer simulations of cardiac defibrillation: a look inside the heart. Comput Visual Sci, Vol. 4, pp. 259-270

Trayanova, N.; Gray, R. A.; Bourn, D. W. & Eason, J. C. (2003). Virtual electrode-induced positive and negative graded responses: new insights into fibrillation induction and defibrillation. J Cardiovasc Electrophysiol, Vol. 14, pp. 756-763

Wang, N-C.; Lee, M-H.; Ohara, T.; Okuyama, Y.; Fishbein, G. A.; Lin, S-F.; Karagueuzian, H. S. & Chen, P-S. (2001). Optical mapping of ventricular defibrillation in isolated swine right ventricles: demonstration of a postshock isoelectric window after near-threshold defibrillation shocks. Circulation, Vol. 104, pp. 227-233

Yashima, M.; Kim, Y-H.; Armin, S.; Wu, T-J.; Miyauchi, Y.; Mandel, W. J., Chen, P-S. & Karagueuzian, H. S. (2003). On the mechanism of the probabilistic nature of ventricular defibrillation threshold. Am J Physiol Heart Circ Physiol, Vol. 284, pp. H249-H255

2

The Role of the Purkinje System in Defibrillation

Edward J Vigmond[1], Patrick M. Boyle[1] and Makarand Deo[2]
[1]*University of Calgary*
[2]*University of Michigan*
[1]*Canada*
[2]*U.S.A.*

1. Introduction

Only relatively recently have we begun to understand how defibrillation shocks work on the mechanistic level (Cheng et al., 1999; Trayanova & Skouibine, 1998). Virtual electrode polarization has offered a plausible mechanism for explaining far field effects of defibrillation shocks. However, this body of work has not considered the role of the specialized cardiac conduction system, the Purkinje System (PS), in the defibrillation process.

Despite its crucial role in activation, relatively little is known about the role of the PS in defibrillation. This is due to several factors which make recording from it challenging: The PS is a fine structure lying on the endocardium which makes it difficult to see and impale with microelectrodes. While Langendorf preparations allow easy access to the epicardium for optical recordings, the PS lies on the endocardium and is, therefore, much harder to access while maintaining the integrity of the ventricles. Depending on species, the PS penetrates various depths into the myocardium, masking midmyocardial activation. Plunge electrodes are one option for recording from the midmyocardium, but amplifier saturation immediately following large shocks would lose important information. Since the PS fibres are fine, the signals produced by them are very small and get easily swamped by signals from the myocardium. This is true for both electrical and optical recordings. Computer modelling, therefore, offers an attractive platform for studying the role of the PS in defibrillation, since the electrical activity everywhere in the system is known and can be visualized.

2. Description of the Purkinje System

The specialized conduction system begins at the atrioventricular node with the bundle of His. The His bundle runs through the ventricular septum, and bifurcates into the left and right Tawara branches, which further subdivide into major fascicles and later form a network on the endocardial surface. There are three major fascicles in the left ventricle, and two in the right.

A large portion of the conduction system is located within the ventricular cavities and is termed free running. Fibres that run within the ventricular walls are very difficult to visualize, requiring histological examination. Referring to the PS network as a tree is incorrect since, unlike true tree structures, fibres follow paths which join back together and at the final level,

forming more of a mesh-like topology. This may give redundancy to the network so that a part of the PS may fail without comprising sinus activation.
Segments of the PS run as bundles wrapped in collagen sheaths. This is easily seen in the bundle of His, which is a large trunk of many fibres. At branch points of thicker fibre bundles, individual fibres do not bifurcate. However, in the distal PS, where a network segment may be formed from a few fibres, individual fibres may branch. Longitudinal coupling is very strong, while lateral connections are sparser.
The PS is electrically isolated from the myocardium except for the termini of the network, where Purkinje-Myocyte Junctions (PMJs) are formed. While the PS can be selectively stained and visualized on the endocardium, determining PMJ locations is difficult. PMJs may be located well within the ventricular wall, which means that histological examination is necessary. Currently, the number of functional PMJs is not well characterized. Although the density of the PS on the endocardium appears high, the number of penetrating segments is unknown, as is the number of PMJs that successfully transmit pulses (Morley et al., 2005).
There are significant species differences in the degree of transmural penetration of terminal PS fibres. Species can roughly be grouped into three categories (Canale et al., 1986): Group 1 comprises the ungulates which have deeply penetrating fibres, reaching almost to the epicardium. Group 2 includes primates and carnivores which have PS termini that penetrate about 1/3 of the way through the wall. Group 3 contains rodents with very little penetration of the PS into the myocardial wall. This factor may be especially important for interpreting experimental results between species.

3. Modeling methods

Modelling the reaction of the of the ventricles and PS to defibrillation shocks is a computationally demanding task since the timestep during the defibrillation pulse must be very small. This is because high field strengths induce rapid changes in model parameters, and numerical instabilities may develop Vigmond et al. (2008). Lastly, ionic models are developed under normal physiological conditions. Defibrillation shocks are outside the bounds of the models developed so additional measures need be taken such as adding an ionic current to properly account for high voltage responses Ashihara & Trayanova (2004).
The bidomain equations are the most complete macroscopic description of cardiac tissue, even being predictive of polarization patterns(Sepulveda et al., 1989) induced by extracellular stimulation. They can be cast into a elliptical and parabolic equation:

$$\nabla \cdot (\bar{\sigma}_i + \bar{\sigma}_e) \nabla \phi_e = -\nabla \cdot \bar{\sigma}_i \nabla V_m - I_e \quad (1)$$

$$\nabla \cdot \bar{\sigma}_i \nabla V_m = -\nabla \cdot \bar{\sigma}_i \nabla \phi_e + \beta I_m \quad (2)$$

where subscripts i and e denote intra- or extracellular quantities respectively, ϕ is potential, $\bar{\sigma}$ is the conductivity tensor, I_e is an applied extracellular stimulus current, β is the surface to volume ratio, and I_m is the transmembrane current. Another set of ordinary differential equations is required to model the flow of the ions across the cell membrane and is embedded in I_m. These equations can be solved using an operator splitting method where extracellular potential (Eqn. 1), ionic currents, and the transmembrane voltage (Eq. 2 are solved sequentially (Vigmond et al., 2008).

The system is solved by using the finite element method. In our simulations, rabbit ventricular geometry (Vetter & McCulloch, 1998) was discretized at approximately 350 μm resolution resulting in about 550,000 nodes comprising the myocardium and another 300,000 nodes comprising the cavities and a surrounding bath. The PS was modelled as a network of one dimensional cubic Hermite finite elements added within the myocardial mesh (Vigmond & Clements, 2007). Two methods have been used to generate PSs for computer modelling studies: One approach is more generic and does not rely on mapping a particular PS. The endocardia of the two ventricles are unrolled and the PS drawn on according to basic physiological principles outlined in the preceding section (Vigmond & Clements, 2007). A fractal method could be used to further increase the endocardial mesh density (Ijiri et al., 2008). The second approach uses high resolution imaging to reconstruct the free running PS (see Fig. 1). This may further be augmented by staining the PS to reveal the endocardial mesh. With either method, the insertion of the PS into the myocardium must follow a rule-based method since the PS cannot be imaged within the myocardium, but requires careful histological examination, electron microscopy or genetic tagging (Miquerol et al., 2004). to reveal its transmural course (Ono et al., 2009). Furthermore, while the endocardial network appears dense, the number of functional PMJs is far less (Morley et al., 2005). The one-dimensional cubic Hermite finite elements are only electrically connected to the myocardium at end points through gap junctions. Due to their higher polynomial order, cubic Hermite elements possess the property that they can enforce current continuity at junctions, as well as at PMJs. Discretization of the PS was at the cellular length level with discrete gap junctions.

Since the discretization of the finite element model is much coarser than the actual physical PMJ structure, a phenomenological approach is followed whereby a single PS terminus stimulates a volume of myocardium. The current flowing from the PS into a myocardial node is given by

$$i_{PMJ} = \frac{1}{R_{PMJ}}(V_m^{PS} - V_m^{myo}) \tag{3}$$

and i_{PMJ} is treated as an intracellular stimulus by the myocardium.

From the PS perspective, the currents are handled as explicit boundary conditions:

$$i_L = \frac{1}{K\,R_{PMJ}} \sum_j (V_m^{PS} - V_{m,j}^{myo}) i_L = \tag{4}$$

where j is the set of myocardial nodes coupled to a PS terminus, and K is a scaling factor which accounts for the current amplification by transitional cells which occurs at scales finer than that discretized. By setting R_{PMJ} and K, it is possible to recreate asymmetric propagation across the PMJ with an anterograde transmission delay on the order of 5 ms and retrograde transmission delay on the order of 1 ms as observed experimentally Huelsing et al. (1998); Wiedmann et al. (1996).

4. Role in fibrillation

It is important to first understand the role of the PS in fibrillation. It has been implicated as a major player in the initiation and maintenance of fibrillation. First, the PS can be a source of focal firing. Chemical ablation of the PS by Lugol's solution, to selectively remove the endocardial layer and the PS embedded within it, has been shown to greatly diminish repetitive endocardial focal discharges and eliminate sustained VF (Wu et al., 2009). Part of this comes from the intrinsic nature of the Purkinje cells, which are resistant to ischemia because of large glycogen stores (Streit, 1987). This is especially important in long duration VF, at which point much of the myocardium has been compromised.

Second, the PS can provide alternative pathways for reentrant pathways. This is supported by experiments wherein chemical ablation of the PS has also been shown to reduce the inducibility of ventricles to VF(Armiger & Knell, 1988; Dosdall et al., 2008) In agreement, computer simulations have also shown an increase in VF vulnerability to large shocks when a PS is present (Deo et al., 2009). Several factors were identified which were responsible for the arrhythmogenic influence of the PS: 1) The presence of a PS produces more activations, which directly lead to reentrant activity. 2) The frequency of scroll waves is increased since the PS accelerates conduction. This acceleration may be visible as a breakthrough occurring ahead of the wavefront, or it may not be visible since the breakthroughs become coincident with the wavefront. This latter synchronization of activity starts to occur after several cycles. 3) Refractory tissue forms small islands around the PMJs, which induce more wavebreaks when a wavefront tries to propagate through the region. Finally, 4) the PS can provide escape pathways for wavefronts which would otherwise die by running into refractory tissue.

The PS affects fibrillation in many ways. Exposure to a large shock may disrupt pathways through the PS to terminate reentry, or ectopically firing PS cells may be reset. Disruption by an external shock may, therefore, influence reentrant activity but exactly how these factors relate remains to be elucidated.

5. Response to electric fields

The response of myocardial tissue to a strong electric shock depends on the orientation of the cells with respect to the electric field and how conductivity changes with respect to the direction of the electric field. This is seen in the expression for the generalized activating function, S (Sobie et al., 1997):

$$S = \mathbf{G_i} : \nabla(\nabla\phi_e) + (\nabla \cdot \mathbf{G_i}) \cdot \nabla\phi \qquad (5)$$

where the colon signifies the matrix inner product. Looking at the two terms, activation can result from a gradient in the electric field, or from the irrotational portion of the conductivity field. Conductivity must be defined as a spatially-dependent tensor since its directional properties are determined by cellular orientation, which varies throughout the heart. This directional dependence arises from gap junction connectivity, which allows current to most easily flow longitudinally and experiences the highest resistance flowing across laminar sheets (Legrice et al., 1997).

The PS is essentially a network of one dimensional cables which repeatedly bifurcate and unify. In addition to the complex topology, the PS fibres undergo sudden changes in direction, as well as have termini which abruptly end. These properties all get reflected in the conductivity tensor. The complicated path of the fibres ensures that at least part of the PS is aligned in such a way as to be excited by the applied electric field. The end of the fibre is an abrupt discontinuity to zero conductivity outside of the fibre. Terminal fibre segments which are aligned with the electric field will, therefore, have transmembrane potentials induced. Ends which face the cathode will be depolarized while ends facing the anode will be hyperpolarized.

The effect of field stimulation is shown in Fig. 1, where an MRI-derived isolated rabbit PS is exposed to shocks. The normal activation pattern is shown for reference, where it can be seen that it takes more than 30 ms for the entire network to be excited. When a shock is applied, many regions are excited simultaneously, not just one. This greatly abbreviates the excitation time of the tree and consequently, will result in near synchronous activation of the myocardium.

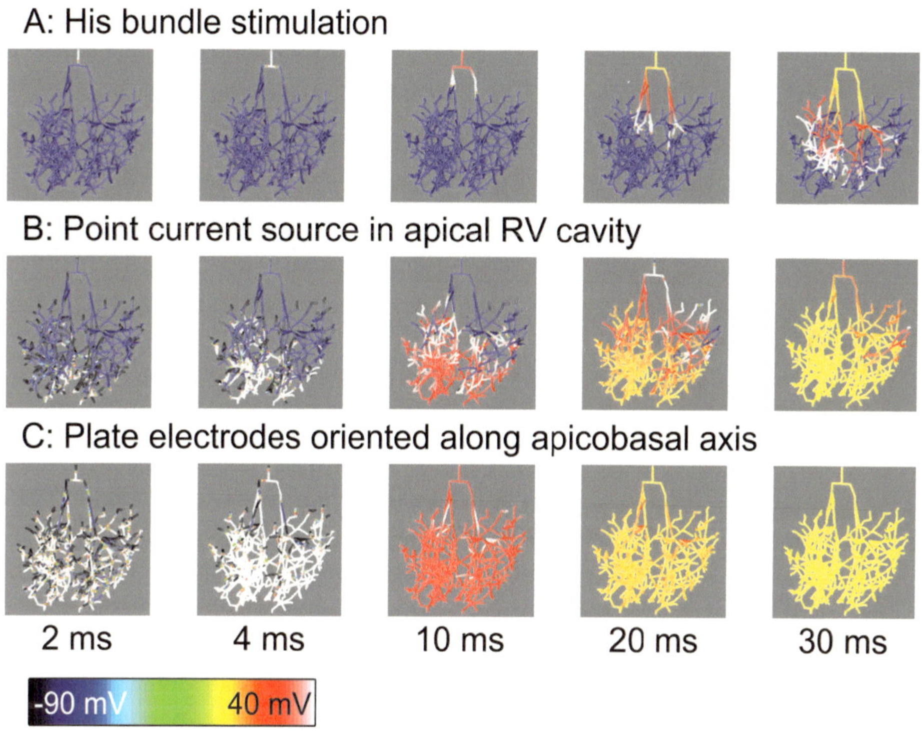

Fig. 1. Response of MRI-derived rabbit Purkinje System to electric fields. **A**: Normal activation starting at the proximal His bundle. **B**: 2.5 ms 125 mA point current source in the right ventricle **C**: 3 ms uniform 5 V/cm field oriented along the major axis of the heart. Color indicates transmembrane voltage. Times are given relative to stimulus onset.

Even on the cellular level, the PS reacts differently to high voltage shocks compared to ventricular myocytes. Using a papillary muscle preparation, Li et al. (1993) found that above a field strength of 20 V/cm, shocks induced a baseline shift and high frequency bursting in PS cells. In contrast, the ventricular myocytes entered a refractory state immediately after large shocks.

Thus, the PS is easily excited by electric field. Due to its one-dimensional nature and complex fibre trajectories, some part of it is always in a position to be excited by the field. This leads to rapid activation of the PS and, hence, of the myocardium connected through the PMJs. This

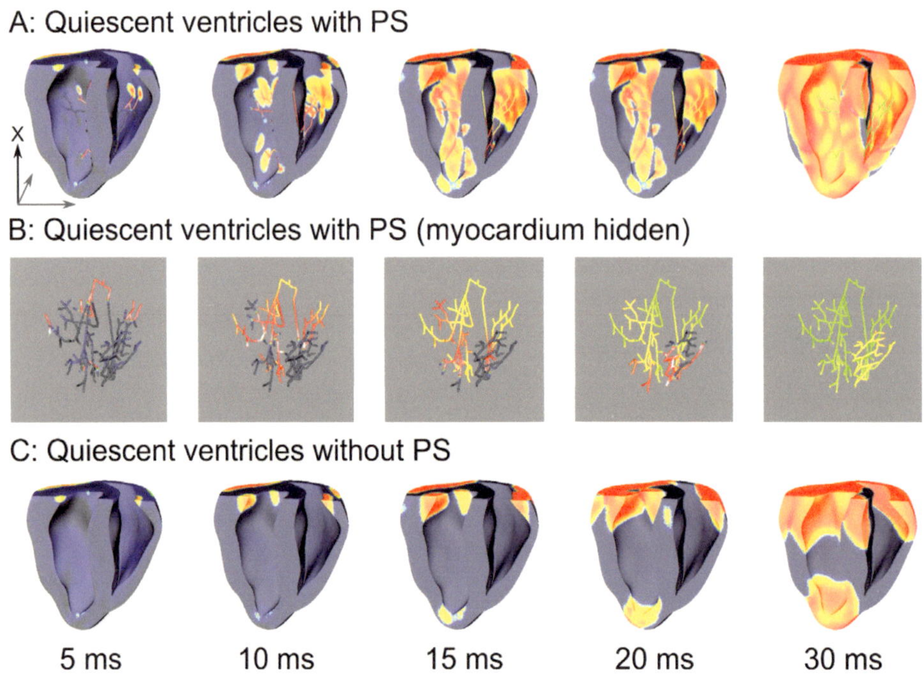

Fig. 2. **Response of the quiescent ventricles and PS to a** 2.5 V/cm **shock.** Field orientation is along the long axis, as shown in A. When the PS is present, additional far-field activations can be seen on the endocardial surface.

will tend to be antiarrhythmic since the excitable gaps, which allow activity to keep exciting recovered tissue, will be more quickly consumed.

6. Quiescent ventricle studies

Simulations of the application of defibrillation-strength shocks to the quiescent ventricles with and without PS allow for the contribution of the PS to be identified. When stimulation is applied, large polarization gradients form in segments of the PS that are parallel to the electric field. The myocardium is also subject to excitation by direct and virtual electrode stimuli, but activation patterns in the two tissues do not necessarily coincide since PS fibres do not always run in the same direction as underlying ventricles cells. Furthermore, current flow in PS fibres is physically constrained and excitation spreads rapidly through the network, so even very weak shocks produce rapid excitation of the entire network. Thus, under the right circumstances, the contribution of the PS to the response of the quiescent ventricles can be remarkable.

Consider Fig. 2, where a 2.5 V/cm field is applied along the long axis of the heart (from apex to base). Far-field excitations on the endocardial surface due to anterograde transmission of shock-induced activity in the PS is clearly visible (A); the presence of these effects is due to rapid propagation in the PS (B) and the relative lack of myocardial excitation from the field, which can be seen explicitly in the ventricles-only response (C). Consequently, the total ventricular activation time (t_{act}) is dramatically abbreviated.

	X			Y			Z		
	PS^+	PS^-	% ↓	PS^+	PS^-	% ↓	PS^+	PS^-	% ↓
–2.5 V/cm	55.7	100.1	44.3	29.3	29.8	1.6	28.4	29.1	2.2
+2.5 V/cm	41.1	63.1	34.8	26.1	26.9	3.2	28.2	29.4	4.1
–5 V/cm	43.1	67.0	35.6	28.3	28.4	0.1	28.2	28.3	0.3
+5 V/cm	33.6	57.3	41.4	24.6	24.8	1.0	27.5	27.7	0.7
–7.5 V/cm	37.3	42.4	12.1	28.2	28.2	0.2	28.5	28.3	0.5
+7.5 V/cm	30.7	38.3	19.9	22.6	23.2	2.2	27.6	27.7	0.3
–10 V/cm	30.0	36.1	17.0	28.4	28.3	0.3	28.1	28.0	0.5
+10 V/cm	30.1	34.5	12.6	22.4	22.4	0.0	27.8	27.9	0.2

Table 1. **Total activation time (t_{act}) with and without PS.** t_{act} was measured between the beginning of the shock and complete ventricular activation for four shock strengths in six directions, as described in the text.

In terms of t_{act}, the contribution of the PS to the response of the quiescent ventricles is only significant in cases where myocardial tissue in the vicinity of Purkinje-myocardial junctions (PMJs) is not excited by the shock. For the simulations discussed here, three orthogonal orientations were tested–along the long axis (X), across the septum (Y), and along the septum. As shown in the tabulated results for all simulations (Tab. 1), significant t_{act} abbreviation was only observed for shocks in the X direction.

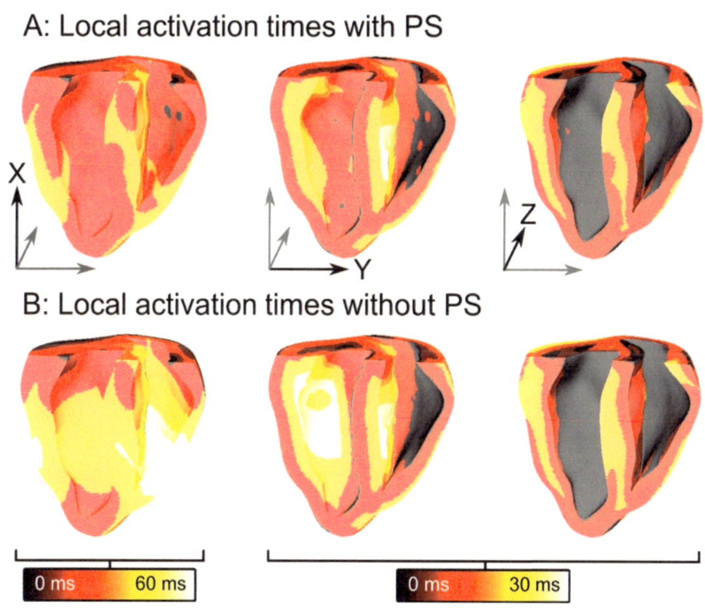

Fig. 3. **Local activation times for different field orientations,** $2.5V/cm$ **shock.** Early activations due to PS activation make the biggest difference for shocks in the X direction, where myocardium near the PS is not significantly activated by the field. For shocks in the Y and Z differences, the PS causes some regions to activate much earlier (i.e. LV endocardial free-wall for Y), but overall activation time is not significantly abbreviated.

Interestingly, while the PS did not have a significant effect on t_{act} for shocks in the Y and Z directions, it did sometimes alter the pattern of local activation. For example, as shown in

Fig. 3, a weak shock in the Y direction resulted in much earlier activation of the LV endocardial free-wall due to PS excitations. Although t_{act} did not differ between simulations with and without the PS in this case, the modified order of activation could have consequences on subsequent beats due to gradients in refractoriness that might arise from local heterogeneity.

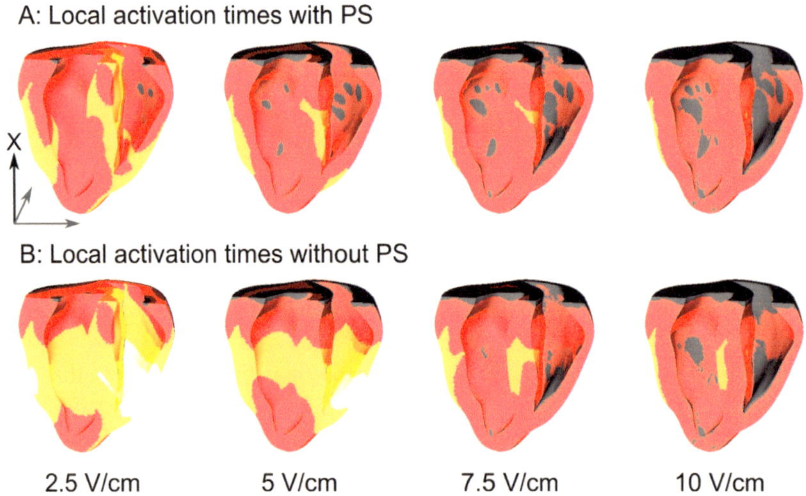

Fig. 4. **Local activation times for different field strengths along the long axis.** As shock strength increases, the role of the PS in the response of the quiescent ventricles is diminished, since the field causes excitation in a larger amount of myocardium. For the strongest shock (10 V/cm) only a few regions near PMJs, particularly in the septal region, contribute to t_{act} abbreviation. Stronger shocks abbreviate the activation delay between coupled PS and ventricular cells.

Increasing shock strength resulted in larger regions of myocardial polarization from the field, which effectively reduced the importance of the PS contribution in the response; this accounts for the diminishing returns in t_{act} abbreviation for shocks in the X direction, which is obvious in Tab. 1. As shown in Fig. 4, for the strongest shocks along the long axis simulated in this study, the primary source of t_{act} abbreviation was early activation of the septum, which is not easily excited by such shocks.

Interestingly, increased shock strength seemed to hasten the local effects of PS on endocardium. For example, in Fig. 4A, consider the dark regions on the endocardial surfaces, which are associated with early activation due to PS excitation. As the strength of stimulation increases (left to right), these regions become darker and larger, suggesting an abbreviation of anterograde transmission delay, perhaps due to the larger gradients in polarization. These observations were confirmed by inspecting voltages at the junctional voltage level (not shown), where the delay between coupled PS and ventricular cell upstroke was found to be almost uniformly shorter for larger shocks.

7. Isoelectric window

In general, shocks above a certain minimal strength result in sustained reentry; however, there is also a threshold for a maximum strength above which reentry is not induced. This Upper Limit of Vulnerability (ULV) is an important measure since it tends to correspond to the Defibrillation Threshold (DFT)–the minimum shock strength necessary to halt ventricular fibrillation(Chen, Shibata, Dixon, Martin & Ideker, 1986). The ULV is particularly valuable as an easier to find surrogate measurement for DFT. Thus, insights on the ULV will provide insight on the DFT, which is of direct clinical importance.

Following failed defibrillation shocks near the ULV, there is a period of time during which new activity is not seen on the epicardium.(Chen, Shibata, Dixon, Wolf, Danieley, Sweeney, Smith & Ideker, 1986) This Isoelectric Window (IW) can be considerable, on the order of tens of milliseconds. It ends when activations break through on the epicardium and reentry resumes. Many long-standing questions surround this phenomenon: What is the nature of concealed activity during the IW? What is the mechanism that allows it to remain hidden for such a long time? Some researchers have argued that the PS plays an important role;(Dosdall et al., 2010) others have proposed the tunnel propagation theory, which suggests that cardiac surfaces are driven into refractory states and post-shock activity is confined to a thin transmural space with no excitable path to the epicardium.(Ashihara et al., 2008; Constantino et al., 2010) Some time later, the surface tissue recovers from refractoriness and activations break through. While the computer simulations carried out to construct this hypothesis were carefully constructed, it must be noted that they did not include a model of the PS.

For the purpose of comparison, we performed a set of simulations with the PS. A cross-shock protocol was applied with the second shock near the ULV to identify possible contributions of the PS during the IW. First, the ventricles were excited, either by transmembrane stimulation at the apex or by His bundle current injection. The former emulates experimental preparations while the latter results in a more physiological excitation pattern. During ventricular repolarization, a shock with appropriate strength and timing to induce arrhythmia was delivered by parallel plates, with the extracellular electric field oriented along the short axis of the heart.

7.1 Effects of varying coupling intervals and shock strengths on IW

Fig. 5 shows IW duration within the window of vulnerability for various combinations of shock timing–i.e. the coupling interval (CI)–and strength. For the AP+PS pre-shock configuration (A), the average IW decreased from 36 to 21 ms as CI increased from 145 to 155 ms. Similar IW gradients were seen for decreasing CI within the AP-PS (B) and His (C) configurations, from 49 to 34 ms and from 37 to 19 ms, respectively.

A similar trend was observed for increasing shock strength. In the AP+PS and His cases, where IW duration was determined by the time between the shock and the first PS-to-myocardial activation, the average IW decreased with increasing shock strength. For AP+PS, shocks ranging from 3.3 to 9 V/cm produced average IWs between 33 and 23 ms; for increasing shock strengths within the His configuration, IWs decreased from 31 to 20 ms. In the AP-PS configuration, where IW duration was determined by the spread of shock-induced activations in the apical region, average IW was reduced from 47 to 34 ms as shock strength increased from weakest to strongest. In the AP+PS and His cases, the PS was actively involved in the generation of first post-shock activity, so it was unsurprising that the IW was shorter than in AP-PS, where the PS was absent. This observation supports the hypothesis that the PS plays an important role in the immediate response to defibrillation shocks.

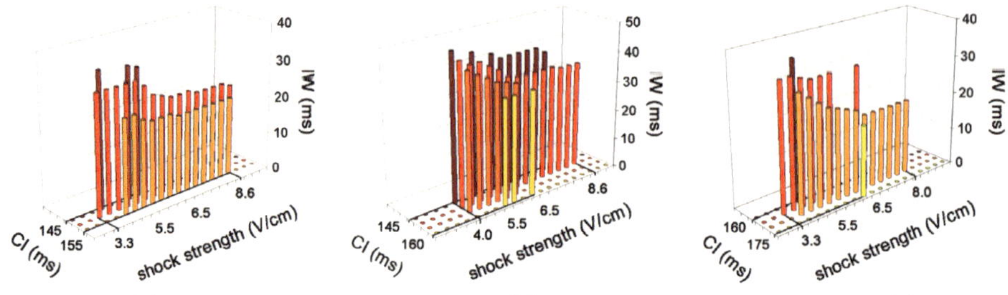

Fig. 5. IW duration for various combinations of shock strength and timing for three reentry induction protocols: (A) apical pacing with the PS (AP+PS), (B) apical pacing without the PS (AP-PS), and (C) His pacing. In general, longer CIs lead to shorter IWs.

7.2 First post-shock activation and the IW period

Activations were always observed in the PS immediately following the shock. During AP+PS runs, the first post-shock myocardial activation emanated from the PS 11 ms after the shock. After 15 ms, significant endocardial activation had occurred, as shown in Fig. 6(a). This is shorter than clinically-observed IWs due to the significant delay during which excitation propagates from the site of transmission to the epicardium. Fig. 6(b) shows the appearance of PS activations on the epicardium 23 ms after the shock; in most shocks applied to models with the PS during the vulnerable period, this pattern of excitation led to the first epicardial breakthrough. Note that the epicardial activation site is immediately opposite the endocardial PS insertion point. Mechanistically, the first PS activation initiated an endocardial rotor, which led to an epicardial activation (black arrow in Fig. 6); the underlying pattern of transmural activation is clearly shown.

As discussed earlier in this chapter, the distinct physiology and geometry of the PS lead to different polarization patterns than in the myocardium; in these simulations, the earliest post-shock activation was always observed within the PS. Excitation spread rapidly through the network and coupled myocardial tissue was activated by anterograde transmission. Thus, the first post-shock ventricular activation always emanated from the PS. In simulations without the PS, large gradients were induced near the apical region, leading to post-shock wavefronts.

Most experimental studies that reported an IW after defibrillation-level shocks mapped only epicardial or endocardial surfaces. Recently, Dosdall et al. (Dosdall et al., 2007) observed epicardial and subepicardial activations in pigs soon after shocks. Since the PS in pigs exhibits full transmural insertion (Chattipakorn et al., 2003), it is plausible that these mapped activations were first post-shock excitations provided by the PS. Furthermore, the earliest myocardial activations recorded were preceded by Purkinje potentials, which is in agreement with our findings. To the best of our knowledge, this is the first attempt to map PS activations following defibrillation. While limited spatial resolution prevented the authors from stating a clear conclusion, the results suggest that our simulation results are a step in the right direction. Other studies have observed endocardial or intramural activations that broke through to the epicardium 42 ms post-shock in sheep hearts (Evans & Gray, 2004). Given the fact that the PS terminates in the subendocardium in sheep,(Ansari et al., 1999) these observations are also

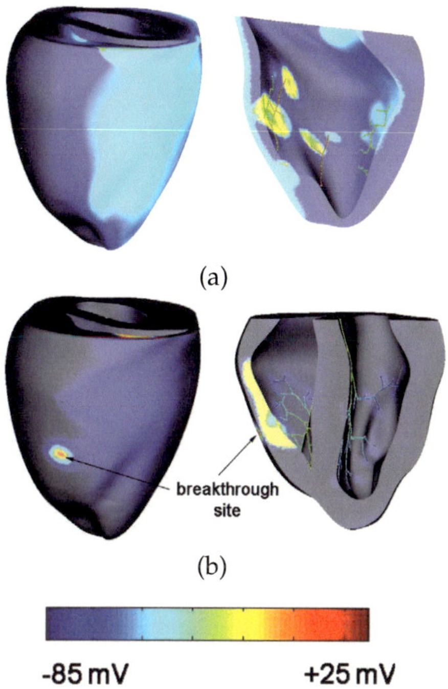

Fig. 6. Earliest postshock activation. (a) The first activation emanating from the PS 15 ms after the shock is clearly seen in the endocardial cross-section. (b) After 23 ms, the PS activation provides a focal breakthrough on the epicardium. Note the breakthrough site (arrow) is situated opposite the PS insertion point. Transmural depolarization due to the earliest postshock activation is evident. The right panel of (a) shows the LV endocardial free wall while the right panel of (b) shows a cross-section perpendicular to the septum with the posterior surface hidden.

consistent with our findings. Our study involves a smaller heart size, which explains the reduced IW durations compared to experimental values discussed here.

In our simulations, the PS was always strongly excited by the shock. In some cases, we observed midwall excitations similar to those observed in tunnel propagation studies.(Ashihara et al., 2008; Constantino et al., 2010) These were isolated by surface refractoriness, with excitable tissue confined to intramural paths. However, activations that originated in the PS broke through more quickly than purely myocardial midwall excitations, as shown in Fig. 7. Rapid conduction in the PS ensured that this happened consistently.

To further test our hypothesis that the PS was the source of epicardial breakthroughs following the IW, we changed the transmural insertion depth of PS endpoints. Figure 8 shows that the IW duration is dramatically reduced when the PS penetrates to the subepicardial layer. This is consistent with the PS being the primary source of post-shock epicardial activations due to rapid field-induced activations: deeper penetration brings PS fibres closer to the epicardium, so it makes sense that the IW is shorter. We observed that IW duration varied from 12 ms (full insertion) to 30 ms (no insertion). Epicardial breakthrough sites remained the same in all simulations for a given insertion depth; these sites were consistently situated opposite PS

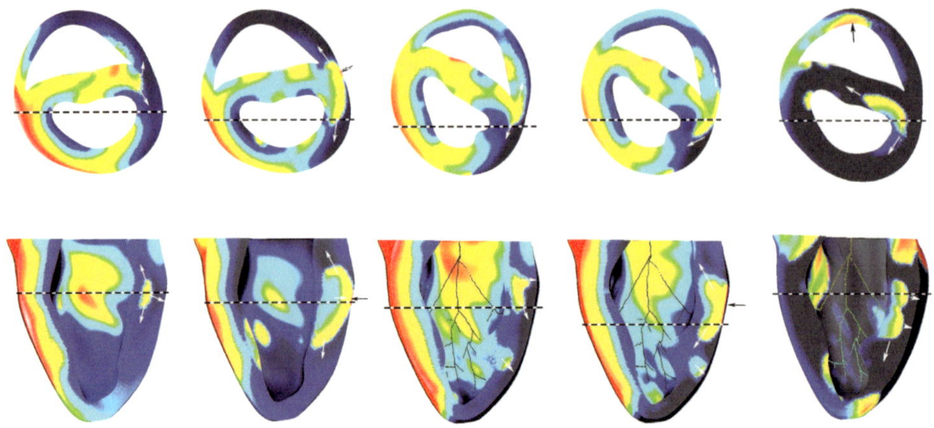

Fig. 7. Transmural postshock activations in the septum (top) and LV free wall (bottom). White arrows indicate the propagation pathways of transmural wavefronts; black arrows indicate epicardial breakthrough sites (a)-(d) or PS-induced propagating activity (e). In (a) and (b), the response to a 10 ms shock is shown in the absence of the PS. Activations originate in the septum and propagate through the free wall. In (c) and (d), similar activations are seen following a 5 ms shock using the AP+PS configuration. Wavefronts originating from PS transmission arrive at the epicardium before shock-induced myocardial wavefronts. (e) shows the response to an even shorter shock (3 ms) for the same configuration. Dashed lines represent cross-section planes relative to the top and bottom views. V_m is shown with the same color scheme used in Fig. 1.

insertion points. While IW abbreviation was indisputable for the fully-penetrating PS, it was less clear for cases where the PS terminated in the midwall. Notably, these cases were subject to a higher degree of variability from sample to sample, which could be the result of surface polarization blocking PS activity.

In our model, rapid conduction through the PS was the source of the epicardial breakthrough terminating the IW. However, there are several limitations and differences with Trayanova's work. We only considered monophasic defibrillation shocks while her group considered biphasic shocks which would lead to different postshock surface states. Our modelling of the PS cell response to large shocks may not be accurate. This is true for all ionic models where behavior outside of the physiological voltage range is not well characterized. If PS conduction became compromised due to a field induced conduction block, or refractory myocardium prevented anterograde transmission across the PMJs, then the tunnel propagation mechanism could account for the IW. In reality, it is likely that both mechanisms play a role, depending on circumstances.

8. Defibrillation

A limited set of computer simulations has been performed with ventricles including a model of the PS(Deo et al., 2009). With an 8 V/cm defibrillation shock, ventricles with a PS were successfully defibrillated while those without a PS were not. The most obvious difference

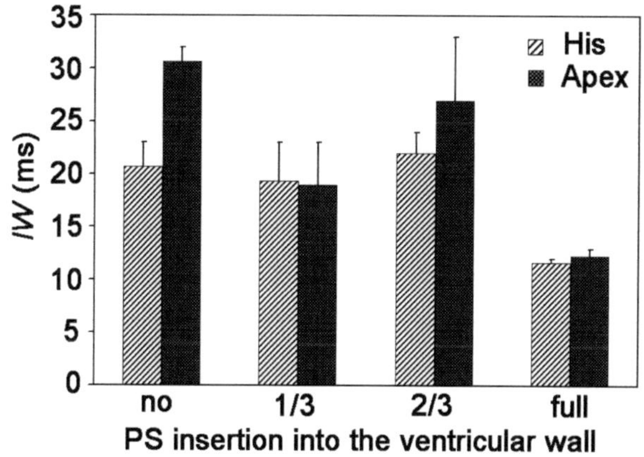

Fig. 8. Effect of PS insertion depth on IW duration. The IW was longest for surface-bound PS and shortest in the case of fibre endpoints that penetrated to the sub-epicardial layer. Error bars correspond to maximum deviation from mean values ($n = 6$).

between the two situations was the more rapid and widespread activation of the epicardium which eliminated excitable gaps. Without the PS, an excitable gap persisted under the anode, allowing reentry to be reinduced. Thus, the PS aided in defibrillation. Experimentally, application of Lugol's solution to the endocardium results in a doubling of DFT(Damiano et al., 1986), suggesting that the PS facilitates defibrillation at lower field strengths.

9. Summary

Based on experimental findings, which are supported by our modelling studies, we conclude that the PS plays a major role in defibrillation. Due to its cable-like nature and complicated geometry, it is excited in many places by an applied electric field, which leads to rapid activation of the entire network. Any excitable gaps are quickly consumed and reentry cannot be reestablishing. This effect is less prominent as shock strength is increased since more myocardium is directly excited by the shock. The complex postshock propagation pattern present with a PS may also play a role in rapid ventricular activation to stop fibrillation.

10. References

Ansari, A., Yen Ho, S. & Anderson, R. H. (1999). Distribution of the Purkinje fibres in the sheep heart, *The Anatomical Record* 254(1): 92–97.

Armiger, L. C. & Knell, C. M. (1988). Fine structural alteration in the atrioventricular junctional conduction tissues of the dog heart during severe ischaemia., *J Submicrosc Cytol Pathol* 20(4): 645–656.

Ashihara, T., Constantino, J. & Trayanova, N. A. (2008). Tunnel propagation of postshock activations as a hypothesis for fibrillation induction and isoelectric window., *Circ Res* 102(6): 737–745.
URL: *http://dx.doi.org/10.1161/CIRCRESAHA.107.168112*

Ashihara, T. & Trayanova, N. A. (2004). Asymmetry in membrane responses to electric shocks: insights from bidomain simulations., *Biophys J* 87(4): 2271–2282.
URL: *http://dx.doi.org/10.1529/biophysj.104.043091*

Canale, E., Campbell, G., Smolich, J. & Campbell, J. (1986). *Cardiac muscle:*, Vol. II, Springer-Verlag, Berlin-Heidelberg-New York-Tokyo, chapter 7, pp. 60–103.

Chattipakorn, N., Fotuhi, P. C., Chattipakorn, S. C. & Ideker, R. E. (2003). Three-dimensional mapping of earliest activation after near-threshold ventricular defibrillation shocks., *J Cardiovasc. Electrophysiol.* 14: 65–69.

Chen, P. S., Shibata, N., Dixon, E. G., Martin, R. O. & Ideker, R. E. (1986). Comparison of the defibrillation threshold and the upper limit of ventricular vulnerability., *Circulation* 73(5): 1022–1028.

Chen, P. S., Shibata, N., Dixon, E. G., Wolf, P. D., Danieley, N. D., Sweeney, M. B., Smith, W. M. & Ideker, R. E. (1986). Activation during ventricular defibrillation in open-chest dogs. evidence of complete cessation and regeneration of ventricular fibrillation after unsuccessful shocks., *J Clin Invest* 77(3): 810–823.
URL: *http://dx.doi.org/10.1172/JCI112378*

Cheng, Y., Mowrey, K. A., Wagoner, D. R. V., Tchou, P. J. & Efimov, I. R. (1999). Virtual electrode-induced reexcitation: A mechanism of defibrillation., *Circ Res* 85(11): 1056–1066.

Constantino, J., Long, Y., Ashihara, T. & Trayanova, N. A. (2010). Tunnel propagation following defibrillation with icd shocks: hidden postshock activations in the left ventricular wall underlie isoelectric window., *Heart Rhythm* 7(7): 953–961.
URL: *http://dx.doi.org/10.1016/j.hrthm.2010.03.026*

Damiano, R. J., Smith, P. K., Tripp, H. F., Asano, T., Small, K. W., Lowe, J. E., Ideker, R. E. & Cox, J. L. (1986). The effect of chemical ablation of the endocardium on ventricular fibrillation threshold., *Circulation* 74(3): 645–652.

Deo, M., Boyle, P., Plank, G. & Vigmond, E. (2009). Arrhythmogenic mechanisms of the purkinje system during electric shocks: a modelling study., *Heart Rhythm* 6(12): 1782–1789.
URL: *http://dx.doi.org/10.1016/j.hrthm.2009.08.023*

Dosdall, D. J., Cheng, K.-A., Huang, J., Allison, J. S., Allred, J. D., Smith, W. M. & Ideker, R. E. (2007). Transmural and endocardial purkinje activation in pigs before local myocardial activation after defibrillation shocks., *Heart Rhythm* 4(6): 758–765.
URL: *http://dx.doi.org/10.1016/j.hrthm.2007.02.017*

Dosdall, D. J., Osorio, J., Robichaux, R. P., Huang, J., Li, L. & Ideker, R. E. (2010). Purkinje activation precedes myocardial activation following defibrillation after long-duration ventricular fibrillation., *Heart Rhythm* 7(3): 405–412.
URL: *http://dx.doi.org/10.1016/j.hrthm.2009.11.025*

Dosdall, D. J., Tabereaux, P. B., Kim, J. J., Walcott, G. P., Rogers, J. M., Killingsworth, C. R., Huang, J., Robertson, P. G., Smith, W. M. & Ideker, R. E. (2008). Chemical ablation of the purkinje system causes early termination and activation rate slowing of long-duration ventricular fibrillation in dogs., *Am J Physiol Heart Circ Physiol* 295(2): H883–H889.
URL: *http://dx.doi.org/10.1152/ajpheart.00466.2008*

Evans, F. G. & Gray, R. (2004). Shock-induced epicardial and endocardial virtual electrodes leading to ventricular fibrillation via reentry, graded responses and transmural activation, *J Cardiovasc. Electrophysiol.* 15: 79–87.

Huelsing, D. J., Spitzer, K. W., Cordeiro, J. M. & Pollard, A. E. (1998). Conduction between isolated rabbit purkinje and ventricular myocytes coupled by a variable resistance., *Am J Physiol* 274(4 Pt 2): H1163–H1173.

Ijiri, T., Ashihara, T., Yamaguchi, T., Takayama, K., Igarashi, T., Shimada, T., Namba, T., Haraguchi, R. & Nakazawa, K. (2008). A procedural method for modeling the purkinje fibers of the heart., *J Physiol Sci* 58(7): 481–486.
URL: *http://dx.doi.org/10.2170/physiolsci.RP003208*

Legrice, I. J., Hunter, P. J. & Smaill, B. H. (1997). Laminar structure of the heart: a mathematical model., *Am J Physiol* 272(5 Pt 2): H2466–H2476.

Li, H. G., Jones, D. L., Yee, R. & Klein, G. J. (1993). Defibrillation shocks produce different effects on purkinje fibers and ventricular muscle: implications for successful defibrillation, refibrillation and postshock arrhythmia., *J Am Coll Cardiol* 22(2): 607–614.

Miquerol, L., Meysen, S., Mangoni, M., Bois, P., van Rijen, H., Abran, P., Jongsma, H., Nargeot, J. & Daniel Gros (2004). Architectural and functional asymmetry of the His-Purkinje system of the murine heart., *Cardiovasc Res* 63: 77-86.

Morley, G. E., Danik, S. B., Bernstein, S., Sun, Y., Rosner, G., Gutstein, D. E. & Fishman, G. I. (2005). Reduced intercellular coupling leads to paradoxical propagation across the purkinje-ventricular junction and aberrant myocardial activation., *Proc Natl Acad Sci U S A* 102(11): 4126–4129.
URL: *http://dx.doi.org/10.1073/pnas.0500881102*

Ono, N., Yamaguchi, T., Ishikawa, H., Arakawa, M., Takahashi, N., Saikawa, T. & Shimada, T. (2009). Morphological varieties of the purkinje fiber network in mammalian hearts, as revealed by light and electron microscopy., *Arch Histol Cytol* 72(3): 139–149.

Sepulveda, N. G., Roth, B. J. & Wikswo, J. P. (1989). Current injection into a two-dimensional anisotropic bidomain., *Biophys J* 55(5): 987–999.
URL: *http://dx.doi.org/10.1016/S0006-3495(89)82897-8*

Sobie, E. A., Susil, R. C. & Tung, L. (1997). A generalized activating function for predicting virtual electrodes in cardiac tissue., *Biophys J* 73(3): 1410–1423.
URL: *http://dx.doi.org/10.1016/S0006-3495(97)78173-6*

Streit, J. (1987). Effects of hypoxia and glycolytic inhibition on electrical properties of sheep cardiac purkinje fibres., *J Mol Cell Cardiol* 19(9): 875–885.

Trayanova, N. & Skouibine, K. (1998). Modeling defibrillation: effects of fiber curvature., *J Electrocardiol* 31 Suppl: 23–29.

Vetter, F. & McCulloch, A. (1998). Three-dimensional analysis of regional cardiac function: a model of rabbit ventricular anatomy., *Prog Biophys Mol Biol* 69(2-3):157–183.

Vigmond, E. J. & Clements, C. (2007). Construction of a computer model to investigate sawtooth effects in the purkinje system., *IEEE Trans Biomed Eng* 54(3): 389–399.
URL: *http://dx.doi.org/10.1109/TBME.2006.888817*

Vigmond, E. J., dos Santos, R. W., Prassl, A. J., Deo, M. & Plank, G. (2008). Solvers for the cardiac bidomain equations., *Prog Biophys Mol Biol* 96(1-3): 3–18.
URL: *http://dx.doi.org/10.1016/j.pbiomolbio.2007.07.012*

Wiedmann, R. T., Tan, R. C. & Joyner, R. W. (1996). Discontinuous conduction at purkinje-ventricular muscle junction., *Am J Physiol* 271(4 Pt 2): H1507–H1516.

Wu, T.-J., Lin, S.-F., Hsieh, Y.-C., Chiu, Y.-T. & Ting, C.-T. (2009). Repetitive endocardial focal discharges during ventricular fibrillation with prolonged global ischemia in isolated rabbit hearts., *Circ J* 73(10): 1803–1811.

3

Analysis of the Lead Sensitivity Distribution in Implantable Cardioverter Defibrillator

Jesús Requena-Carrión[1], Juho Väisänen[2], Jari Hyttinen[2] and Juan J. Vinagre-Díaz[1]
[1]*University Rey Juan Carlos*
[2]*Tampere University of Technology*
[1]*Spain*
[2]*Finland*

1. Introduction

Most current Implantable Cardioverter Defibrillators (ICD) use intracardiac leads for electrogram (EGM) sensing and defibrillation (Belott & Reynolds, 2007). Intracardiac leads consist of several electrodes that for the basic functionality of ventricular tachyarrhythmia detection and termination, are inserted transvenously into the right ventricle (Gradaus et al., 2003; Swerdlow et al., 2007). In addition to intracardiac electrodes, ICD also use the casing of the implant as an indifferent, distant electrode.

In ICD technology, three main intracardiac lead configurations are distinguished based on the combination of electrodes that they use, namely unipolar, dedicated bipolar and integrated bipolar. Unipolar leads, so-called because they use the casing of the implant as an indifferent electrode, consist of a single electrode located in the right ventricle, whereas bipolar leads, both dedicated and integrated, consist of two closely spaced electrodes located in the right ventricle. In general, unipolar lead configurations are used for cardiac defibrillation, while bipolar lead configurations are used for EGM sensing, i.e. they provide with the EGM signals from which heart rhythm can be extracted.

Previous studies indicate that lead configuration can affect EGM sensing and ICD performance. For instance, it is well known that fundamental EGM features such as wave duration, wave amplitude and power spectrum, depend on the configuration of the recording leads (DeCaprio et al., 1977; Jenkins, 1992; Langberg et al., 1988; Parsonnet et al., 1980). Also, differences in ventricular fibrillation detection and redetection times have been reported when comparing ICD dedicated and integrated bipolar leads (Cooklin et al., 1999; Frain et al., 2007; Goldberger et al., 1998; Natale et al., 1996). Other studies have addressed the effects on EGM sensing, of artifacts originating from non-ventricular bioelectric sources. For example, inappropriate ICD discharges have been ascribed to myopotentials oversensing (Deshmukh & Anderson, 1998; Kowalski et al., 2008; Sandler & Kutalek, 1994; Schulte et al., 2001). Pacing stimulus artifacts, which are often associated to ICD undersensing, have been found to be greater in integrated than in dedicated bipolar leads (Menz et al., 1998). Finally, an optimized lead design for atrial sensing has been proposed, in order to facilitate rejection of artifacts such as R-waves and myopotentials (Nash et al., 2005). Therefore, the existing evidence indicates that by carefully designing ICD intracardiac leads, EGM sensing and hence ICD overall performance can be further improved.

The effects of lead configuration on ICD sensing performance can be explored through the notion of lead sensitivity distribution, also known as lead field. The lead sensitivity distribution describes the ability of leads to measure the electrical activity generated by bioelectric organs and tissues in the body and hence, it can help to identify the sources of bioelectric artifacts and to quantify their effects. In addition to this, the analysis of the lead sensitivity distribution can contribute to widen the range of functionality of ICD systems by providing with an estimation of lead spatial resolution. The quantification of the lead spatial resolution could be of great interest, especially in those scenarios where the underlying cardiac pathology is caused by local physiological abnormalities such as myocardial ischemia (Asbach et al., 2006; Bunch & Day, 2008; Williams et al., 2008), or when the underlying pathology can be related to tissue spatial heterogeneities (Zaitsev et al., 2000).

The sensitivity distributions of two unipolar and two bipolar ICD intracardiac lead configurations have been investigated in a previous study (Requena-Carrión et al., 2009). By combining a detailed numerical model of the human thorax and finite difference methods (FDM), the sensitivity distribution at the ventricles of each lead configuration was obtained. The sensitivity distribution also allowed to quantify the spatial resolution of each lead configuration, and significant differences in sensing between different lead configurations were found. However, a more complete picture of EGM sensing in ICD should account for the measurement of the activity of other bioelectric sources that could affect ICD performance, such as myopotentials. The analysis of the sensitivity of intracardiac leads at other bioelectric sources in the human body would improve our understanding on how electrophysiological artifacts affect EGM sensing and therefore, it would help to devise new strategies to reject such artifacts by means of designing new lead configurations.

In this study, the sensitivity distribution of four ICD intracardiac lead configurations is calculated at the ventricles, the atria and near skeletal muscles. For that purpose, a detailed computational model of the human thorax is used in combination with numerical methods. Additionally, a discrimination index which is based on the sensitivity distribution is used for quantifying differences in sensing at the ventricles, atria and near muscles. This discrimination index takes the accumulated sensitivity of ICD leads at the ventricles, where the signals of interest are originated, and compares it with the accumulated sensitivity at the other bioelectric sources.

2. Principles of bioelectric signals measurement

Bioelectric measurement models consist of two basic elements, namely a bioelectric source and a volume conductor (Malmivuo & Plonsey, 1995). The bioelectric source is the biological tissue or organ that generates electric currents for regulating a physiological function, whereas the volume conductor is the conducting medium in which the bioelectric source resides. Well-known examples of bioelectric sources are the heart, the brain and the skeletal muscle; the human body as a whole, on the other hand, behaves electrically as a volume conductor.

As a consequence of the activity of bioelectric sources, a time-varying voltage gradient is induced across the volume conductor. This voltage gradient can be measured by means of measurement leads, which consist of at least one pair of electrodes in contact with the volume conductor. From the point of view of the measurement leads, the time-varying measured voltage $u(t)$ can be modeled mathematically as a weighted linear combination of the currents

$\mathbf{J}(t, v)$ generated by the bioelectric source V:

$$u(t) = \int_V \mathbf{L}(v) \cdot \mathbf{J}(t, v) dv. \tag{1}$$

In this equation $\mathbf{L}(v)$ denotes the lead sensitivity distribution and it describes the ability of the lead to measure the bioelectric currents $\mathbf{J}(t, v)$ generated by the source at $v \in V$. In general, since the lead sensitivity distribution will be larger in some regions of the bioelectric source than in others, the contribution to the total measured voltage will vary from one region within the bioelectric source to another. As a consequence, it can be said that the lead sensitivity distribution focus the measurement on selected regions within the bioelectric source and therefore, the lead sensitivity distribution will define a characteristic lead spatial resolution.
Whenever more than one bioelectric source reside within the volume conductor, by virtue of the superposition principle the total voltage measured by the leads can be expressed as the sum of the voltages induced by each source independently. For example, if two sources V_1 and V_2 exist, the total voltage $u(t)$ will be expressed as:

$$u(t) = u_1(t) + u_2(t) = \int_{V_1} \mathbf{L}(v) \cdot \mathbf{J}(t, v) dv + \int_{V_2} \mathbf{L}(v) \cdot \mathbf{J}(t, v) dv, \tag{2}$$

where $u_1(t)$ and $u_2(t)$ are the voltages generated by sources V_1 and V_2, respectively. In this scenario, the lead sensitivity distribution will determine the contribution of each region V_1 and V_2 to the total measured voltage. If, for instance, $\mathbf{L}(v)$ is much larger in V_1 than in V_2, the contribution of V_1 to the total measured voltage $u(t)$ will be expected to be higher than the contribution of V_2. Consequently, the lead sensitivity distribution, in addition to define the lead spatial resolution, will also allow to investigate the ability of a measurement lead to discriminate between different bioelectric sources.
Since the lead sensitivity distribution depends on both the volume conductor and the design and arrangement of the measurement leads, different leads will be characterized by different measurement properties. Based on the analysis of the lead sensitivity distribution, several techniques have been devised in the literature for investigating how current lead systems measure bioelectric phenomena. One of the earliest and most popular methods is the analysis of iso-sensitivity surfaces, which consists of depicting the surfaces in the bioelectric source where the magnitude of the lead sensitivity distribution remains constant. This analysis method was used by Rush and Driscoll for describing electroencephalographic (EEG) leads (Rush & Driscoll, 1969) and by Arzbaecher et al. for investigating the sensitivity of precordial and esophageal electrocardiographic (ECG) leads (Arzbaecher et al., 1979).
The sensitivity distribution has also been the basis for quantifying the lead spatial resolution. Based on the estimation of iso-sensitivity surfaces, Malmivuo et al. proposed the half sensitivity volume (HSV), which was defined as the bioelectric region enclosed by the surface where the sensitivity magnitude drops to half of the maximum sensitivity (Malmivuo et al., 1997). By using the HSV, the spatial resolutions of EEG and magnetoencephalography systems were compared. Also, by combining sensitivity distribution models and numerical simulations of cardiac dynamics, Requena-Carrión et al. proposed the resolution volume (ResV) for quantifying lead spatial resolution (Requena-Carrión et al., 2007). The ResV was defined as the bioelectric region that contributes to a given fraction of the measured signal power, and it was used for quantifying the spatial resolution of surface ECG leads (Requena-Carrión et al., 2007) and intracardiac leads in ICD (Requena-Carrión et al., 2009). Finally, Väisänen et al. further explored the notion of lead spatial resolution by proposing

ICD Casing	Height (mm)	64
	Width (mm)	51
	Depth (mm)	15
Helix	Length (mm)	2
	Diameter (mm)	3
Ring	Length (mm)	3
	Diameter (mm)	3
Right ventricular coil	Length (mm)	57
	Diameter (mm)	3
Interelectrode spacing	Helix-Ring (mm)	8
	Helix-Coil (mm)	12

Table 1. Electrode specifications.

the region of interest sensitivity ratio (ROISR), defined as the ratio between the average sensitivities of any two regions within the bioelectric source (Väisänen et al., 2008). The ROISR allowed to quantify the specificity of EEG (Väisänen et al., 2008) and surface ECG measurements (Väisänen & Hyttinen, 2009).

In summary, the lead sensitivity distribution constitutes both a useful theoretical tool for understanding the nature of bioelectric signals, and a useful practical tool for describing quantitatively the sensing properties of measurement leads. In this study, the sensitivity distribution will be used to quantify and compare the ability of four ICD intracardiac leads to measure ventricular bioelectrical events and reject bioelectrical artifacts from the atria and near muscles. For that purpose, the sensitivity distribution of each lead configuration under investigation will be analyzed and in addition to this, a measure of discrimination based on the sensitivity distribution will be proposed.

3. Methods

3.1 Intracardiac ICD leads

The measurement properties of four ICD intracardiac lead configurations (two unipolar, one dedicated bipolar and one integrated bipolar) were investigated. In order to define the geometry and the anatomical location of the electrodes that formed each intracardiac lead, a commercial ICD system was used as a reference model. This system consisted of two elements, namely the Medtronic Secura ICD (Medtronic, 2008) and the Medtronic Sprint Quattro Secure ventricular lead (Medtronic, 2010). The Medtronic Secura ICD is a single chamber ICD which is used in combination with a right ventricular lead for analyzing heart rhythm and providing defibrillation, cardioversion and both bradycardia and antitachycardia pacing therapies. As for the Medtronic Sprint Quattro Secure, it is a quadripolar ventricular lead designed for pacing, sensing, cardioversion and defibrillation therapies.

The Secura ICD is intended to be located in the pectoral region. Its casing, which can be used as an indifferent, distant electrode, has the physical dimensions shown in Table 1. As for the Sprint Quattro Secure ventricular lead, it consists of a helix electrode located at the tip of the lead, followed consecutively by a ring electrode, a right ventricular coil and a superior vena cava coil. The helix and the ring electrode are used for EGM sensing and pacing, while both coils in combination with the ICD casing are used for defibrillation. Since this study focuses

Unipolar *A*	helix to casing
Unipolar *B*	coil to casing
Dedicated bipolar	helix to ring
Integrated bipolar	helix to coil

Table 2. Intracardiac leads definition.

on bioelectric measurement of ventricular events, the electrodes that were considered were the helix, the ring and the right ventricular coil. The physical dimensions and relative distances of the electrodes that were considered for this study are shown in Table 1.
Based on the aforementioned electrode specifications, the four intracardiac ICD leads were defined as follows (Table 2): the unipolar *A* lead used the casing of the implant and the helix electrode; the unipolar *B* lead used the casing of the implant and the right ventricular coil; the dedicated bipolar lead used the helix and the ring electrodes and finally, the integrated bipolar lead used the helix electrode and the right ventricular coil.

3.2 Computational model of the human thorax

A realistic 3D computational model of the bioelectric properties of the human thorax was implemented for calculating the lead sensitivity distributions. This computational model was defined based on the widely used Visible Human Man dataset, and consisted of a $341\times594\times394$ cubic grid with a 1 mm$\times$1 mm$\times$1 mm resolution (Sachse et al., 1998). The human thorax model was segmented into 20 different organ and tissue types, including the atria, the ventricles and near muscles, and they were assigned resistivity values previously reported in the literature (Gabriel et al., 1996).
Lead sensitivity distributions were calculated in the realistic human thorax by applying the principle of reciprocity (Malmivuo & Plonsey, 1995), which states that when a lead is reciprocally energized, the current field that is induced in the volume conductor corresponds to the lead sensitivity distribution. An FDM approach was developed for calculating the current field induced in the realistic human thorax when each electrode pair was reciprocally energized. The FDM solver was based on the Incomplete Cholesky Preconditioner and Conjugate Gradient (Takano, 2002) and was executed on an AMD 3000+ 64Bit, 2 GB RAM, 200GB SATA RAID computer.

3.3 Discrimination power

Lead sensitivities at the ventricles were compared to lead sensitivities at the atria and near muscles. For that purpose, two discrimination indices based on the notion of ROISR (Väisänen et al., 2008) were defined as follows:

$$di_{AV} = \frac{\int_{atria} |\mathbf{L}(v)| dv}{\int_{ventricles} |\mathbf{L}(v)| dv} \qquad (3)$$

$$di_{MV} = \frac{\int_{muscle} |\mathbf{L}(v)| dv}{\int_{ventricles} |\mathbf{L}(v)| dv}$$

The discrimination index di_{AV} allowed to compare the accumulated sensitivities at the atria with the accumulated sensitivities at the ventricles, whereas the di_{MV} allowed to compare the accumulated sensitivities at near skeletal muscles with the accumulated sensitivities at the ventricles. A logarithmic transformation was subsequently applied to both indices:

$$\begin{aligned} DI_{AV} &= 20\log_{10}\left(di_{AV}\right) \\ DI_{MV} &= 20\log_{10}\left(di_{MV}\right) \end{aligned} \tag{4}$$

Consequently, the lower the value of a discrimination index for a given lead, the lower the sensitivity of that lead to the corresponding non-ventricular source (atria or skeletal muscle) and therefore, the lower the effects of bioelectric artifacts from that source.

4. Results

The analysis of the sensitivity distribution of each intracardiac lead reveals that, irrespective of the lead configuration and design, sensitivity is always higher at the close proximity of the electrodes and decreases with the distance. Specifically, as shown in Figures 1 and 2, the sensitivity of configurations using the signal provided by the helix electrode, i.e. unipolar *A*, dedicated bipolar and integrated bipolar, is highest near the ventricular apex, into which the helix electrode is usually inserted; similarly, the sensitivity across the ventricular septum is significantly higher in configurations using the right ventricular coil, i.e. unipolar *B* and integrated bipolar configurations. Figures 1 and 2 also show that the sensitivity of unipolar configurations decreases more slowly with the distance to the electrodes than the sensitivity of bipolar configurations and therefore, unipolar measurements are more uniform throughout the heart than bipolar measurements. In other words, bipolar configurations concentrate their measurements more than unipolar configurations.

As a consequence of the previous observation, since intracardiac ICD leads are inserted into the right ventricle, their sensitivity at the ventricular myocardium is higher than at the atrial myocardium. However, it is worth noting that the sensitivity distribution at the atria depends on the configuration of the lead. As seen in Figures 1 and 2, in the case of unipolar configurations the sensitivity distribution at the atria is of roughly the same order of magnitude as the sensitivity distribution at the ventricles, whereas in the case of bipolar configurations, the sensitivity distribution drops several orders of magnitude. In addition to this, by comparing bipolar configurations it can be concluded that the sensitivity at the atria is higher in the case of integrated bipolar than in the case of dedicated bipolar. Finally, by invoking the same physical principle according to which lead sensitivity decreases with the distance to the electrodes, since ICD are usually implanted in the pectoral area, the sensitivity at the pectoral muscle will be higher for unipolar leads, in which the casing of the implant acts as the indifferent electrode.

By calculating the discrimination indices DI_{AV} and DI_{MV}, the previous qualitative observations based on the analysis of the sensitivity distribution can be quantitatively contrasted. As Table 3 shows, the accumulated sensitivity of bipolar leads is several orders of magnitude higher at the ventricles than at the other non-ventricular bioelectric sources, namely the atria and near muscles. In addition to this, it can be noticed that dedicated bipolar configurations have a higher discrimination power than integrated bipolar configurations. Unipolar configurations, on the contrary, are characterized by a lower discrimination power, especially against muscular artifacts due to the proximity to the casing of the ICD. In general, it can be concluded from this analysis that the unipolar *B* configuration using the right ventricular coil and the casing of the implant, is the most vulnerable intracardiac configuration, whereas the dedicated bipolar configuration is the most robust configuration against bioelectric artifacts.

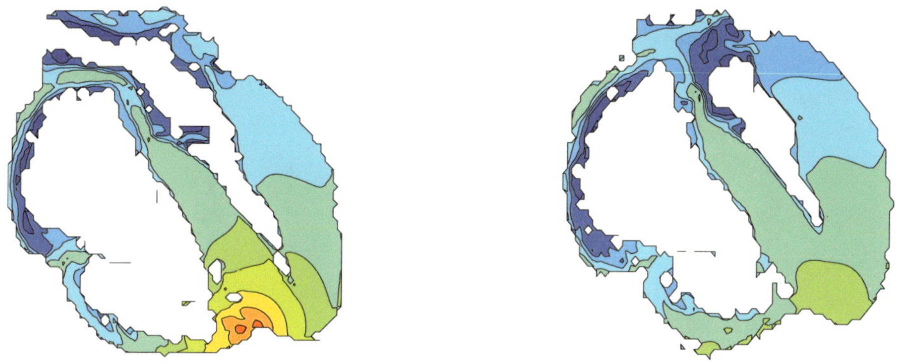

Unipolar *A* configuration (helix to casing)

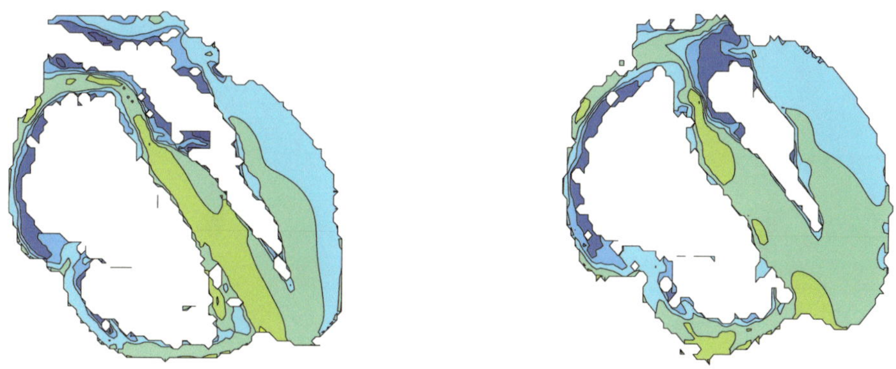

Unipolar *B* configuration (coil to casing)

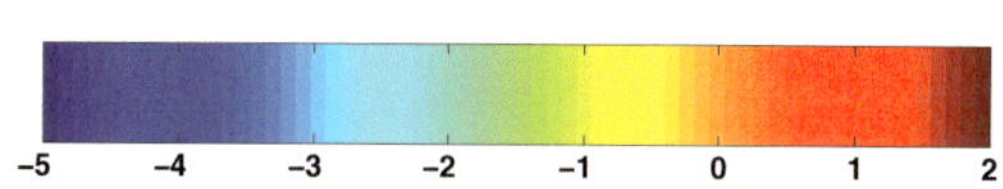

Fig. 1. Sensitivity distributions of unipolar intracardiac configurations at two cross-sections of the heart (arbitrary units, logarithmic scale).

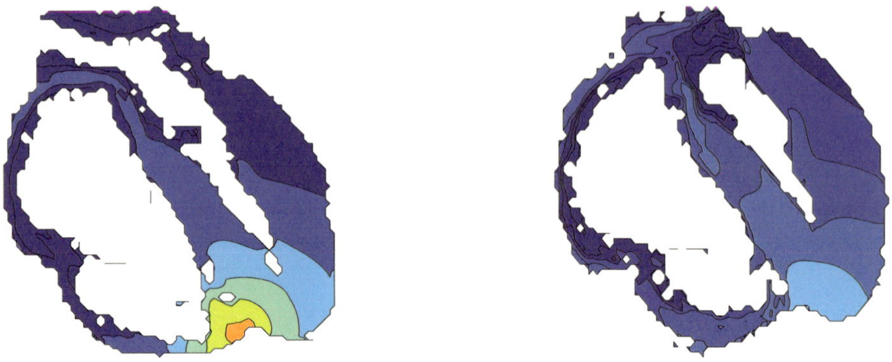

Dedicated bipolar configuration (helix to ring)

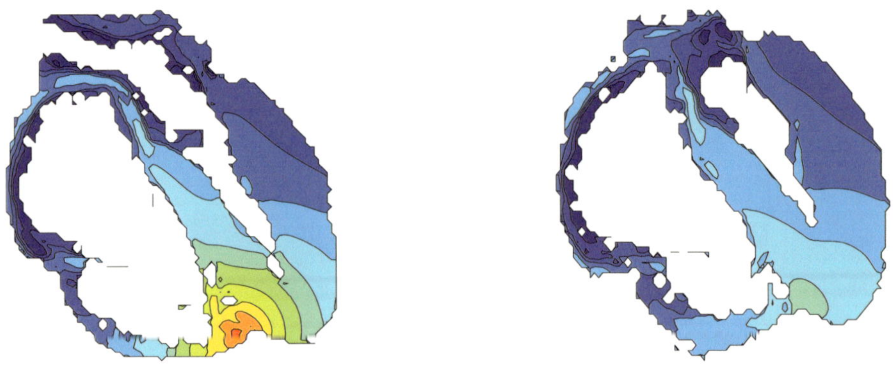

Integrated bipolar configuration (helix to coil)

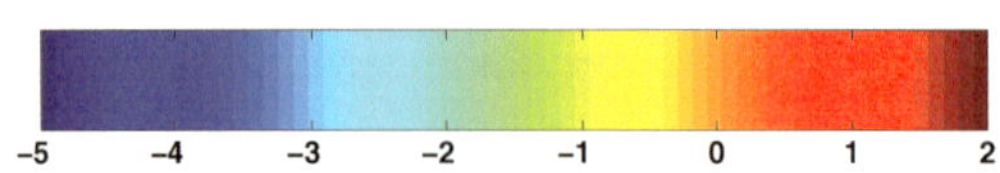

Fig. 2. Sensitivity distributions of bipolar intracardiac configurations at two cross-sections of the heart (arbitrary units, logarithmic scale).

	Discrimination power (dB)	
	DI_{AV}	DI_{MV}
Unipolar *A*	-33	-13
Unipolar *B*	-15	-2
Dedicated bipolar	-61	-57
Integrated Bipolar	-48	-50

Table 3. Discrimination power against atrial and muscular artifacts.

5. Conclusions

Current ICD tachyarrhythmia detection algorithms use heart rhythm criteria to determine whether patients are suffering from a life-threatening arrhythmia. In order to extract heart rhythm, ICD currently estimate the duration of the RR interval on a beat-to-beat basis by sensing ventricular activations in EGM signals, which are continuously recorded by intracardiac leads. As a consequence, ICD overall performance depends on the ability of intracardiac leads to measure ventricular bioelectric events and reject other biolectric events of non-ventricular origin, which include myopotentials (Deshmukh & Anderson, 1998; Kowalski et al., 2008; Sandler & Kutalek, 1994; Schulte et al., 2001) and pacing stimulus artifacts (Menz et al., 1998).

It is widely acknowledged that lead design can affect EGM sensing and therefore ICD performance. On the basis that bipolar configurations are more specific to ventricular events than unipolar configurations, current ICD use bipolar leads, either dedicated or integrated, for EGM sensing, while unipolar-like leads are mainly used for cardiac defibrillation. In a previous study, the sensitivity distribution of two unipolar and two bipolar intracardiac ICD leads were investigated in a numerical model of the ventricles (Requena-Carrión et al., 2009). This study showed quantitatively that bipolar leads concentrate their measurements more than unipolar leads and therefore, provide with ventricular events at a more local level than unipolar leads, which are characterized by global measurements.

In the present study, the investigation previously developed in (Requena-Carrión et al., 2009) has been extended by including the analysis of the sensitivity distribution at the atria and near muscles. Four intracardiac leads based on a current ICD commercial system have been studied in a computational model of the human thorax. Our analysis supports the view that bipolar configurations concentrate their measurement on a local level, while unipolar configurations provide with global measurements. In addition to this, we have been able to analyze qualitatively the sensitivity distribution at the ventricular and atrial myocardium, showing that the sensitivity distribution of unipolar configurations is roughly of the same order of magnitude at the atria and at the ventricles, whereas the sensitivity distribution of bipolar configurations drops several orders of magnitude from the ventricles to the atria. In order to analyze quantitatively the sensitivity to non-ventricular bioelectric sources, we have proposed a discrimination index that compares the accumulated sensitivity at the ventricles with the accumulated sensitivity at other non-ventricular bioelectric sources. Our results reveal that bipolar configurations are more specific to ventricular sources than unipolar configurations and hence, less vulnerable to bioelectric artifacts.

The notion of lead sensitivity distribution can provide with a useful insight into the nature of bioelectric signals. In combination with numerical methods, the sensitivity distribution can help to analyze the performance of current leads and can assist in the design of future leads.

6. Acknowledgments

The authors would like to thank Dr. -Ing. Gunnar Seeman of Karlsruhe Institute of Technology for kindly providing with the detailed numerical model of the human thorax that was used in this study.

7. References

Arzbaecher, R. C., Jenkins, J. M., Collins, S. & Berbari, E. (1979). Atrial electrical activity: The view from the esophagus, *IEEE/EMBS Frontiers of Engineering in Health Care*, pp. 314–318.

Asbach, S., Weiss, I., Wenzel, B., Bode, C. & Sehender, M. (2006). Intrathoracic far-field electrocardiogram allows continuous monitoring of ischemia after total coronary occlusion, *Pacing and Clinical Electrophysiology* 29(12): 1334–1340.

Belott, P. H. & Reynolds, D. W. (2007). Permanent pacemaker and implantable cardioverter-defibrillator implantation, *in* Ellenbogen, K. A., Kay, G. N., Lau, C. P. & Wilkoff, B. L. (eds), *Clinical cardiac pacing, defibrillation, and resynchronization therapy*, Saunders/Elsevier, Philadephia, pp. 561–651.

Bunch, T. J. & Day, J. D. (2008). The diagnostic evolution of the cardiac implantable electronic device: The implantable monitor of ischemia, *Journal of Cardiovascular Electrophysiology* 19(3): 282–284.

Cooklin, M., Tummala, R. V., Peters, R. W., Shorofsky, S. R. & Gold, M. R. (1999). Comparison of bipolar and integrated sensing for redetection of ventricular fibrillation, *American Heart Journal* 138(1 Pt 1): 133–136.

DeCaprio, V., Hurzeler, P. & Furman, S. (1977). A comparison of unipolar and bipolar electrograms for cardiac pacemaker sensing, *Circulation* 56(5): 750–755.

Deshmukh, P. & Anderson, K. (1998). Myopotential sensing by a dual chamber implantable cardioverter defibrillator: Two case reports, *Journal of Cardiovascular Electrophysiology* 9(7): 767–772.

Frain, B. H., Ellison, K. E., Michaud, G. F., Koo, C. H., Buxton, A. E. & Kirk, M. M. (2007). True bipolar defibrillator leads have increased sensing latency and threshold compared with the integrated bipolar configuration, *Journal of Cardiovascular Electrophysiology* 18(2): 192–195.

Gabriel, S., Lau, R. W. & Gabriel, C. (1996). The dielectric properties of biological tissues: II. Measurements in the frequency range 10 hz to 20 Ghz, *Physics in Medicine and Biology* 41: 2251–2269.

Goldberger, J. J., Horvath, G., Donovan, D., Johnson, D., Challapalli, R. & Kadish, A. H. (1998). Detection of ventricular fibrillation by transvenous defibrillating leads: integrated versus dedicated bipolar sensing, *Journal of Cardiovascular Electrophysiology* 9: 677–688.

Gradaus, R., Breithardt, G. & Bocker, D. (2003). ICD leads: design and chronic dysfunctions, *Pacing and Clinical Electrophysiology* 26(2 Pt 1): 649–657.

Jenkins, J. M. (1992). Impact of electrode placement and configuration on performance of morphological measures of intraventricular electrograms, *IEEE Computers in Cardiology*, pp. 367–370.

Kowalski, M., Ellenbogen, K. A., Wood, M. A. & Friedman, P. L. (2008). Implantable cardiac defibrillator lead failure or myopotential oversensing? An approach to the diagnosis of noise on lead electrograms, *Europace* 10(8): 914–917.

Langberg, J. J., Gibb, W. J., Auslander, D. M. & Griffin, J. C. (1988). Identification of ventricular tachycardia with use of the morphology of the endocardial electrogram, *Circulation* 77(6): 1363–1369.

Malmivuo, J. & Plonsey, R. (1995). *Bioelectromagnetism: Principles and applications of bioelectric and biomagnetic fields*, Oxford University Press, New York.

Malmivuo, J., Suihko, V. & Eskola, H. (1997). Sensitivity distributions of EEG and MEG measurements, *IEEE Transactions on Biomedical Engineering* 44: 196–208.

Medtronic (2008). *Secura VR D224VRC*.

Medtronic (2010). *Sprint Quattro Secure 6947*.

Menz, V., Schwartzman, D., Drachman, D., Michele, J. J. & Dillon, S. M. (1998). Recording of pacing stimulus artifacts by endovascular defibrillation lead systems: Comparison of true and integrated bipolar circuits, *Journal of Interventional Cardiac Electrophysiology* 2: 269–272.

Nash, A., Fröhlig, G., Taborsky, M., Stammwitz, E., Maru, F., Bouwens, L. & Çeliker, C. (2005). Rejection of atrial sensing artifacts by a pacing lead with short tip-to-ring spacing, *Europace* 7(1): 67–72.

Natale, A., Sra, J., Axtell, K., Akhtar, M., Newby, K., Kent, V., Geiger, M. J., Brandon, M. J., Kearney, M. M. & Pacifico, A. (1996). Undetected ventricular fibrillation in transvenous implantable cardioverter-defibrillators. Prospective comparison of different lead system-device combinations, *Circulation* 93(1): 91–98.

Parsonnet, V., Myers, G. H. & Kresh, Y. M. (1980). Characteristics of intracardiac electrograms II: Atrial endocardial electrograms, *Pacing and Clinical Electrophysiology* 3(4): 406–417.

Requena-Carrión, J., Väisänen, J., Alonso-Atienza, F., García-Alberola, A., Ramos-López, F. & Rojo-Álvarez, J. L. (2009). Sensitivity and spatial resolution of transvenous leads in implantable cardioverter defibrillator, *IEEE Transactions on Biomedical Engineering* 56(12): 2773 -2781.

Requena-Carrión, J., Väisänen, J., Rojo-Álvarez, J. L., Hyttinen, J., Alonso-Atienza, F. & Malmivuo, J. (2007). Numerical analysis of the resolution of surface electrocardiographic lead systems, *FIMH*, pp. 310–319.

Rush, S. & Driscoll, D. A. (1969). EEG electrode sensitivity–an application of reciprocity, *IEEE Transactions on Biomedical Engineering* 16(1): 15–22.

Sachse, F. B., Werner, C. D., Meyer-Waarden, K. & Dössel, O. (1998). Applications of the visible man dataset in electrocardiology: Calculation and visualization of body surface potential maps of a complete heart cycle, *Second Users Conference of the National Library of Medicine's Visible Human Project*, pp. 47–48.

Sandler, M. J. & Kutalek, S. P. (1994). Inappropriate discharge by an implantable cardioverter defibrillator: Recognition of myopotential sensing using telemetered intracardiac electrograms, *Pacing and Clinical Electrophysiology* 17(4): 665–671.

Schulte, B., Sperzel, J., Carlsson, J., Dürsch, M., Erdogan, A., Pitschner, H. F. & Neuzner, J. (2001). Inappropriate arrhythmia detection in implantable defibrillator therapy due to oversensing of diaphragmatic myopotentials, *Journal of Interventional Cardiac Electrophysiology* 5: 487–493.

Swerdlow, C. D., Gillberg, J. M. & Olson, W. H. (2007). Sensing and detection, *in* Ellenbogen, K. A., Kay, G. N., Lau, C. P. & Wilkoff, B. L. (eds), *Clinical cardiac pacing, defibrillation, and resynchronization therapy*, Saunders/Elsevier, pp. 75–160.

Takano, N. (2002). Reduction of ECG leads and equivalent sources using orthogonalization and clustering techniques, *Doctoral Thesis 302*, Ragnar Granit Institute, Tampere University of Technology.

Väisänen, J. & Hyttinen, J. (2009). Region of interest sensitivity ratio in analyzing sensitivity distributions of electrocardiographic measurements, *Annals of Biomedical Engineering* 37: 692–701.

Väisänen, J., Väisänen, O., Malmivuo, J. & Hyttinen, J. (2008). New method for analysing sensitivity distributions of electroencephalography measurements, *Medical & Biological Engineering & Computing* 46: 101–8.

Williams, J. L., Mendenhall, G. S. & Saba, S. (2008). Effect of ischemia on implantable defibrillator intracardiac shock electrograms, *Journal of Cardiovascular Electrophysiology* 19(3): 275–281.

Zaitsev, A. V., Berenfeld, O., Mironov, S. F., Jalife, J. & Pertsov, A. M. (2000). Distribution of excitation frequencies on the epicardial and endocardial surfaces of fibrillating ventricular wall of the sheep heart, *Circulation Research* 86: 408–417.

4

Modeling Defibrillation

Gernot Plank[1] and Natalia Trayanova[2]
[1]*Medical University of Graz, Austria*
[2]*Johns Hopkins University, MD, Baltimore*
[1]*Austria*
[2]*USA*

1. Introduction

Cardiac fibrillation is the breakdown of the organized electrical activity in the heart into disorganized self-sustained electrical activation patterns. Fibrillatory episodes when affecting the ventricles, i.e. the main pumping chambers of the heart, result in loss of cardiac output and unless timely intervention is administered, death quickly ensues. The only known effective therapy for lethal disturbances in cardiac rhythm is defibrillation, the delivery of a strong electric shock to the heart. This technique, as accomplished nowadays by automatic, implantable cardioverter-defibrillator (ICD) devices, constitutes the most important means of combating sudden cardiac death. Several multi-center clinical trials have provided consistent evidence that ICD therapy prolongs patient life. This convincing demonstration of efficacy has led to a nearly exponential growth, over the last decade, in the number of patients receiving implantable devices. Currently, around 0.2 million ICDs are implanted every year throughout the world.

Although ICD therapy has proved to be efficient and reliable in preventing sudden cardiac death (Bardy et al., 1993), with success rates clearly superior to other therapeutic options such as pharmacological anti-arrhythmia therapy (Zipes et al., 1997), it is far from ideal. There are several known adverse effects secondary to the administration of electrical shocks, the most prominent are linked to electroporation (DeBruin & Krassowska, 1998), (i.e. the formation of pores in the cellular membrane that allow the free and indiscriminate redistribution of ions, enzymes and large molecules between intracellular and interstitial space), and its after-effects which are indirectly caused by the high field strengths required to terminate arrhythmias such as ventricular fibrillation (VF) with sufficiently high probability. Moreover, psychological effects on patients play an important role. Conscious patients may perceive shock delivery as extremely painful which leads to traumatization and reduction in quality of life. Although pain may be tolerable in those cases where shock delivery saves human lives, this is less likely in those cases where inadequate shocks are delivered due to high voltage component malfunctions of the device. A recent meta-analysis of industrial reports (Maisel, 2006) concluded that such malfunctions are much more frequent than expected, with thousands of patients being affected. Further, clinical data from ICD trials suggested that 6 out of 7 shocks delivered can be classified as inadequate, indicating the amount of over-treatment in the ICD population is significant (Zipes et al., 1997). Therefore, despite the impressive clinical success and efficacy of ICD implant, the therapy is clearly suboptimal due to these numerous adverse side effects and as such research on defibrillation mechanisms remains to be an important topic. Achieving defibrillation reliably with shocks of much lower energy than those delivered by ICD devices today, would constitute a major step forward. Advancing our understanding towards a full appreciation of the mechanisms by which a shock interacts with the heart is the most promising approach to achieve this goal.

1.1 Experimental approaches to investigate defibrillation mechanisms

Elucidating the biophysical underpinnings of defibrillation mechanisms has been a long and arduous process. The key to understanding the cardiac defibrillation process is to uncover those mechanisms by which electric current delivered to the heart during shock delivery traverses myocardial structures and interacts with the wavefronts of fibrillation. The quest for uncovering these mechanistic links between applied electric fields and evoked membrane responses has proved to be enormously challenging. In no small part these difficulties can be attributed to the lack of suitable experimental methodologies which would allow to observe electrical events occurring before, during and after shock delivery with sufficiently high spatio-temporal resolution. Early studies relied on recordings of extracellular potentials following the defibrillation shock, since overwhelming electrical artifacts had prevented researchers from recording during and shortly after the shock. Although these pioneering electrical mapping studies provided some insights which laid the basis for developing the first theories such as the upper limit of vulnerability (ULV) hypothesis, there was no direct experimental evidence to prove the putative mechanisms. A major breakthrough occur ed with the introduction of potentiometric dyes, which allowed to record electrical events before, during and after shock delivery at a higher spatio-temporal resolution. The ability of these optical mapping techniques to provide optical fluorescence signals, V_{opt}, which are proportional to the transmembrane voltage, $\propto V_m$, proved to be a further advantage. Unlike extracellularly recorded electric potentials, Φ_e, which integrate contributions of bioelectric activity in the vicinity of a recording site via the volume conductor in which the heart is immersed, V_m provides a more direct measure for shock-induced membrane responses, although optical signals are not purely local representations of V_m at a recording site either, since fluorescence detectors collect photons emerging from within a certain scattering volume (Bishop et al., 2007). Although optical mapping setups allow to elegantly visualize shock-induced changes in tissue polarizations, these observations are confined to record electrical activity from cardiac surfaces only. However, in a complex three-dimensional anatomical structure such as the heart electrical events occur throughout the entire myocardium including the depth of the myocardial walls. Therefore, the restricted capabilities of current optical mapping techniques to detect events which may occur in deeper layers of the myocardial wall without any signature at the surfaces (Ashihara et al., 2008), poses a severe limitation, rendering investigations of defibrillation mechanisms by experimental means alone a challenging endeavor.

1.2 Role of computer modeling

The absence of experimental methodology for observing shock-induced membrane polarizations in 3D inspired the theoretical community to develop and refine computer models of the cardiac defibrillation process. Since there is insufficient direct experimental evidence which would allow a direct verification of model predictions in the depth of the myocardium, computer models are compared against optical maps recorded at the ventricular surfaces. Assuming that model formulations are valid quantitatively correct representation of cardiac bioelectricity, models which correctly predict experimental observations at the

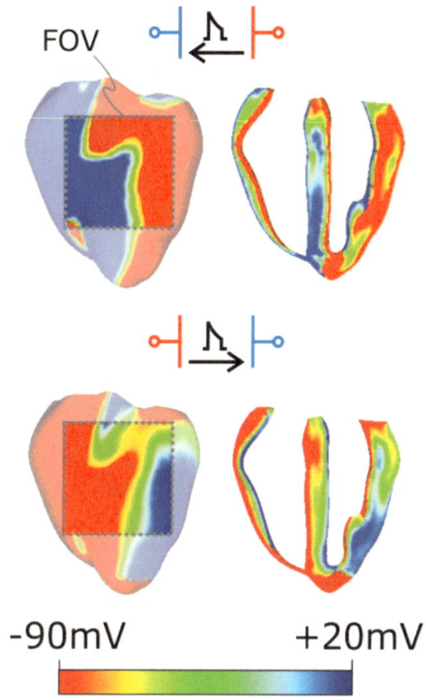

Fig. 1. Left panel: In most experimental setups the field of view (FOV) of optical recordings, as indicated by a gray dashed rectangle, is confined to the surface. Shown are polarization patterns at the end of the shock delivered via plate electrodes, with the cathode being located next to the left ventricle (top) and the right ventricle (bottom). Right panel: Computer models allow to observe shock-induced changes in polarization throughout the entire myocardium, revealing important shock-induced changes in electrical state of the tissue, such as shape, size and location of the post-shock excitable gap (blue regions).

surfaces could be used with some confidence to take a look inside the depth of myocardial walls, thus allowing to bridge the gap between experimental observations recorded at epicardial and endocardial surfaces (Fig. 1).

In earlier computational studies of defibrillation mechanisms monodomain models were employed. Such monodomain formulations do not account explicitly for current flow in the extracellular domains. This simplification reduces model complexity and computational costs at the cost of biophysical accuracy. Although monodomain models were well established for studying impulse propagation in the heart, their suitability in the context of simulating the process of defibrillation quickly turned out to be of limited value. Theoretical considerations based on the monodomain equations predicted shock-induced changes in transmembrane voltage, ΔV_m, only along tissue boundaries and around conductive discontinuities in the heart, leaving the bulk of the myocardium essentially unaffected. However, such predictions contradicted experimental findings which had established that a critical mass of the tissue of $\sim 95\%$ (Adgey et al., 2005; Ideker et al., 1991) has to be affected by a sufficiently strong gradient of > 5 V/cm (Frazier et al., 1989; Zhou et al., 1993) to be effective. To resolve this dilemma the theoretical community put forward the more comprehensive bidomain model which explicitly accounts for current flow in both the intracellular and interstitial domains. The bidomain model proved quickly to be an invaluable powerful tool for studying defibrillation mechanisms, providing the sought after "missing link" (Roth & Krassowska, 1998) between externally applied electric field and membrane responses in the tissue bulk. Using a bidomain model Sepulveda and coworkers (Sepulveda et al., 1989) demonstrated in a seminal study that shock-induced changes in membrane polarizations can be much more complex than previously anticipated. Their simulation results suggested that the tissue response in the vicinity of a strong unipolar stimulus involved the simultaneous occurrence of both positive (depolarizing) and negative (hyperpolarizing) effects in close proximity, if the anisotropy ratios between intracellular and interstitial space comprising the myocardium are unequal, i.e. both spaces are anisotropic, but to a different degree. In the absence of unequal anisotropy ratios, as it is the case with monodomain models which inherently assume equal anisotropies, no polarizations of opposite polarity can occur (Fig. 2). This prediction of the existence of

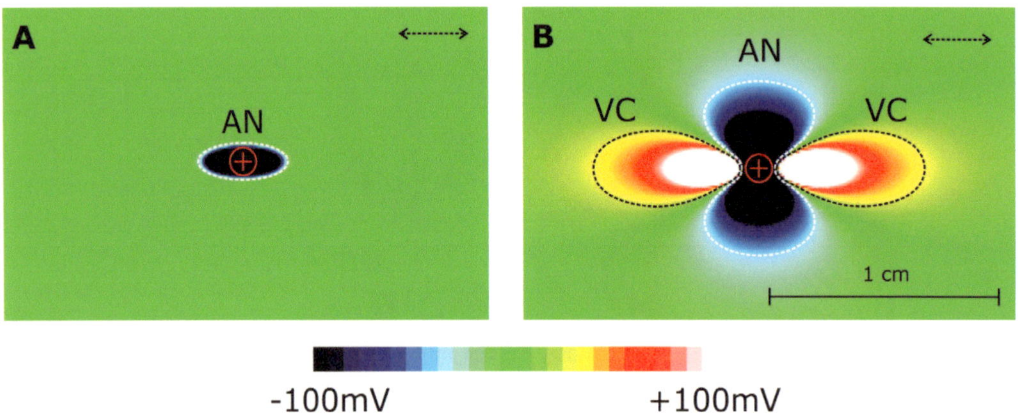

Fig. 2. Unequal anisotropy ratios between intracellular and interstitial space is a necessary condition for the existence of bulk VEPs. A) A unipolar anodal stimulus is delivered to the center of a tissue sheet of equal anisotropy ratios. Shock induced polarizations of only one polarity (hyperpolarizing) are observed and the tissue affected by the shock is limited the immediate vicinity of the electrode. B) The exact same shock delivered to tissue of unequal anisotropy ratios induced polarizations of both polarities and the area of tissue affected extends far beyond the electrotonic space constant. Dashed lines indicate the longitudinal axis of myocyte orientation.

"virtual electrodes" departed from the established view that tissue responses should only be depolarizing if the stimulus is cathodal, or hyperpolarizing if the stimulus is anodal. Optical mapping studies that followed convincingly confirmed these theoretical predictions (Wikswo Jr et al., 1995). Since, "virtual electrode polarization" (VEP) has been documented in experiments involving various stimulus configurations (Efimov, Aguel, Cheng, Wollenzier & Trayanova, 2000; Efimov et al., 1997; Efimov, Gray & Roth, 2000; Evans et al., 2002; Knisley et al., 1999).

1.3 Current understanding of defibrillation mechanisms

Conceptually, defibrillation can be considered to be a two-step process. First, the applied shock drives currents that traverse the myocardium and cause complex polarization changes in transmembrane potential distribution (Sobie et al., 1997). Secondly, post-shock active membrane reactions are invoked that eventually result either in termination of fibrillation in the case of shock success, or in reinitiation of fibrillatory activity in the case of shock failure. Using computer models to analyze the etiology of VEP patterns during the shock application phase revealed that shape, location, polarity, and intensity of shock-induced VEP are determined by both the cardiac tissue structure as well as the configuration of the applied field (Knisley et al., 1999; Rodriguez et al., 2005; Sobie et al., 1997). Based on theoretical considerations VEPs can be classified either as "surface VEP", which penetrates the ventricular wall over a few cell layers, or as "bulk VEP" where polarizations arise throughout the ventricular wall (Entcheva et al., 1999; Trayanova et al., 1998). Analysis of the bidomain equations revealed that a necessary condition for the existence of the bulk VEP is the presence of unequal anisotropies in the myocardium. Sufficient conditions include either spatial non-uniformity in applied electric field, or non-uniformity in tissue architecture, such as fiber curvature, fiber rotation, fiber branching and anastomosis, and local changes in tissue conductivity due to resistive heterogeneities (Plank et al., 2005) (Fig. 3).

The cellular response depends on VEP magnitude and polarity as well as on pre-shock state of the tissue. APD can be either extended (by positive VEP) or shortened (by negative VEP) to a degree that depends on VEP magnitude and shock timing, with strong negative VEP completely abolishing (de-exciting) the action potential thus creating post-shock excitable gaps. As demonstrated in bidomain modeling studies (Ashihara et al., 2008; Roth, 1995), the post-shock VEP pattern is also the major determinant of the origin of post-shock activations. In those regions where shock-induced virtual anodes and virtual cathodes are in close proximity, a "break" excitation at shock-end (i.e, the "break" of the shock) can be elicited. The virtual cathode serves as an electrical stimulus eliciting a regenerative depolarization and a propagating wave in the newly created excitable area. Whether or not break excitations arise depends on whether the transmembrane potential gradient across the border spans the threshold for regenerative depolarization (Cheng, Mowrey, Van Wagoner, Tchou & Efimov, 1999). The finding of break excitations, combined with the fact that positive VEP can result in "make" excitations (where "make" refers to the onset of a shock) in regions where tissue is at or near diastole, resulted in a novel understanding of how a strong stimulus can trigger the development of new activations.

According to VEP theory, mechanisms for shock success or failure are multifactorial depending mainly on post-shock distribution of V_m as well as timing and speed of propagation of shock-induced wavefronts. Whether the depolarization of the post-shock excitable gap is achieved in time critically depends on number and conduction velocity of post-shock activations, as well as the available time window which is bounded by the instant at which refractory borders enclosing the excitable regions recover excitability. All factors depend, ultimately, on shock strength. Increasing shock strength results in higher voltage gradients across borders between regions of opposite polarity, leading to more break-excitations (Cheng, Mowrey, Van Wagoner, Tchou & Efimov, 1999) which then start to traverse the post-shock excitable gap earlier (Skouibine et al., 2000a) and at a faster velocity (Cheng, Mowrey, Van Wagoner, Tchou & Efimov, 1999), as well as extending refractoriness to a larger degree (Knisley et al., 1994).

2. Computationally modeling defibrillation and shock-induced arrhythmogenesis

Comprehensive mechanistic insight into defibrillation remains a major scientific frontier and the 3D bidomain model is an important tool to complement and interpret experimental observations. The quest to unravel how shocks could succeed in terminating fibrillation or how they could re-instate arrhythmia has driven the technological aspects of computer simulations of 3D bidomain activity. In order to be able to simulate electrical processes

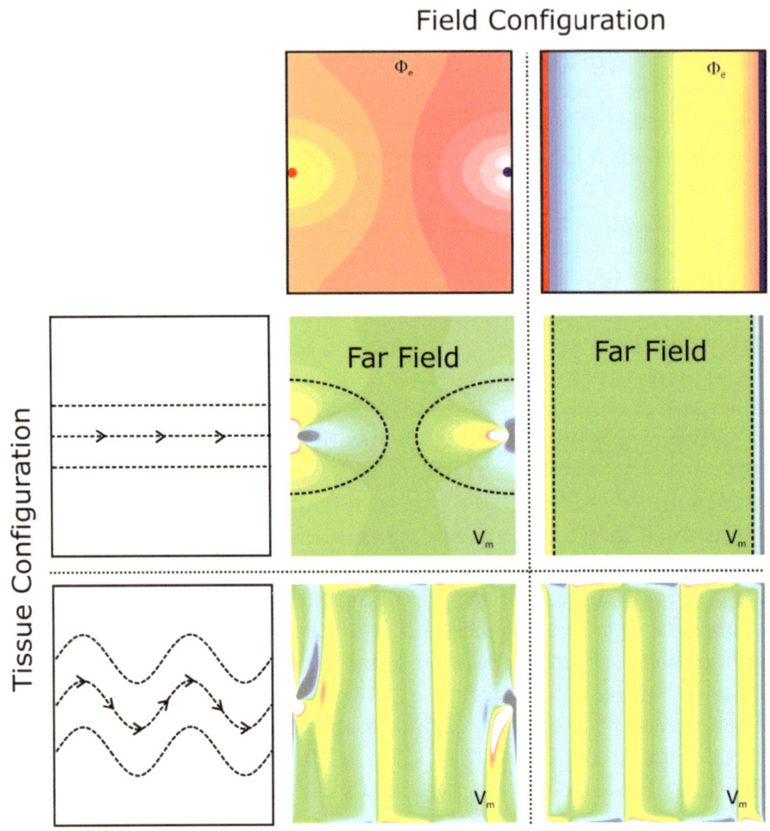

Fig. 3. An important insight learned from the bidomain model is that the etiology of VEPs is determined by both field configuration as well as tissue structure. Shown are shock-induced polarization patterns as a function of field and tissue configuration. Top panels: Shown are the extracellular electric potentials Φ_e as induced by two point-like electrodes (left) and line-like electrodes (right). Red(blue) indicates cathodal (anodal) stimulus. Left panels: Two tissue configurations are shown, a homogeneous configuration with straight fibers only (top), and a configuration where fiber orientation varies as a function of space (bottom). Preferred longitudinal axes of the tissue is indicated by dashed lines. Central panels: Shock-induced polarization patterns for all possible combinations between field and tissue configuration. In the case of plate electrodes with a homogeneous tissue structure only surface polarizations close to the electrode locations are observed. The bulk of the tissue remains essentially unaffected.

driven by the delivery of shocks to the ventricles, computational research has managed to overcome tremendous difficulties associated with obtaining solutions of very large systems of unknowns, involving stiff equations and computational meshes of irregular geometry. A brief overview of the computational approaches involved in conducting simulations of shock administration and post-shock arrhythmogenesis is presented below.

2.1 Simulating cardiac bioelectric activity at the tissue and organ level

Computer models of cardiac biolelectric activity are built upon first principles which represent the movement of ions in within the myocardial tissue. A building block of central importance are cardiac myocytes which make up the tissue. A myocyte is of roughly cylindrical shape, $\sim 100\mu m$ long and 10-20μm in diameter. The intracellular spaces of adjacent myocytes are interconnected by specialized connexins referred to as gap junctions (Desplantez et al., 2007). The connexin expression over the cell is heterogeneous with a higher density of gap junctions at the intercalated discs located at the cell ends (along the long axis of the cell) and a lower density along the lateral boundaries (Gourdie et al., 1991; Hoyt et al., 1989), and different connexins of varying conductance are expressed in different regions of the heart (Severs et al., 2008). As a consequence of the elongated cellular geometry as well as the directionally varying gap junction density current flows more readily along the longitudinal axes of the cells than transverse to it. This property is referred to as anisotropy. Cardiac tissue is composed of two spaces: an intracellular space formed by the interconnected network of myocytes, and the cleft spaces between myocytes referred to as interstitial space which is made up of the extracellular matrix and the interstitial fluid. The extracellular matrix consists of networks of collagen fibers which determine the passive mechanical properties of the myocardium. Electrically, it is assumed that the preferred directions are co-aligned between the two spaces, but that the conductivity ratios between the principal axes are unequal between the two domains (Clerc, 1976; Hooks et al., 2007; Roberts & Scher, 1982; Roth, 1997). All parameters influencing the electrical properties of the tissue, such as density and conductance of gap junctions, cellular geometry, orientation and cell packing density, and the composition of the interstitial space, are heterogeneous and may vary at all size scales, from the cellular level up to the organ. As a consequence, direction and speed of a propagating electric wave is constantly modified by interactions with discontinuous spatial variations in material properties at various size scales. At a finer size scale below the space constant, λ, of the tissue, i.e. $<$1mm, the tissue is best characterized as a discrete network in which the electrical impulse propagates in a discontinuous manner (Kleber & Rudy, 2004; Spach & Heidlage, 1995). At a larger more macroscopic size scale ($\gg \lambda$) the tissue behaves as a continuous functional syncytium where the effects of small-scale discontinuities are assumed to play a minor role.

Theoretically, the idea of modeling an entire heart by using models of a single cell as the basic building block is conceivable. However, the associated computational costs are prohibitive with current computing hardware, since a single heart consists of roughly 5 billion cells. Although a few high resolution modeling studies have been conducted where small tissue preparations were discretized at a sub-cellular resolution (Hooks et al., 2007; Roberts et al., 2008; Spach & Heidlage, 1995), in general the spatial discretization steps were chosen based on the spatial extent of electrical wave fronts and not on the size scales of the tissue's micro-structures. For this sake cardiac tissue is treated as a continuum for which appropriate material parameters have to be determined which translate the discrete cellular matrix into an electrically analog macroscopic representation. In principle, this is achieved by averaging material properties over suitable length scales such that both potential and current solution match between homogenized and discrete representation. A rigorous mathematical framework for this procedure is provided by homogenization theory which has been applied by several authors to the bidomain problem (Hand et al., 2009; Henriquez, 1993; Neu & Krassowska, 1993; Pennacchio M. et al., 2006). Homogenization is a two-step process where the intracellular and interstitial domain are homogenized in a first step and the two respective domains are spread out and overlapped to fill the entire tissue domain. This concept of interpenetrating domains states that everywhere within the entire myocardial volume intracellular space, extracellular space and the cellular membrane coexist (Fig. 4).

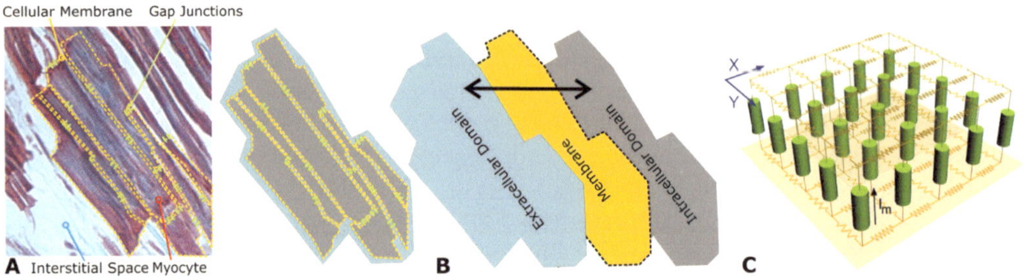

Fig. 4. a) Cardiac tissue is made up of discrete myocytes which are interconnected via gap junctions. b) Discrete structures in both the intracellular as well as the interstitial space are homogenized to arrive at a continuum representation, which matches electrical properties between discrete microscopic size scale and continuous macroscopic size scale. Further, both homogenized domains are overlapped, separated by a membrane at each point in space (interpenetrating domains). c) Discrete representation of both conductive domains and membrane, as discretized by a finite difference approach.

2.2 Governing equations

The bidomain equations(Plonsey, 1988) describe the electrical behavior of cardiac tissue as a syncytium, where all tissue parameters are accounted for in an averaged sense. The domains of interest, intracellular and extracellular, and the cellular membranes which physically separate the two domains, are distributed over the entire tissue volume. The bidomain equations state that currents that enter the intracellular or extracellular spaces by crossing the cell membrane represent the sources for the intracellular potential, ϕ_i, and the extracellular potential, ϕ_e,

$$\nabla \cdot \boldsymbol{\sigma_i} \nabla \phi_i = \beta I_m \tag{1}$$

$$\nabla \cdot \boldsymbol{\sigma_e} \nabla \phi_e = -\beta I_m - I_e \tag{2}$$

$$I_m = C_m \frac{\partial V_m}{\partial t} + I_{ion}(V_m, \boldsymbol{\eta}) - I_{stim} \tag{3}$$

$$V_m = \phi_i - \phi_e, \tag{4}$$

where $\boldsymbol{\sigma_i}$ and $\boldsymbol{\sigma_e}$ are the intracellular and extracellular conductivity tensors, respectively, β is the bidomain membrane surface to volume ratio, I_m is the transmembrane current density, I_{stim} is the current density of the transmembrane stimulus used to initiate an action potential, I_e is the current density of the extracellular stimulus, C_m is the membrane capacitance per unit area, V_m is the transmembrane potential, and I_{ion} is the density of the total current flowing through the membrane ionic channels, pumps and exchangers, which depends on V_m and a set of state variables, $\boldsymbol{\eta}$. At the tissue boundaries, electrical isolation is assumed, which is accounted for by imposing no-flux boundary conditions on ϕ_e and ϕ_i.

If, however, cardiac tissue is surrounded by a conductive medium, such as blood in the ventricular cavities or a perfusing bath (Tyrode solution) in which the heart is submerged, then Laplace equation has to be additionally solved

$$\nabla \cdot \sigma_b \nabla \phi_e = 0, \tag{5}$$

where σ_b is the isotropic conductivity of the conductive medium. In this case no-flux boundary conditions are assumed at the boundaries of the conductive medium, whereas continuity of the normal component of the extracellular current and continuity of ϕ_e are enforced at the tissue-bath interface. The no-flux boundary conditions for ϕ_i remain the same.
For most applications the bidomain equations are recast into other forms by substituting eq.(4) into (1) and (2) and executing algebraic transformations. Several ways to recast the bidomain equations have been proposed; a systematic overview of the different linear transformations is found in (Hooke et al., 1994). A widely used transformation is to add eqs. (1) and (2) and replace ϕ_i by $V_m + \phi_e$ (Pollard et al., 1992)

$$\nabla \cdot (\boldsymbol{\sigma_i} + \boldsymbol{\sigma_e}) \nabla \phi_e = -\nabla \cdot \boldsymbol{\sigma_i} \nabla V_m - I_e \tag{6}$$

$$\nabla \cdot \boldsymbol{\sigma_i} \nabla V_m = -\nabla \cdot \boldsymbol{\sigma_i} \nabla \phi_e + \beta I_m, \tag{7}$$

which retains V_m and ϕ_e as the independent variables. For comparison of tissue and organ level simulations with experimental data this is advantageous since ϕ_e can be measured via electrical mapping techniques and optical mapping techniques allow to record signals $V_{opt} \propto V_m$.

2.3 Computational considerations

Large-scale computational studies employing the bidomain model in general, and defibrillation studies in particular, have remained a challenge even though computer speed and memory have dramatically increased. There are numerous factors which render any numerical solution of the bidomain equations computationally challenging. First, the upstroke of the action potential is very fast, lasting only $\sim$ 1ms. These fast transients translate into a steep propagating wavefront in space where the depolarization wavefront extends only a few hundreds of μm. As a consequence, both spatially fine-grained computational grids and a high temporal resolution is required to faithfully capture wavefront propagation. Further, the discretized domain of interest has to be chosen large enough to support reentrant wave propagation when studying the formation, maintenance and termination of cardiac arrhythmias. With constraints on spatial discretization as mentioned above, the results is a large system, on the order of 0.1 to 100 million degrees of freedom. Finally, the maximum time step which can be taken to advance the solution of the bidomain equations in time is limited, either by stability (Courant et al., 1928) or accuracy constraints. Since the physiological processes of interest take place over seconds or minutes, temporal step size limits necessitate a large number of time steps, typically in the range from tens to hundreds of thousands.
Beyond the high computational load imposed by bidomain simulations in general, there are numerous additional methodological challenges which need to be addressed when using computer models for studying the delivery of defibrillation shocks. To model the effect of extracellularly applied fields, the use of unstructured grids for anatomically realistic models of the heart is mandatory as to allow smooth representation of the organ's surfaces. Jagged boundaries, which inevitably form along the organ surfaces when regular structured or block structured grids are employed, cause spurious polarizations upon delivery of a defibrillation-strength shock. Further, even finer spatial discretization may be required since large transmembrane voltage gradients are induced by the shock; for instance, in a passive 2D bidomain study (Aguel et al., 1999) a voltage drop of 1V over a distance as short as 100 μm has been reported. Another serious difficulty is the use of state-of-the-art ionic models which incorporate now up to several tens of state variables of ever increasing stiffness. These models are developed and tested within the normal physiological range of action potentials,

however, during the shock administration transmembrane voltages may rise significantly beyond this range, even when ionic models are augmented with additional currents such as electroporation currents (DeBruin & Krassowska, 1998) or hypothetical potassium currents (Cheng, Tung & Sobie, 1999). Although these currents kick in at elevated transmembrane voltages to cap the rise of V_m at a few hundreds of mV, transmembrane voltages still rises well beyond the physiological range which could potentially entail undesirable behavior of the model equations. Moreover, due to the even faster transients in state variables during shock onset enforce, even smaller time steps may be required, making computations during the shock very burdensome. Typically, modifications are required to render an ionic model suitable for defibrillation studies (Ashihara & Trayanova, 2004; Skouibine et al., 2000b). Finally, due to the nature of defibrillation, where shock success depends on a multitude of parameters such as shock strength and timing, pulse shape and polarity or electrode geometry and location, a large number of simulations is required to sweep the parameter space. For instance, a standard problem is to determine the window of vulnerability for a given electrode configuration, that is, for which range of shock strength and coupling intervals the tissue is vulnerable to arrhythmia induction. Such studies involve the construction of vulnerability grids where N timings and M shock strengths have to be tested. Therefore a total of $N \times M$ shocks need to be computed and $N \times M$ simulations of post-shock evolution need to be performed to determine arrhythmia inducibility for each combination.

2.4 Spatial discretization

Various spatial discretization techniques have been applied to the cardiac bidomain problem, most notably the finite difference method (FDM) (Potse et al., 2006; Skouibine et al., 2000a), the finite volume method (FVM) (Harrild & Henriquez, 1997; Trew, Le Grice, Smaill & Pullan, 2005) and the finite element method (FEM) (Rogers & McCulloch, 1994; Vigmond et al., 2002), although other non-standard techniques such as the interconnected cable model have been employed successfully as well (Leon & Roberge, 1991; Wang et al., 1996). In general, the FDM is easiest to implement, but the method does not accommodate complex boundaries as naturally as the FEM or the FVM do. Although suggestions were made to overcome this limitation by employing the phase-field approach (Fenton et al., 2005) or other generalizations (Buist et al., 2003; Trew, Smaill, Bullivant, Hunter & Pullan, 2005), the FDM looses its most appealing advantage, the ease of implementation. FEM and FVM are both very well suited for spatial discretizations of complex geometries with smooth representations of the boundaries, which is a key feature when polarization patterns induced via extracellularly applied currents are to be studied. Both FVM and FEM have been used to model electrical activity in anatomical realistic models of the atria (Harrild & Henriquez, 2000; Seemann et al., 2006; Vigmond et al., 2004; Virag et al., 2002) as well as the ventricles (Ashihara et al., 2008; Plank et al., 2009; Potse et al., 2006; Ten Tusscher et al., 2007). Mesh generation requirements are similar for both techniques, that is, the domain of interest has to be tessellated into a set of non-overlapping and conformal geometric primitives (Fig. 5). With the FVM, quadrilaterals in 2D (Harrild & Henriquez, 1997) and hexahedral elements in 3D (Harrild & Henriquez, 2000; Trew, Le Grice, Smaill & Pullan, 2005) have been preferred, whereas with the FEM, triangles and quadrilaterals were used in 2D and tetrahedral (Plank et al., 2009) or hexahedral elements in 3D (Munteanu et al., 2009; Seemann et al., 2006). Typically, monolithic meshes consisting of one element type only were used, but exception exist (Prassl et al., 2009; Rocha et al., 2011) where hybrid meshes consisting of tetrahedra, hexahedra, pyramids and prisms were used. Further, most FEM studies relied on the Galerkin FEM where linear test functions with tetrahedral elements (Franzone et al., 2006; Sundnes et al., 2006; Vigmond et al., 2002), isoparametric trilinear test functions with hexahedral elements (Munteanu et al., 2009) or cubic-hermite hexahedral elements (Rogers & McCulloch, 1994; Saucerman et al., 2004) were used.

Independently of the spatial discretization technique, the choice of space step, h, is of major importance. It is known since very early modeling studies that the solution of the bidomain equations does depend, to a certain degree, on h, even with very fine spatial discretizations (Pollard et al., 1993). This sensitivity has to be attributed to the non-linearity and stiffness of the reaction term which entails an extremely fast upstroke of the cardiac action potential, lasting $\sim$ 1 ms only. When propagating, a fast upstroke in time translates into a steep wavefront in space. Depending on tissue conductivity and cellular excitability, physiological conduction velocities range between 0.2 - 0.7 m/s within the myocardium which translates an upstroke duration of 1 ms duration into a wavefront that extends 200-700 μm in space. Under pathological situations where tissue conductivity and/or excitability is reduced, conduction velocity may be substantially slower, leading to wavefronts where the spatial extent may be even below 100 μm. The spatial extent of a wavefront along a direction ζ is proportional to the space constant, λ_ζ,

$$\lambda_\zeta = \sqrt{\frac{1}{\beta}\frac{\sigma_{i\zeta}\sigma_{e\zeta}}{\sigma_{i\zeta}+\sigma_{e\zeta}}}. \tag{8}$$

It has been shown that for sufficiently small effective discretizations, $H_\zeta = \lambda_\zeta / h_\zeta < 0.15$, solutions converge with deviations in conduction velocity <1% (Pollard et al., 1993). In practice, a trade-off has to be made between accuracy and computational tractability. In tissue and organ scale modeling studies a standard choice for h, or for an average discretization $\bar{h}$ when unstructured grids are considered, is 250μm, but finer (Plank et al., 2009) as well as coarser discretizations (Ashihara et al., 2008; Saucerman et al., 2004) have been reported as well. With very coarse discretizations, h >500 μm, and physiologically realistic models of cellular dynamics simulations deviate substantially from results obtained at finer resolutions. Conduction velocities at such coarse grids are underestimated to different degrees as a function of direction, leading to wavefront distortions (Clayton et al., 2011), even conduction block may occur as a numerical side effect due to spatial undersampling.

2.5 Construction of models of cardiac anatomy

In order to construct geometrically-realistic models of cardiac anatomy, such information must be first obtained via various different imaging modalities, to then be processed and used in model construction. In the past decade or so, efforts have been focused towards developing techniques to construct 3D computational cardiac models directly from non-invasive 3D imaging modalities such as magnetic resonance (MR). In the last few years, the advent of stronger magnets and refined scanning protocols has significantly increased the resolution of anatomical MR scans, such that small mammalian hearts now can have MR voxel dimensions of $\approx 20 - 25$ μm (Burton et al., 2006; Plank et al., 2009). An example of a high resolution anatomical MR scan of a rabbit heart with voxel resolution $\approx$ 25 μm isotropic is shown in Fig. 5. As a result of this increase in attainable resolution, anatomical MR imaging is now capable of providing a wealth of information regarding fine-scaled cardiac structural complexity. Such MR data is currently allowing accurate identification of microscopic features such as the coronary vasculature, extracellular cleft spaces and the free-running Purkinje system, as well as macroscopic structures such as trabeculations and papillary muscles. In addition, information regarding the organization of cardiomyocytes into cardiac fibers

(Streeter et al., 1969), as well as the laminar structure of the myocardial wall (LeGrice et al., 1995) is required to account for orthotropic tissue properties. Such data is unattainable with normal anatomical MR imaging, however, the eigenaxes of the tissue can be estimated in 3D using diffusion-tensor MR imaging (DT-MRI).

This information must then be processed and transformed into a usable format to facilitate the generation of anatomically-detailed computational cardiac models. A first processing step is to faithfully extract the complex geometrical information present in the image stacks. This procedure, referred to as segmentation, involves labeling voxels based-on their association with different regions, types of tissue, objects or boundaries within the image. Ideally, computational algorithms are employed, which automatically segment regions of interest within the image with little or no manual input. For generating a computational model it is required to discriminate those voxels in the MR data set which belong to cardiac 'tissue' from those which represent non-tissue or 'background', effectively translating a gray-scale MR image data set into a binary black/white (0/1) image mask.

In a final step, classified objects in the binarized image stacks are tessellated into finite element meshes. The construction of such meshes is a highly non-trivial task. Recent advances in image-based mesh generation techniques allow the direct construction of finite element meshes using segmented image stacks as input (Prassl et al., 2009). Although the exceptionally high resolution of such data sets currently being obtained can provide unprecedented insight regarding intact cardiac anatomical structure, faithfully transferring this information into a finite element mesh that is both of good quality and is computationally tractable, is a significant challenge. A widely used approach is based on a recently published image-based unstructured mesh generation technique (Prassl et al., 2009) or its commercial implementation Tarantula (`www.meshing.at, CAE-Software Solutions, Eggenburg, Austria`). This method uses a modified dual mesh of an Octree applied directly to segmented 3D image stacks. The algorithm operates fully automatically with no requirements for interactivity and generates accurate volume-preserving representations of arbitrarily complex geometries with smooth surfaces. The generated unstructured meshes are hybrid, hexahedra-dominant, boundary fitted, locally refined, conformal finite element meshes (see Fig. 5, middle panel). The smooth nature of the surfaces ensures general applicability of the meshes generated, in particular for studies involving the application of strong external stimuli, since the smooth, unstructured grids lack jagged boundaries that can introduce spurious currents due to tip effects, as is the case for structured grids. To reduce the overall computational load of the meshes, unstructured grids can be generated adaptively such that the spatial resolution varies throughout the domain. Fine discretizations with little adaptivity can be used to model the myocardium thus minimizing undesired effects of grid granularity on propagation velocity, whilst coarser elements that grow in size with distance from myocardial surfaces are generated to represent a surrounding volume conductor (e.g. tissue bath or torso for example). Using adaptive mesh generation techniques facilitates the execution of bidomain simulations with a minimum of overhead due to the discretization of a surrounding volume conductor.

2.6 Numerical schemes

Among the possible castings of the bidomain equations, the one presented as (6) and (7) is the most popular. In the most general case, where a conducting medium is in contact with the

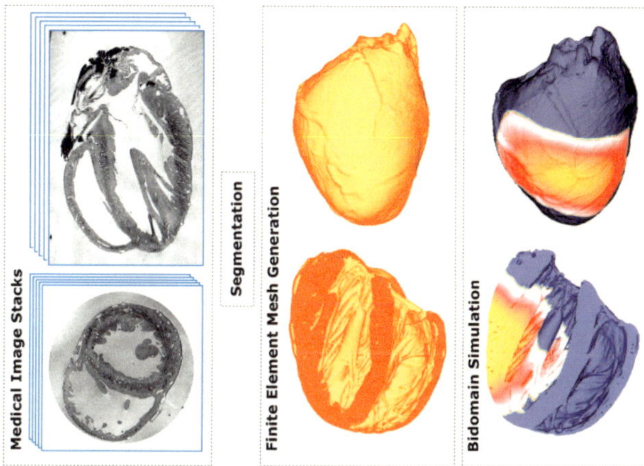

Fig. 5. Image based mesh generation pipeline for constructing geometrically detailed models of cardiac anatomy. Medical image stacks are segmented and fed into an image-based mesh generation algorithm which tessellates classified objects in the image stack into finite element meshes which are suitable for being used in bidomain simulations.

myocardium, the bidomain equations are written as

$$\begin{bmatrix} -\nabla \cdot (\boldsymbol{\sigma}_i + \boldsymbol{\sigma_e}) \nabla \phi_e \\ -\nabla \cdot \sigma_b \nabla \phi_e \end{bmatrix} = \begin{bmatrix} \nabla \cdot \boldsymbol{\sigma_i} \nabla V_m \\ I_e \end{bmatrix} \tag{9}$$

$$\frac{\partial V_m}{\partial t} = \frac{1}{\beta C_m} \left(\nabla \cdot \boldsymbol{\sigma}_i \nabla V_m + \nabla \cdot \boldsymbol{\sigma_i} \nabla \phi_e \right) - \frac{1}{C_m} I_{ion}(V_m, \boldsymbol{\eta}) \tag{10}$$

$$\frac{d\boldsymbol{\eta}}{dt} = g(V_m, \boldsymbol{\eta}) \tag{11}$$

Numerically, the bidomain equations can be solved as a coupled system (Vigmond et al., 2002) or alternatively, operator splitting techniques are applied (Keener & Bogar, 1998) to decouple the computing scheme into three components, an elliptic partial differential equation (PDE), a parabolic PDE, and a set of non-linear ODEs. It has been shown that the decoupled scheme converges quickly against the coupled scheme by employing a Block Gauss-Seidel iteration (Pennacchio & Simoncini, 2002). However, in most studies the components are essentially treated as independent. Solutions are then found by leap-frogging between the decoupled components where either V_m in (9) or Φ_e in (10) are considered as constant. In (Vigmond et al., 2002) it has been found that with small error tolerances the differences between coupled and decoupled approaches are negligible.
Discretizing the decoupled bidomain equations leads to a three-step scheme, which involves a solution of the parabolic PDE, the elliptic PDE and the non-linear system of ODEs at each time step. The inner loop of this scheme is given by

$$V_m^{k^*} = V_m^k + \frac{\Delta t}{\beta C_m} \left[\theta \nabla \cdot \left(\boldsymbol{\sigma_i} \nabla V_m^{k^*} \right) + (1-\theta) \nabla \cdot \left(\boldsymbol{\sigma_i} \nabla V_m^k \right) \right] \tag{12}$$

$$\boldsymbol{\eta}_f^{k+1} = \boldsymbol{\eta}_f^k e^{-\frac{\Delta t}{\tau}} + \boldsymbol{\eta}_\infty \left(1 - e^{-\frac{\Delta t}{\tau}} \right) \tag{13}$$

$$\boldsymbol{\eta}_s^{k+1} = \boldsymbol{\eta}_s^k + \boldsymbol{g}(V_m^{k^*}, \boldsymbol{\eta}_s^k)\Delta t \tag{14}$$

$$V_m^{k+1} = V_m^{k^*} - \frac{\Delta t}{C_m} I_{ion}(V_m^{k^*}, \boldsymbol{\eta}^{k+1}) \tag{15}$$

$$-\nabla \cdot \left((\boldsymbol{\sigma_i} + \boldsymbol{\sigma_e})\nabla\Phi_e^{k+1}\right) = \nabla \cdot \left(\boldsymbol{\sigma_i}\nabla V^{k+1}\right) \tag{16}$$

$$-\nabla \cdot \left(\sigma_b \nabla\Phi_e^{k+1}\right) = I_e, \tag{17}$$

where the reaction and diffusion part of the parabolic PDE is split by employing a Strang or a Gudunov scheme (Qu & Garfinkel, 1999; Sundnes et al., 2005). The parabolic portion (12) is solved either by choosing $\theta = 0.5$, which results in a Crank-Nicholson scheme, or $\theta = 0.0$, which results in an explicit forward Euler scheme. Depending on the choice of θ the overall system is solved then either with a fully explicit scheme, or an implicit-explicit (IMEX) scheme. The ODE integration approach in (13)-(14) is based on the Rush-Larsen method (Rush & Larsen, 1978) where an analytical solution was used to update the fast gating variables, $\boldsymbol{\eta}_f$, where τ and η_∞ are functions of the rate coefficients which govern channel gating, and an explicit Euler step to update all other slower state variables, $\boldsymbol{\eta}_s$ (Maclachlan et al., 2007; Plank et al., 2008).

Typically, additional Dirichlet boundary conditions have to be enforced for the elliptic PDE to eliminate the Nullspace, otherwise the elliptic system is singular. This is usually achieved by adding a grounding electrode, i.e. choosing nodes in the mesh where ϕ_e is set to zero, which serves as the reference potential when simulating the shock, as it is the case in a real physical setup.

2.7 Linear solvers

Although the PDEs are solved most efficiently with direct methods, this is possible for small grids only (Plank et al., 2007; Vigmond et al., 2002); otherwise memory demands increase quickly which, in turn, significantly increases the required number of operations per solver step. Although direct methods have been implemented to run in parallel environments (Amestoy et al., 2001; Li & Demmel, 2003), typically they are harder to parallelize due to the fine-grained parallelism, which is communication-intense. For large systems, iterative methods are mandatory.

When executing bidomain simulations on sequential computers, the main computational burden can be attributed to the solution of the elliptic problem and the set of ODEs. Typically, with simple ionic models, the elliptic problem contributes more than 90% to the overall workload, whereas with recent ionic models involving very stiff ODEs (Cortassa et al., 2006; Iyer et al., 2004), the ODE solution may even begin to dominate the computations. The parabolic problem is typically less of a concern. On coarser meshes, where time steps are limited by the ODEs, simple forward Euler steps can be employed to update V_m. In this case, the contributions of the diffusional component (PDE) and the local membrane component to changes in V_m can be updated separately, which renders the PDE linear. On finer grids, semi-implicit Crank-Nicholson schemes perform well. Even when relatively cheap iterative solvers are employed, the parabolic portion can be updated efficiently due to the diagonal dominance of the linear system.

For large systems, on the order of several hundreds of thousands of unknowns, parallel computing approaches are necessary to reduce execution times. The parallel computing context alleviate the problem of solving the set of ODEs. State variables in an ionic model do not diffuse, which qualifies the ODEs as an embarrassingly parallel problem. No communication between processors is required to update the state variable and thus the parallel scaling of the ODE portion is linear. The parabolic problem is efficiently solved in parallel as well (Niederer S. et al., 2011). Either only a forward Euler step is required (essentially a matrix-vector product for which good scalability is expected), or the well-posed diagonally-dominant linear system is solved efficiently with relatively cheap iterative methods, such as preconditioned conjugate-gradient (CG). Typically, with an incomplete LU (ILU) preconditioner for the iterative CG solver the parabolic problem can be solved in less than 10 iterations.

The elliptic PDE is the most challenging problem. Standard iterative solvers like ILU-CG typically require several hundreds of iterations to converge, which makes this solution significantly more expensive than that of the parabolic system, although both systems share the same sparsity pattern. The parallel scaling of standard iterative solvers is fairly good (Plank et al., 2007); for instance, a parallel ILU-CG solver, where the system is decomposed by a Block Jacobi preconditioner with ILU(0), i.e. an incomplete LU factorization with zero fill-in levels that preserves the sparsity pattern of the original matrix, used as a subblock preconditioner, exhibits good parallel scaling (Plank et al., 2007). With fewer number of processors, ILU(N) with N levels of fill-in tends to be more efficient, however, with an increasing number of processors the efficiency of the preconditioning deteriorates since the preconditioner is applied to the main diagonal block only. This can be circumvented by employing overlapping block preconditioners such as additive Schwarz methods, however, they increase the communication burden, which, depending on the particular hardware, may be undesirable.

It has been demonstrated in several recent studies (Austin et al., 2006; Plank et al., 2007; Weber dos Santos et al., 2004) that multilevel preconditioners for CG methods both significantly improve the overall performance and show reasonable parallel efficiency (better than 80%) for up to 128 processors. A generally applicable algebraic multigrid preconditioner (AMG) in conjunction with an iterative Krylov solver reduces the number of iterations per solver step by almost two orders of magnitude compared to ILU-CG. Although a single iteration with AMG is significantly more expensive than with ILU, the reduction in number of iterations clearly favors a multilevel approach. In (Plank et al., 2007), a speedup of 6 was reported. Using AMG-CG is, to date, the most efficient method for solving the elliptic portion of the bidomain equations. The method is particularly well suited for defibrillation studies since it is computationally efficient and handles unstructured grids straightforwardly.

3. References

Adgey, A. A. J., Spence, M. S. & Walsh, S. J. (2005). Theory and practice of defibrillation: (2) defibrillation for ventricular fibrillation., *Heart* 91(1): 118–125.

Aguel, F., DeBruin, K. A., Krassowska, W. & Trayanova, N. A. (1999). Effects of electroporation on the transmembrane potential distribution in a two-dimensional bidomain model of cardiac tissue, 10: 701–714.

Amestoy, P., Duff, I. S., L'Excellent, J.-Y. & Koster, J. (2001). Mumps: A general purpose distributed memory sparse solver, *PARA '00: Proceedings of the 5th International Workshop on Applied Parallel Computing, New Paradigms for HPC in Industry and Academia*, Springer-Verlag, London, UK, pp. 121–130.

Ashihara, T., Constantino, J. & Trayanova, N. A. (2008). Tunnel propagation of postshock activations as a hypothesis for fibrillation induction and isoelectric window., *Circ Res* 102(6): 737–45.

Ashihara, T. & Trayanova, N. (2004). Asymmetry in membrane responses to electrical shocks: insight from bidomain simulations, 87: 2271–2282.

Austin, T. M., Trew, M. L. & Pullan, A. J. (2006). Solving the cardiac bidomain equations for discontinuous conductivities., *IEEE Trans Biomed Eng* 53(7): 1265–72.

Bardy, G. H., Hofer, B., Johnson, G., Kudenchuk, P. J., Poole, J. E., Dolack, G. L., Gleva, M., Mitchell, R. & Kelso, D. (1993). Implantable transvenous cardioverter-defibrillators., *Circulation* 87(4): 1152–68.

Bishop, M., Rodriguez, B., Qu, F., Efimov, I., Gavaghan, D. & Trayanova, N. (2007). The role of photon scattering in optical signal distortion during arrhythmia and defibrillation, *Biophys. J.* 93: 3714–3726.

Buist, M., Sands, G., Hunter, P. & Pullan, A. (2003). A deformable finite element derived finite difference method for cardiac activation problems., *Ann Biomed Eng* 31(5): 577–88.

Burton, R., Plank, G., Schneider, J., Grau, V., Ahammer, H., Keeling, S., Lee, J., Smith, N., Gavaghan, D., Trayanova, N. & Kohl, P. (2006). 3-d models of individual cardiac histo-anatomy: tools and challenges, *Ann NY Acad Sci* 1380: 301–319.

Cheng, D. K.-L., Tung, L. & Sobie, E. A. (1999). Nonuniform responses of transmembrane potential during electric field stimulation of single cardiac cells, 277: H351–H362.

Cheng, Y., Mowrey, K. A., Van Wagoner, D. R., Tchou, P. J. & Efimov, I. R. (1999). Virtual electrode induced re-excitation: a mechanism of defibrillation, 85: 1056–1066.

Clayton, R. H., Bernus, O., Cherry, E. M., Dierckx, H., Fenton, F. H., Mirabella, L., Panfilov, A. V., Sachse, F. B., Seemann, G. & Zhang, H. (2011). Models of cardiac tissue electrophysiology: progress, challenges and open questions., *Prog Biophys Mol Biol* 104(1-3): 22–48.

Clerc, L. (1976). Directional differences of impulse spread in trabecular muscle from mammalian heart, *Journal of Physiology* 255: 335–346.

Cortassa, S., Aon, M. A., O'Rourke, B., Jacques, R., Tseng, H. J., Marban, E. & Winslow, R. L. (2006). A computational model integrating electrophysiology, contraction, and mitochondrial bioenergetics in the ventricular myocyte., *Biophys J* 91(4): 1564–89.

Courant, R., Friedrichs, K. & Lewy, H. (1928). Über die partiellen Differenzengleichungen der mathematischen Physik, *Mathematische Annalen* 100(1): 32–74.

DeBruin, K. A. & Krassowska, W. (1998). Electroporation and shock-induced transmembrane potential in a cardiac fiber during defibrillation strength shocks, 26: 584–596.

Desplantez, T., Dupont, E., Severs, N. J. & Weingart, R. (2007). Gap junction channels and cardiac impulse propagation., *J Membr Biol* 218(1-3): 13–28.

Efimov, I. R., Aguel, F., Cheng, Y., Wollenzier, B. & Trayanova, N. A. (2000). Virtual electrode polarization in the far field: implications for external defibrillation, 279: H1055–H1070.

Efimov, I. R., Cheng, Y., Biermann, M., Van Wagoner, D. R., Mazgalev, T. N. & Tchou, P. J. (1997). Transmembrane voltage changes produced by real and virtual electrodes during monophasic defibrillation shock delivered by an implantable electrode, 8: 1031–45.

Efimov, I. R., Gray, R. A. & Roth, B. J. (2000). Virtual electrodes and deexcitation: new insights into fibrillation induction and defibrillation, 11: 339–353.

Entcheva, E., Trayanova, N. A. & Claydon, F. J. (1999). Patterns of and mechanisms for shock-induced polarization in the heart: a bidomain analysis., *IEEE Trans Biomed Eng* 46(3): 260–70.

Evans, F. G., Ideker, R. E. & Gray, R. A. (2002). Effect of shock-induced changes in transmembrane potential on reentrant waves and outcome during cardioversion of isolated rabbit hearts, 13: 1118–1127.

Fenton, F. H., Cherry, E. M., Karma, A. & Rappel, W. J. (2005). Modeling wave propagation in realistic heart geometries using the phase-field method., *Chaos* 15(1): 13502.

Franzone, P. C., Deuflhard, P., Erdmann, B., Lang, J. & Pavarino, L. F. (2006). Adaptivity in space and time for reaction-diffusion systems in electrocardiology, *SIAM J. Sci. Comput.* 28(3): 942–962.

Frazier, D. W., Wolf, P. D., Wharton, J. M., Tang, A. S., Smith, W. M. & Ideker, R. E. (1989). Stimulus-induced critical point. mechanism for electrical initiation of reentry in normal canine myocardium, *J Clin Invest* 83: 1039–52.

Gourdie, R. G., Green, C. R. & Severs, N. J. (1991). Gap junction distribution in adult mammalian myocardium revealed by an anti-peptide antibody and laser scanning confocal microscopy., *J Cell Sci* 99 (Pt 1): 41–55.

Hand, P. E., Griffith, B. E. & Peskin, C. S. (2009). Deriving Macroscopic Myocardial Conductivities by Homogenization of Microscopic Models., *Bull Math Biol* .

Harrild, D. & Henriquez, C. (2000). A computer model of normal conduction in the human atria., *Circ Res* 87(7): E25–36.

Harrild, D. M. & Henriquez, C. S. (1997). A finite volume model of cardiac propagation., *Ann Biomed Eng* 25(2): 315–34.

Henriquez, C. S. (1993). Simulating the elctrical behavior of cardiac tissue using the bidomain equations, *Critical Reviews in Biomedical Engineering* 1(1): 1–77.

Hooke, N., Henriquez, C. S., Lanzkron, P. & Rose, D. (1994). Linear algebraic transformations of the bidomain equations: implications for numerical methods., *Math Biosci* 120(2): 127–45.

Hooks, D. A., Trew, M. L., Caldwell, B. J., Sands, G. B., LeGrice, I. J. & Smaill, B. H. (2007). Laminar arrangement of ventricular myocytes influences electrical behavior of the heart., *Circ Res* 101(10): e103–12.

Hoyt, R. H., Cohen, M. L. & Saffitz, J. E. (1989). Distribution and three-dimensional structure of intercellular junctions in canine myocardium., *Circ Res* 64(3): 563–74.

Ideker, R. E., Wolf, P. D., Alferness, C., Krassowska, W. & Smith, W. M. (1991). Current concepts for selecting the location, size and shape of defibrillation electrodes, *Pacing Clin Electrophysiol* 14: 227–40.

Iyer, V., Mazhari, R. & Winslow, R. L. (2004). A computational model of the human left-ventricular epicardial myocyte., *Biophys J* 87(3): 1507–25.

Keener, J. P. & Bogar, K. (1998). A numerical method for the solution of the bidomain equations in cardiac tissue., *Chaos* 8(1): 234–241.

Kleber, A. G. & Rudy, Y. (2004). Basic mechanisms of cardiac impulse propagation and associated arrhythmias., *Physiol Rev* 84(2): 431–88.

Knisley, S. B., Trayanova, N. A. & Aguel, F. (1999). Roles of electric field and fiber structure in cardiac electric stimulation, 77: 1404–1417.

Knisley, S., Smith, W. & Ideker, R. (1994). Prolongation and shortening of action potentials by electrical shocks in frog ventricular muscle., *Am J Physiol* 266(6 Pt 2): H2348–58.

LeGrice, I., Smaill, B., Chai, L., Edgar, S., Gavin, J. & Hunter, P. (1995). Laminar structure of the heart: ventricular myocyte arrangement and connective tissue architecture in the dog., *Am. J. Physiol.* 269: H571–H582.

Leon, L. J. & Roberge, F. A. (1991). Directional characteristics of action potential propagation in cardiac muscle. A model study., *Circ Res* 69(2): 378–95.

Li, X. & Demmel, J. (2003). SuperLU DIST: A scalable distributed-memory sparse direct solver for unsymmetric linear systems, *ACM Transact ions on Mathematical Software (TOMS)* 29(2): 110–140.

Maclachlan, M. C., Sundnes, J. & Spiteri, R. J. (2007). A comparison of non-standard solvers for ODEs describing cellular reactions in the heart., *Comput Methods Biomech Biomed Engin* 10(5): 317–26.

Maisel, W. (2006). Pacemaker and ICD generator reliability: meta-analysis of device registries., *JAMA* 295: 1929–1934.

Munteanu, M., Pavarino, L. & Scacchi, S. (2009). A scalable Newton-Krylov-Schwarz method for the bidomain reaction-diffusion system, *SIAM J. Sci. Comput.* .

Neu, J. & Krassowska, W. (1993). Homogenization of syncytial tissue, *Critical Reviews in Biomedical Engineering* 21(2): 137–199.

Niederer S., Mitchell L., Smith N. & Plank G. (2011). Simulating human cardiac electrophysiology on clinical time scales, *Front Physiol* 2:14.

Pennacchio M., Savare G. & Colli Franyone P. (2006). Multiscale modeling for the bioelectric activity of the heart., *SIAM J. Math. Anal* 37(4): 1333–1370.

Pennacchio, M. & Simoncini, V. (2002). Efficient algebraic solution of reaction-diffusion systems for the cardiac excitation process, *J Comp Appl Math* 145: 49–70.

Plank, G., Burton, R., Hales, P., Bishop, M., Mansoori, T., Bernabeau, M., Garny, A., Prassl, A., Bollensdorf, C., Mason, F., Rodriguez, B., Grau, V., Schneider, J., Gavaghan, D. & Kohl, P. (2009). Generation of histo-anatomically representative models of the individual heart: tools and application, *Phil Trans Roc Soc* .

Plank, G., Leon, L.J., Kimber, S. & Vigmond, E. J. (2005). Defibrillation depends on Conductivity Fluctuations and the Degree of Disorganization in Reentry Patterns, *J Cardiovasc Electrophysiol* 16(2):205–16.

Plank, G., Liebmann, M., Weber dos Santos, R., Vigmond, E. J. & Haase, G. (2007). Algebraic Multigrid Preconditioner for the Cardiac Bidomain Model, *IEEE TBME* 54(4):585–96.

Plank, G., Zhou, L., Greenstein, J. L., Cortassa, S., Winslow, R. L., O'Rourke, B. & Trayanova, N. A. (2008). From mitochondrial ion channels to arrhythmias in the heart: computational techniques to bridge the spatio-temporal scales., *Philos Transact A Math Phys Eng Sci* 366(1879): 3381–409.

Plonsey, R. (1988). Bioelectric sources arising in excitable fibers (ALZA lecture)., *Ann Biomed Eng* 16(6): 519–46.

Pollard, A. E., Burgess, M. J. & Spitzer, K. W. (1993). Computer simulations of three-dimensional propagation in ventricular myocardium. Effects of intramural fiber rotation and inhomogeneous conductivity on epicardial activation., *Circ Res* 72(4): 744–56.

Pollard, A. E., Hooke, N. & Henriquez, C. S. (1992). Cardiac propagation simulation., *Crit Rev Biomed Eng* 20(3-4): 171–210.

Potse, M., Dube, B., Richer, J., Vinet, A. & Gulrajani, R. M. (2006). A comparison of monodomain and bidomain reaction-diffusion models for action potential propagation in the human heart., *IEEE Trans Biomed Eng* 53(12 Pt 1): 2425–35.

Prassl, A. J., Kickinger, F., Ahammer, H., Grau, V., Schneider, J. E., Hofer, E., Vigmond, E. J., Trayanova, N. A. & Plank, G. (2009). Automatically generated, anatomically accurate meshes for cardiac electrophysiology problems., *IEEE Trans Biomed Eng* 56(5): 1318–30.

Qu, Z. & Garfinkel, A. (1999). An advanced algorithm for solving partial differential equation in cardiac conduction., *IEEE Trans Biomed Eng* 46(9): 1166–8.

Roberts, D. E. & Scher, A. M. (1982). Effect of tissue anisotropy on extracellular potential fields in canine myocardium in situ., *Circ Res* 50(3): 342–51.

Roberts, S. F., Stinstra, J. G. & Henriquez, C. S. (2008). Effect of nonuniform interstitial space properties on impulse propagation: a discrete multidomain model., *Biophys J* 95(8): 3724–37.

Rocha, B. M., Kickinger, F., Prassl, A. J., Haase, G., Vigmond, E. J., Santos, R. W., Zaglmayr, S. & Plank, G. (2011). A macro finite-element formulation for cardiac electrophysiology simulations using hybrid unstructured grids., *IEEE Trans Biomed Eng* 58(4): 1055–65.

Rodriguez, B., Li, L., Eason, J. C., Efimov, I. R. & Trayanova, N. A. (2005). Differences between left and right ventricular chamber geometry affect cardiac vulnerability to electric shocks., *Circ Res* 97(2): 168–75.

Rogers, J. M. & McCulloch, A. D. (1994). A collocation–Galerkin finite element model of cardiac action potential propagation., *IEEE Trans Biomed Eng* 41(8): 743–57.

Roth, B. J. (1995). A mathematical model of make and break electrical stimulation of cardiac tissue by a unipolar anode or cathode, *IEEE Transactions on Biomedical Engineering* 42: 1174–1184.

Roth, B. J. (1997). Electrical conductivity values used with the bidomain model of cardiac tissue., *IEEE Trans Biomed Eng* 44(4): 326–8.

Roth, B. J. & Krassowska, W. (1998). The induction of reentry in cardiac tissue. The missing link: How electric fields alter transmembrane potential., *Chaos* 8(1): 204–220.

Rush, S. & Larsen, H. (1978). A practical algorithm for solving dynamic membrane equations., *IEEE Trans Biomed Eng* 25(4): 389–92.

Saucerman, J. J., Healy, S. N., Belik, M. E., Puglisi, J. L. & McCulloch, A. D. (2004). Proarrhythmic consequences of a KCNQ1 AKAP-binding domain mutation: computational models of whole cells and heterogeneous tissue., *Circ Res* 95(12): 1216–24.

Seemann, G., Hoper, C., Sachse, F. B., Dossel, O., Holden, A. V. & Zhang, H. (2006). Heterogeneous three-dimensional anatomical and electrophysiological model of human atria., *Philos Transact A Math Phys Eng Sci* 364(1843): 1465–81.

Sepulveda, N. G., Roth, B. J. & Wikswo, Jr, J. P. (1989). Current injection into a two-dimensional anisotropic bidomain., *Biophys J* 55(5): 987–99.

Severs, N. J., Bruce, A. F., Dupont, E. & Rothery, S. (2008). Remodelling of gap junctions and connexin expression in diseased myocardium., *Cardiovasc Res* 80(1): 9–19.

Skouibine, K., Trayanova, N. A. & Moore, P. (2000a). Success and failure of the defibrillation shock: insights from a simulation study, 11: 785–796.

Skouibine, K., Trayanova, N. A. & Moore, P. K. (2000b). A numerically efficient model for simulation of defibrillation in an active bidomain sheet of myocardium, 166: 85–100.

Sobie, E. A., Susil, R. C. & Tung, L. (1997). A generalized activating function for predicting virtual electrodes in cardiac tissue., *Biophys J* 73(3): 1410–23.

Spach, M. S. & Heidlage, J. F. (1995). The stochastic nature of cardiac propagation at a microscopic level. Electrical description of myocardial architecture and its application to conduction., *Circ Res* 76(3): 366–80.

Streeter, D., Spontnitz, H., Patel, D., Ross, J. & Sonnenblick, E. (1969). Fiber orientation in the canine left ventricle during diastole and systole, *Circ. Res.* 24: 339–347.

Sundnes, J., Lines, G. T. & Tveito, A. (2005). An operator splitting method for solving the bidomain equations coupled to a volume conductor model for the torso., *Math Biosci* 194(2): 233–48.

Sundnes, J., Nielsen, B. F., Mardal, K. A., Cai, X., Lines, G. T. & Tveito, A. (2006). On the Computational Complexity of the Bidomain and Monodomain Models of Electrophysiology, *Ann. of Biomed. Eng.* 34(7): 1088–1097.

Ten Tusscher, K. H., Hren, R. & Panfilov, A. V. (2007). Organization of ventricular fibrillation in the human heart., *Circ Res* 100(12): e87–101.

Trayanova, N., Skouibine, K. & Aguel, F. (1998). The role of cardiac tissue structure in defibrillation., *Chaos* 8(1): 221–233.

Trew, M. L., Smaill, B. H., Bullivant, D. P., Hunter, P. J. & Pullan, A. J. (2005). A generalized finite difference method for modeling cardiac electrical activation on arbitrary, irregular computational meshes., *Math Biosci* 198(2): 169–89.

Trew, M., Le Grice, I., Smaill, B. & Pullan, A. (2005). A finite volume method for modeling discontinuous electrical activation in cardiac tissue., *Ann Biomed Eng* 33(5): 590–602.

Vigmond, E. J., Aguel, F. & Trayanova, N. A. (2002). Computational techniques for solving the bidomain equations in three dimensions., *IEEE Trans Biomed Eng* 49(11): 1260–9.

Vigmond, E. J., Tsoi, V., Kuo, S., Arevalo, H., Kneller, J., Nattel, S. & Trayanova, N. (2004). The effect of vagally induced dispersion of action potential duration on atrial arrhythmogenesis., *Heart Rhythm* 1(3): 334–44.

Virag, N., Jacquemet, V., Henriquez, C. S., Zozor, S., Blanc, O., Vesin, J. M., Pruvot, E. & Kappenberger, L. (2002). Study of atrial arrhythmias in a computer model based on magnetic resonance images of human atria., *Chaos* 12(3): 754–763.

Wang, S., Leon, L. J. & Roberge, F. A. (1996). Interactions between adjacent fibers in a cardiac muscle bundle., *Ann Biomed Eng* 24(6): 662–74.

Weber dos Santos, R., Plank, G., Bauer, S. & Vigmond, E. (2004). Parallel multigrid preconditioner for the cardiac bidomain model., *IEEE Trans Biomed Eng* 51(11): 1960–8.

Wikswo Jr, J. P., Lin, S.-F. & Abbas, R. A. (1995). Virtual electrodes in cardiac tissue: a common mechanism for anodal and cathodal stimulation, 69: 2195–2210.

Zhou, X., Daubert, J. P., Wolf, P. D., Smith, W. M. & Ideker, R. E. (1993). Epicardial mapping of ventricular defibrillation with monophasic and biphasic shocks in dogs., *Circ Res* 72(1): 145–160.

Zipes, D. P., Wyse, D. G., Friedman, P. L., Epstein, A. E., Hallstrom, A. P., Greene, H. L., Schron, E. B. & Domanski, M. (1997). A comparison of antiarrhythmic-drug therapy with implantable defibrillators in patients resuscitated from near-fatal ventricular arrhythmias. The Antiarrhythmics versus Implantable Defibrillators (AVID) Investigators., *N Engl J Med* 337(22): 1576–83.

Part 2

Challenges in Clinical Defibrillation

5

What Can We Do Before Defibrillation?

Chunsheng Li, Shuo Wang and Junyuan Wu
Beijing Chaoyang Hospital, Affiliated to Capital Medical University, China

1. Introduction

The introduction of closed-chest massage by Kouwenhoven, Jude and Knickerbocker in 1960 was one of the key components of resuscitation that made recovery from sudden cardiac arrest (SCA) a realistic possibility, both in hospital and in the community.

The guidelines for cardiopulmonary resuscitation (CPR) of American Heart Association (AHA) were progressing from 1992. The 1992 guidelines for CPR and emergency cardiac care (ECC) described early access, early CPR, early defibrillation, and early advanced cardiovascular life support (ACLS), namely the 'chain of survival', as essential components of a series of actions designed to reduce the mortality associated with SCA.

The 2000 guidelines for CPR and ECC reported that the intervals of collapse to conventional CPR and collapse to defibrillation were most powerful factors in determining survival from cardiac arrest. 2005 guidelines for CPR and ECC have reported that survival rates from witnessed cardiac arrest due to shockable rhythm (i.e., ventricular fibrillation or pulseless ventricular tachycardia) decrease 7–10% for every minute that passes between collapse and defibrillation if no CPR by bystanders is provided, but the decrease in survival rates is more gradual and average 3–4% per minute from collapse to defibrillation when bystander conventional CPR is provided.

Now the 2010 guidelines have been announced by AHA. Initiating chest compressions before giving rescue breaths (i.e. C-A-B rather than A-B-C) has been advocated.

In the past five decades, scientific knowledge about arrest pathophysiology and resuscitation mechanisms has increased substantially; it is also a cause of effectively translating the science of resuscitation into clinical care and improving resuscitation outcomes.

2. Recognition of SCA

Immediate recognition of cardiac arrest is the first step of the survival chain. Prompt emergency activation and initiation of CPR requires rapid recognition of SCA.

SCA is death resulting from an abrupt loss of heart function. The victim may or may not have diagnosed heart disease. Most of the cardiac arrests that lead to sudden death occur when the electrical impulses in the diseased heart become rapid (ventricular tachycardia) or chaotic (ventricular fibrillation) or both.

Agonal gasps are common early after SCA and can be confused with normal breathing. It has been recognized as a signal of SCA.

Pulse detection alone is often unreliable, and it may require additional time. Detection of a pulse can be difficult, and even highly trained healthcare providers often incorrectly assess the presence or absence of a pulse when blood pressure is abnormally low or absent.

Healthcare providers should take no more than 10 seconds to determine if a pulse is present. The lay rescuer should activate the emergency response system if he or she finds an unresponsive adult. The lay rescuer should not attempt to check for a pulse and should assume that cardiac arrest is present if an adult suddenly collapses, is unresponsive, and is not breathing or not breathing normally.

3. What can we do before defibrillation?

It's essential to integrate early defibrillation into an effective emergency cardiovascular care system.

- Early Access – quickly calling the Emergency Medical Services (9-1-1) system
- Early CPR – promptly giving cardiopulmonary resuscitation
- Early Defibrillation – having proper equipment and being trained to use it when indicated

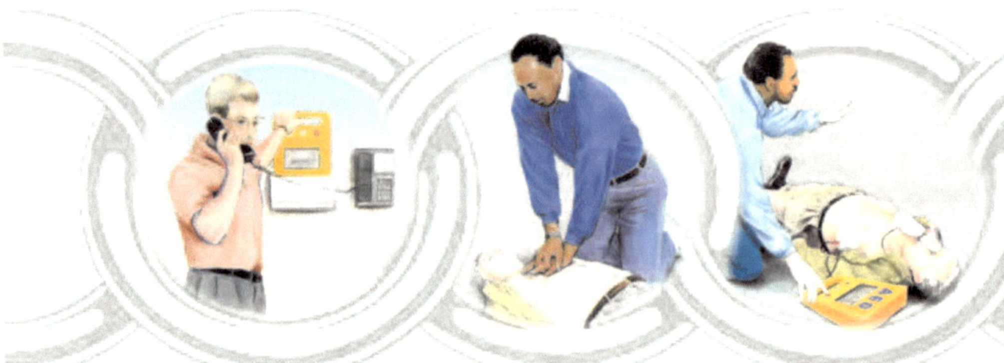

Fig. 1. Adult Chain of Survival.

4. Call EMS

Calling the Emergency Medical Services (9-1-1) system or your local emergency number immediately is the first important help that you can provide to a SCA victim.
When phoning 911 for help, the rescuer should be prepared to answer the dispatcher's questions about location, what happened, number and condition of victims, and type of aid provided. The caller should hang up only when instructed to do so by the dispatcher and should then return to the victim to provide CPR and defibrillation if needed.

5. Early CPR

Victims of cardiac arrest need immediate CPR. CPR provides a small but critical amount of blood flow to the heart and brain. CPR prolongs the time VF is present and increases the likelihood that a shock will terminate VF and allow the heart to resume an effective rhythm and effective systemic perfusion. CPR is especially important if a shock is not delivered for 4, 5 or more minutes after collapse. Defibrillation does not "restart" the heart; defibrillation "stuns" the heart, briefly stopping VF and other cardiac electrical activity. If the heart is still viable, its normal pacemakers may then resume firing and produce an effective ECG rhythm that may ultimately produce adequate blood flow.

Early CPR means giving CPR promptly and properly when necessary. When CPR is performed, mouth-to-mouth breathing and chest compressions circulate blood (and oxygen) to vital organs. This buys time until defibrillation, the next link in the chain of survival, can occur.
The Early CPR link is strengthened when bystanders or callers know CPR and Emergency Medical Dispatchers can give CPR instructions by phone.

6. Chest compressions

Chest compressions consist of rhythmic applications of pressure over the lower half of the sternum. These compressions create blood flow by increasing intrathoracic pressure and directly compressing the heart. Blood flow generated by chest compressions delivers a small but critical amount of oxygen and substrate to the brain and myocardium. In victims of VF SCA, chest compressions increase the likelihood that a shock will be successful.
The rescuer should compress the lower half of the victim's sternum in the center (middle) of the chest, between the nipples. The rescuer should place the heel of the hand on the sternum in the center (middle) of the chest between the nipples and then place the heel of the second hand on top of the first so that the hands are overlapped and parallel.

7. Open the airway: Lay rescuer and healthcare provider

The lay rescuer should open the airway using a head tilt– chin lift maneuver for both injured and noninjured victims. The jaw thrust is no longer recommended for lay rescuers because it is difficult for lay rescuers to learn and perform, is often not an effective way to open the airway, and may cause spinal movement. A healthcare provider should use the head tilt-chin lift maneuver to open the airway of a victim without evidence of head or neck trauma. If a healthcare provider uspects a cervical spine injury, open the airway using a jaw thrust without head extension.

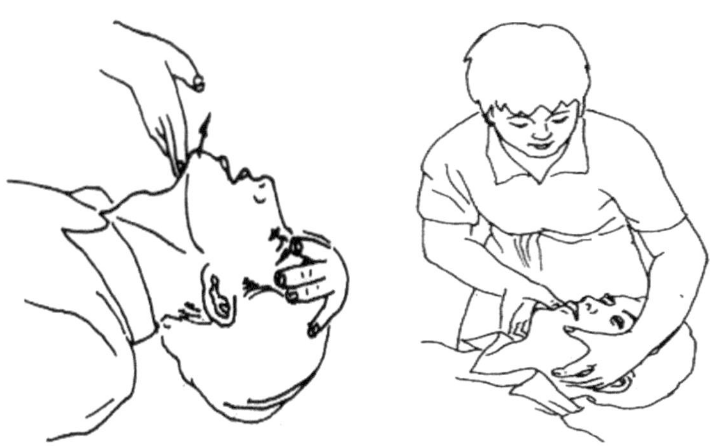

Fig. 2. Open the Airway with head tilt–chin lift maneuver or jaw thrust.

8. Breaths

Give 2 rescue breaths, each over 1 second inspiratory time and tidal volume of about 600 mL, with enough volume to produce visible chest rise. This recommended 1-second duration to make the chest rise applies to all forms of ventilation during CPR, including mouth-to-mouth and bag-mask ventilation and ventilation through an advanced airway, with and without supplementary oxygen.

1. During the first minutes of VF SCA, rescue breaths are probably not as important as chest compressions because the oxygen level in the blood remains high for the first several minutes after cardiac arrest. In early cardiac arrest, myocardial and cerebral oxygen delivery is limited more by the diminished blood flow than a lack of oxygen in the blood. During CPR blood flow is provided by chest compressions. Rescuers must be sure to provide effective chest compressions and minimize any interruption of chest compressions.
2. Both ventilations and compressions are important for victims of prolonged VF SCA, when oxygen in the blood is utilized. Ventilations and compressions are also important for victims of asphyxial arrest, such as children and drowning victims who are hypoxemic at the time of cardiac arrest.
3. During CPR blood flow to the lungs is substantially reduced, so an adequate ventilation-perfusion ratio can be maintained with lower tidal volumes and respiratory rates than normal. Rescuers should not provide hyperventilation (too many breaths or too large a volume). Excessive ventilation is unnecessary and is harmful because it increases intrathoracic pressure, decreases venous return to the heart, and diminishes cardiac output and survival.
4. Avoid delivering breaths that are too large or too forceful. Such breaths are not needed and may cause gastric inflation and its resultant complications.

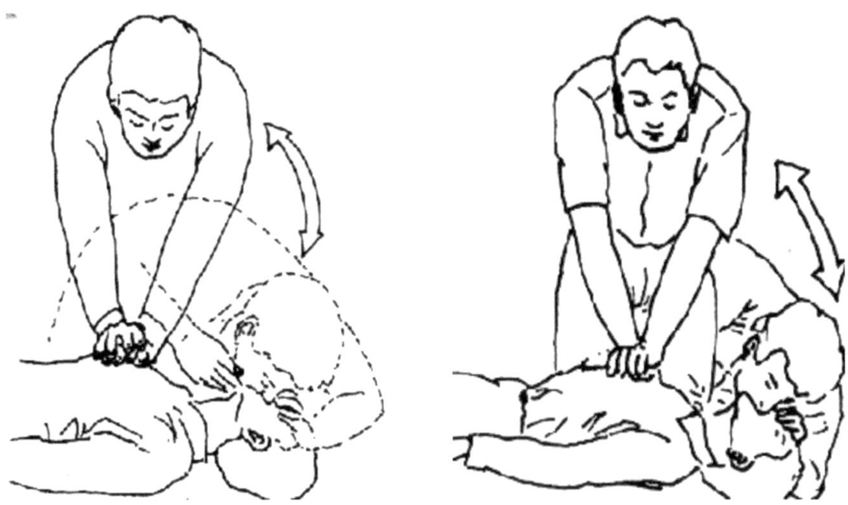

Fig. 3. Compression-ventilation ratio of 30:2CPR can be given by one or two rescuer.

9. Compression-ventilation ratio

A compression-ventilation ratio of 30:2 is recommended. This 30:2 ratio is based on a consensus of experts rather than clear evidence. It is designed to increase the number of compressions, reduce the likelihood of hyperventilation, minimize interruptions in chest compressions for ventilation, and simplify instruction for teaching and skills retention.

10. "A-B-C" to "C-A-B"

The newest development in the 2010 AHA Guidelines for CPR and ECC is a change in the basic life support (BLS) sequence of steps from "A-B-C" (Airway, Breathing, Chest compressions) to "C-A-B" (Chest compressions, Airway, Breathing) for adults and pediatric patients (children and infants, excluding newly borns).

The vast majority of cardiac arrests occur in adults, and the highest survival rates from cardiac arrest are reported among patients of all ages with witnessed arrest and a rhythm of VF or pulseless ventricular tachycardia (VT). In these patients the critical initial elements of CPR are chest compressions and early defibrillation.

In the A-B-C sequence chest compressions are often delayed while the responder opens the airway to give mouth-to-mouth breaths or retrieves a barrier device or other ventilation equipment. By changing the sequence to C-A-B, chest compressions will be initiated sooner and ventilation only minimally delayed until completion of the first cycle of chest compressions

Fewer than 50% of persons in cardiac arrest receive bystander CPR. There are probably many reasons for this, but one impediment may be the A-B-C sequence, which starts with the procedures that rescuers find most difficult: opening the airway and delivering rescue breaths. Starting with chest compressions might ensure that more victims receive CPR and that rescuers who are unable or unwilling to provide ventilations will at least perform chest compressions.

11. Encouraging Hands-Only (chest compression only) CPR

Cardiopulmonary resuscitation is traditionally defined as chest compression and ventilation. The need for chest compressions is unquestionable. The prompt initiation of effective chest compressions is a fundamental aspect of cardiac arrest resuscitation. Providing chest compressions of adequate rate, depth, complete chest recoil, minimizing interruptions and avoiding excessive ventilation are several most important factors of chest compression.

Encouraging Hands-Only (compression only) CPR for the untrained lay rescuer has been advocated by AHA 2010 guidelines. That is not only because Hands-Only CPR is easier to perform by those with no training, but also because it can be more readily guided by dispatchers over the telephone. Performing chest compressions alone is reasonable for trained laypersons if they are incapable of delivering airway and breathing maneuvers to cardiac arrest victims. The provision of chest compressions with ventilations is reasonable for trained laypersons who are capable of giving CPR with ventilations to cardiac arrest victims.

12. CPR or CCR?

Cardiocerebral resuscitation (CCR) is a new approach to the resuscitation of patients with witnessed cardiac arrest and a shockable rhythm developed by the University Of Arizona

Sarver Heart Center Resuscitation Group that significantly improves neurologically intact survival. For ACLS, it advocates either prompt or delayed single defibrillation shock, based on the three-phase time-sensitive model of ventricular fibrillation. Endotracheal intubation is delayed, excessive ventilations avoided, and early administration of epinephrine is advocated. CCR is not recommended for individuals with respiratory arrest. Endotracheal intubation has adverse effects not only due to the relatively long interruptions of chest compressions during placement but also due to the adverse effects of positive pressure ventilation and frequent hyperventilation.

13. Electrical therapies

Integration of AED into a system of care is critical in the Chain of Survival in public places outside of hospitals. To give the victim the best chance of survival, 3 actions must occur within the first moments of a cardiac arrest: activation of the EMS system, provision of CPR, and operation of a defibrillator.

14. AED

Automated external defibrillator （AED） is designed to treat victims of sudden cardiac arrest, where no explicit advanced directive regarding resuscitation is recorded. An AED should be used when a victim is found to be unresponsive and not breathing normally and in a shockable rhythm for example ventricular fibrillation and ventricular tachycardia.

Defibrillation will take priority to cardiopulmonary resuscitation unless there is more than one rescuer, where cardiopulmonary resuscitation can be commenced until the AED is brought to the scene, and its use can be initiated.

15. Sequence of actions when using an AED

The following sequence applies to the use of both semi-automatic and automatic AEDs in a ventricular fibrillation and pulseless ventricular tachycardia victim

1. Follow the adult BLS sequence. Do not delay starting CPR unless the AED is available immediately.
2. As soon as the AED arrives:
   If more than one rescuer is present, continue CPR while the AED is switched on.
   If you are alone, stop CPR and switch on the AED.
   Follow the voice / visual prompts.
   Attach the electrode pads to the patient's bare chest.
   Ensure that nobody touches the victim while the AED is analysing the rhythm.
3. If a shock is indicated:
   Ensure that nobody touches the victim.
   Push the shock button as directed
   Continue as directed by the voice / visual prompts.
   Minimise, as far as possible, interruptions in chest compression.
   If no shock is indicated:
   Resume CPR immediately using a ratio of 30 compressions to 2 rescue breaths.

Continue as directed by the voice / visual prompts.

4. Continue to follow the AED prompts until:
   Qualified help arrives and takes over OR the victim starts to show signs of regaining consciousness, such as coughing, opening eyes, speaking, or moving purposefully and starts to breathe normally or you become exhausted.

16. AED electrode pad placement in adults and/or children

The AEDs in the Trust may have adult and/or child AED electrode pads, depending on the age of the client group in that particular service area.
Adult AED pads are used on individuals above the age of 8 years,

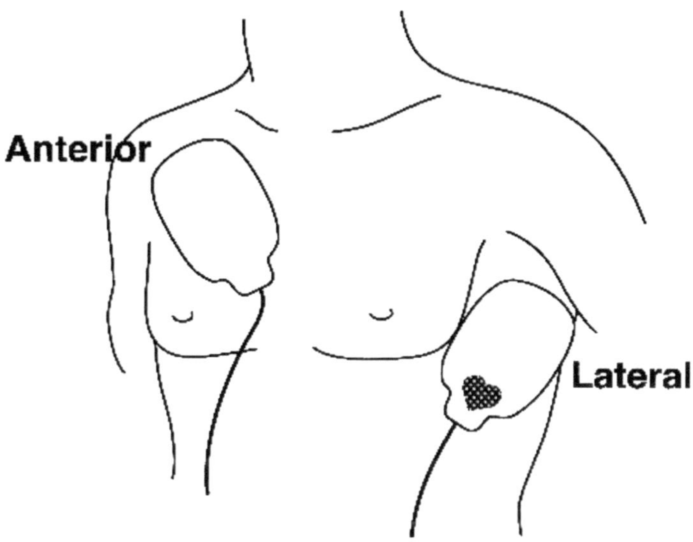

Fig. 4. AED electrode pad placement.

Place one AED pad to the right of the sternum (breast bone), below the clavicle (collar bone). Place the other pad in the left mid-axillary line, in line with the armpit and below the left breast.
It is important that this pad is placed sufficiently laterally and that it is clear of any breast tissue.
Although most AED pads are labelled left and right or carry a picture of their correct placement, it does not matter if their positions are reversed.
It is important if this happens 'in error', the pads should not be removed and replaced because this wastes time and they may not adhere adequately when re-attached.
The victim's chest must be sufficiently exposed to enable correct pad placement. Chest hair will prevent the pads adhering to the skin and will interfere with electrical contact. Shave

the chest only if the hair is excessive, and even then spend as little time as possible on this. Do not delay defibrillation if a razor is not immediately available.
Child reduced energy AED electrode pads are suitable for children 1-8 years of age, these are placed in the anterior posterior position, with one pad, placed in the centre of the chest between the nipples and the other on the back between the scapulae (shoulder bones).

17. Automated rhythm analysis

AEDs have microprocessors that analyze multiple features of the surface ECG signal, including frequency, amplitude, and some integration of frequency and amplitude, such as slope or wave morphology. Filters check for QRS-like signals, radio transmission, or 50- or 60-cycle interference as well as loose electrodes and poor electrode contact. They are extremely accurate in rhythm analysis. Although AEDs are not designed to deliver synchronized shocks (ie, cardioversion for VT with pulses), AEDs will recommend a (nonsynchronized) shock for monomorphic and polymorphic VT if the rate and R-wave morphology exceed preset values.

18. Safety during AED use

1. Defibrillation if the victim is wet
   As long as there is no direct contact between the user and the victim when the shock is delivered, there is no direct pathway that the electricity can take that would cause the user to experience a shock.
   Dry the victim's chest so that the adhesive AED pads will stick and take particular care to ensure that no one is touching the victim when a shock is delivered.
2. Defibrillation in the presence of supplemental oxygen
   If supplemental oxygen is being delivered by a face mask, remove the face mask and place it at least one metre away before delivering a shock. Do not allow this to delay shock delivery.
3. Minimise interruptions in CPR
   The importance of early, uninterrupted chest compressions is emphasised throughout resuscitation guidelines. Interrupt CPR only when it is necessary to analyse the rhythm and deliver a shock.

When two rescuers are present, the rescuer operating the AED applies the electrodes while the other continues CPR. The AED operator delivers a shock as soon as the shock is advised, ensuring that no one is in contact with the victim. Radio-Frequency interference from devices, such as Mobile phones can cause improper AED operation, and should be switched off near life support equipment. The AED electrode pads must completely adhere to the patient's skin, air pockets between the skin and electrode pads can cause patient burns. The AED may prompt the Operator that there is 'Poor Pad Contact', if this occurs; re-check all electrical and patient connections.
Do not use dried out AED electrode pads.
Attach the AED pads only to the patient's bare chest, do not allow the AED electrode pads to touch each other or other ECG electrodes, lead wires, dressings, transdermal patches, etc. Such contact can cause electrical arcing and patient skin burns during defibrillation and it may also divert the defibrillation current away from the heart.

If the AED detects a possible problem with the AED electrode pads or cable, It may alert the Operator with a 'Replace Pads' prompt, if this occurs remove the pads and replace with a new set.

19. Precautions in using AED devices

Do not place AED pads over medication patches such as nitroglycerin. Remove the patch before placing the AED pad.
Do not apply pads over an implanted pacemaker or defibrillator.
Do not use alcohol to wipe the patient's chest before applying the AED pads.
Do not attach pads to any patient unless the patient is unresponsive, no breathing and no pulse.
Do not press the shock button unless until no one is in contact with the patient.
If a child pad is available, use the Child pad for children.
Do not use AED's on infants (NO AEDs are designe) yet for infant patients).

20. Manual defibrillation

At present it is clear that both low-energy and high-energy biphasic waveform shocks are effective, but definitive recommendations for the first and subsequent energy levels for all devices cannot be made because devices vary in waveform and reported shock success. Although both escalating-energy and nonescalating-energy defibrillators are available, there is insufficient data to recommend one approach over another.

21. Which is first, compression or defibrillation?

Prompt defibrillation is recommended if bystanders have ready access to an AED or if police or EMS personnel with AEDs arrive during the electrical phase, that is, the first 4 or 5 min of ventricular fibrillation arrest. During the circulatory phase of ventricular fibrillation arrest (VF 5-10 min), the fibrillating myocardium has used much of its energy stores, and chest compressions that perfuse the heart are necessary and, therefore, advocated prior to and immediately after a defibrillator shock.

22. Criteria for not starting CPR

Scientific evaluation shows that few criteria can accurately predict the futility of CPR. In light of this uncertainty, all patients in cardiac arrest should receive resuscitation unless

- The patient has a valid Do Not Attempt Resuscitation (DNAR) order
- The patient has signs of irreversible death (eg, rigor mortis, decapitation, decomposition, or dependent lividity)
- No physiological benefit can be expected because vital functions have deteriorated despite maximal therapy (eg, progressive septic or cardiogenic shock).

23. References

2005 American Heart Association Guidelines for Cardiopulmonary Resuscitation and Emergency Cardiovascular Care. Circulation 2005; 112:IV1-IV203.

2010 American Heart Association Guidelines for Cardiopulmonary Resuscitation and Emergency Cardiovascular Care: Part 5, 6. Circulation 2010; 122(suppl 2):S298 - S337.

Wang S, Li C, Ji X, et al. Effect of continuous compressions and 30:2 cardiopulmonary resuscitation on global ventilation/perfusion values during resuscitation in a porcine model. Crit Care Med 2010; 38: 2073-2075.

Ewy GA. Cardiocerebral resuscitation: the new cardiopulmonary resuscitation. Circulation 2005; 111:2134–2142.

Kern KB, Hilwig RW, Berg RA, et al: Importance of continuous chest compressions during cardiopulmonary resuscitation: improved outcome during a simulated single lay-rescuer scenario. Circulation 2002:645-649.

6

Pulmonary, Cardiovascular and Mechanical Complications of Implantable Cardioverter Defibrillators (ICDs)

Georgia Hardavella, Georgios Dionellis and Nikolaos Koulouris
1st Department of Respiratory Medicine, Medical School, Athens University, "Sotiria" Athens Chest Diseases Hospital, Athens, Greece

1. Introduction

Automatic implantable cardioverter defibrillators (ICDs) have been used widely for the prevention of recurrent sudden cardiac death and the treatment of life-threatening ventricular tachyarrhythmias in ambulatory patients, since 1980 (Mirowski M et al., 1982). The remarkable efficacy of the ICD has been demonstrated to be 95% at 3 years and this has led to its ever-increasing use (Linl G et al., 2009).

Despite this benefit, there are many potential complications associated with ICDs (Pfeiffer D et al., 1994; Linl G et al., 2009). Nevertheless, the rate of complications related to the ICDs has fallen markedly with the evolution from a large device that required an abdominal pocket and insertion of an epicardial lead system via thoracotomy to the current use of much smaller transvenous pectoral devices (Krohn J et al., 2001; DiMarco JP et al., 2003). The incidence of ICD complications is difficult to determine due to inconsistent definitions and the lack of mandatory reporting. Nevertheless, women are more likely than men to have in-hospital adverse events related to ICD implantation (Peterson PN et al., 2009).

2. Definitions, aims and search strategy

The European Community and the International Standards Organization have provided standard criteria for adverse events observed during trials with implantable medical devices, defining an adverse event as any undesirable clinical occurrence and taking into account the severity and relationship to the implanted device. This does not include any information regarding the underlying technical or clinical cause (Rosenqvist M et al., 1998). Thus, complications are defined as any undesirable clinical occurrence related to the ICD implantation and function including intraoperative mortality and 30 day post-operative mortality.

This chapter aims to perform a systematic review of the published literature to provide the reader with the best available evidence and most current medical knowledge regarding pulmonary, cardiovascular and mechanical complications that occur due to the implantation of ICDs. Moreover, this chapter will attempt to ameliorate the weaknesses inherent in the current medical literature and scientific published medical literature regarding the issue.

Therefore, English language and adult population published literature from 1980 to December 2010 was searched using PubMed, Current Contents, Cochrane Library, Embase, Cinahl, Google Scholar and supplemented by a manual review of bibliographies of all relevant papers. Proceedings from relevant conferences, reference lists, relevant clinical trials and research registers were also searched. English language published literature from 1980 to 2010 was sought utilizing the following search strategy: *implantable cardioverter defibrillators* [MeSH] *and/or pulmonary and/or cardiac and/or mechanical/ device-related complications.* Studies were required to present sole evidence justifying the presence of complications secondary to the ICD. Data from each study was extracted by one author and reviewed by the two others.

3. Pulmonary complications

The majority of pulmonary complications were associated with the placement technique of the ICDs (Kuck KH et al., 2000). Implantation of an ICD involves placement of both the ICD lead system and the pulse generator. Current ICD lead systems are typically placed transvenously via the axillary, subclavian, or cephalic vein. This approach has largely replaced the surgical epicardial lead placement of the ICD which was associated with considerable postoperative morbidity (Chevalier P et al., 1996; Kuck KH et al., 2000) and with pulmonary complications that are unique to thoracotomy such as atelectasis with pneumonia, symptomatic pleural effusions, ARDS (adult respiratory distress syndrome).

In 1985, Lurie AL et al reported complications in a series of 22 patients that underwent ICD placement by thoracotomy. Among them, 77% presented with atelectasis, infiltrates or pleural effusion in the chest radiograph and 13% with pneumothoraces resulting from transvenous lead placement. The authors (Lurie AL et al., 1985) reported these as transient postimplantation complications. Pneumothorax, infections, and bleeding tend to occur soon after implant (Krohn J et al., 2001; Krohn J et al., 2003). As subclavian vein puncture may be associated with pneumothorax in approximately 1% of patients, the cephalic vein should be preferred for nonthoracotomy lead placement (Krohn J et al., 2003).

Pneumothorax occurs uncommonly and is directly related to operator experience, the difficulty of the subclavian puncture, and is almost eliminated using the cephalic cut-down technique. However, these traditional comparisons may become obsolete as the axillary vein cannulation technique (Martin C et al. 1996) threatens to eliminate this controversy. Often the pneumothorax is asymptomatic and noted in routine follow up plain chest radiograph.

Recurrent hemoptysis has been reported as a delayed complication on the grounds of ICD placement (Kao N et al., 1991; Verheyden CN et al., 1994; Dasgupta A et al., 1998; Driscoll JA et al., 2005). Clinicians caring for patients with an ICD should be aware of this complication and consider patch erosion into the bronchus as a cause, albeit rare, in the differential diagnosis of recurrent hemoptysis. Rarely, the patch erosion can be visualised bronchoscopically as the underlying cause of hemoptysis (Dasgupta A et al., 1998). Common radiographical findings can be a pleural infusion and vague infiltrates (Dasgupta A et al., 1998). Patch removal may reveal destruction of a significant part of the underlying bronchus, thereby prohibiting bronchial reconstruction. In patients who have undergone placement of an automatic ICD using pericardial or epicardial defibrillator patches and present with hemoptysis, bronchopericardial fistula should be also suspected (Nolan RL et al., 1999). Air between a defibrillator patch and the heart on chest radiographs or CT is diagnostic.

Infections of the ICD electrodes causing recurrent pneumonias are common and could lead to ARDS if remain uncontrolled. In reported cases, the ICD electrodes grew Methicillin sensitive *Staphylococcus epidermidis/aureus,* Methycillin Resistant *Staphylococcus aureus, Haemophillus Paranfluenzae, Aspergillus fumigatus, Pseudomonas aeruginosa,* while clots on the ICD patch grew *Haemophillus Influenzae (*Dasgupta A et al., 1998; Cook RJ et al., 2004; Pai RK et al., 2004; Ioannides MA et al., 2006; Rusanov A, Spotnitz HM. 2010*);* these pathogens are quite commonly isolated in infections caused by ICD placement. Infection of the patch can ultimately lead to its dislodgement and migration to the lung. Regarding the culture findings, it is difficult to be sure whether there was primary device infection with the pathogens presumably introduced during the ICD placement, a primary pneumonia with subsequent seeding of the ICD patch, or an underlying hematoma formation at the time of patch placement which then secondarily became infected, leading to subsequent erosion and pulmonary complications. Concomitantly, infections have increased the frequency of lead extraction. The frequency of lead infections has also risen faster than expected based solely on the number of implanted leads (Voigt A et al., 2006)

Patients developing severe pneumonias could also present with septic pulmonary embolism secondary to the infection(Cook RJ et al., 2004). This typically produces abnormalities on chest radiography, but its appearance is not uniform (Ryu JH et al., 2003; Huang RM et al., 1989; Rossi SE et al.,2000); multiple bilateral cavitary nodules at the lung periphery are most typical (Wong KS et al., 2002). Characteristic CT findings are discrete nodules in various stages of cavitation with visible feeding vessels (Rossi SE et al., 2000). However, multifocal cavitary lesions in the lung can also be associated with neoplasms, pulmonary infarctions, abscesses, vasculitides, congenital abnormalities, rheumatoid nodules, and pneumoconioses (Ryu JH et al., 2003). Consequently, correlation with the clinical context is important to narrow the broad differential diagnosis.

However, in this context, in 1997 Lick SD et al considered a cavitary lesion in a patient bearing an ICD and presenting with cough, malaise and weight loss commonly suspicious for a cavitary malignant neoplasm. Fiberoptic bronchoscopy was performed and no evidence of a malignant tumour was seen. Surprisingly, a defect was found in the lingular bronchus through which the bronchoscope could pass, opening into a large air-filled cavity, in part bordered by the patch itself. Cultures from the cavity debris grew *Aspergillus* and *Staphylococcus aureus.*

Hemothorax has also been reported as a late pulmonary complication of an ICD placement usually after the onset of pleuritic pain (Kremmers MS et al., 1995; Quigley RL et al., 1996). This complication results from trauma to the great vessels rather than the lung. The risk can be minimised by direct inward and outward passes of the puncture needle rather than a side-to-side potentially lacerating movement (Pavia S, Wilkoff B. 2001).

Air embolism has been reported during deep inspiration at the time of central venous access causing significant air to be drawn into the venous system due to the physiological negative pressure developed (Pavia S, Wilkoff B. 2001). It can be prevented through operator care and using introducers with hemostatic valves. The diagnosis is obvious because it is heralded by a hissing sound as the air is sucked in and with the fluoroscopic confirmation that follows. Patients are surprisingly tolerant of this occurrence. However, respiratory distress, hypotension, and arterial oxygen desaturation may occur depending on the size of the embolus and 100% oxygen should be administered alone with ionotropic support in some cases (Ellenbogen KA, Wood MA. 2005). Aspiration of the embolus from the right heart has also been successful. However, usually no therapy is required, as the air is filtered and consequently absorbed by the lungs.

4. Cardiac complications

Endocarditis secondary to leads' infection is one of the most common cardiac complications of ICDs. The majority of infections are caused by coagulase negative *Staphylococcus* and *Staphylococcus aureus* and rarely *Staphylococcus lugdunensis* (Anguera et al 2005; Liu PY et al., 2010; Chopra A et al., 2010). Although the risk of infection of intracardiac devices is well known, the clinical presentation of this complication can be insidious, delayed in onset and difficult to diagnose. The onset of symptoms can be in the first 6 months (Cacoub P et al., 1998) or in the first few years. Right sided endocarditis on the grounds of *Aspergillus fumigatus* infection has been reported (Cook RJ et al., 2004) as a delayed complication. The infection presented as persistent pulmonary infiltrates and anemia more than 2 years after the implantation of the device. Endocarditis caused by *Staphylococcus capitis* has also been reported and presented with a subacute course (Cone LA et al., 2005). Infrequently, gram negative bacilli can also cause lead infection and endocarditis. *Klebsiella pneumoniae* is a pathogenic gram negative bacillus which has been reported to cause ICD associated endocarditis (Pai RK et al., 2006).

Acute pericardial effusion and tamponade can occur secondary to lead perforation of the heart. This is an infrequent complication of device implantation which may also present as a subacute process days later, or even as a delayed process (Mahapatra S et al., 2005; Khan MN et al., 2005; Henrikson CA et al., 2006).

Some series have suggested an increase in ventricular arrhythmias after the implantation of epicardial patch electrodes (Bocker D et al., 1993). However, one study which randomized 900 patients undergoing coronary artery bypass grafting to an ICD or no ICD found no difference in the incidence of postoperative ventricular or supraventricular arrhythmias between the two groups (Curtis AB et al., 1998).

Many patients who receive an ICD have left ventricular dysfunction. An unresolved question is whether worsening myocardial function would affect the defibrillation threshold. In an animal model, the development of congestive heart failure did not alter defibrillation energy requirements (Friedman PA et al., 1998).

Multiple low energy defibrillation shocks via an endocardial right ventricular electrode cause significant myocardial damage in dogs, manifested as mitochondrial injury and dysfunction (Schirmer U et al., 1997). Although these changes are more apparent in the right ventricle, they are also seen in the left ventricle.

Myocardial necrosis is another cardiac ICD complication. Rapid consecutive shocks from the ICD results in elevation in serum troponin I, reflecting subtle injury to the heart. In one series of 12 patients who received a mean of 6 shocks with a mean cumulative energy of 112 J during ICD implantation, 5 had elevated troponin I levels which peaked within the first 12 hours after the shocks and were normal or near normal by 24 hours (Joglar JA et al., 1999). Only 1 of these patients had an increase in CK-MB and no patient had associated ECG changes.

5. Mechanical complications

Mechanical complications can be divided into lead/device/pocket related and inappropriate defibrillator shocks.

Lead-related problems occur in approximately 5% of patients, including lead dislodgement, fracture, and insulation defects, which can lead to either over- or undersensing. Lead-related problems can occur at any time during long-term follow-up (Kron J et al., 2001; Yap SC et al., 2007) with the vast majority of lead dislodgments occurring within the first post-operative months. With increasing age of the transvenous lead systems, a growing number of lead fractures and insulation defects have to be expected (Mewis C., 1997; Kron J., 2003). Necessity for operative revision is reported for 6% within 1 year of initial implant and up to 15% during 4 years (Kron J et al., 2001). A relation between the incidence of lead-related complications and the number of leads used in ICD systems has been reported (Takahashi T et al.,2002). Lead dislodgments occur significantly more frequently in patients with dual chamber ICDs (12%) and in patients with biventricular ICDs (19%) when compared with single chamber ICDs (3%).

One study evaluated 171 patients who received an epicardial lead system and were followed for 4 years: lead malfunction occurred in 11% of patients and in up to 28% with some systems (Brady PA et al., 1998). The majority of lead malfunctions occurred more than 2 years after implantation; most patients were asymptomatic (58%). Another report evaluated 132 patients who received a transvenous lead system and pectoral implantation and were followed for 30 months (Mehta D et al., 1998). A 13% incidence of erosion of the lead insulation was noted when systems using long transvenous leads and relatively larger generators were used. This problem is caused by pressure of the generator against the lead.

Pocket-related complications including skin erosion, hematoma and seroma, wound infection, or device migration usually occur within the first 6 months after implantation (Gold MR et al., 1996).

Device-related complications include migration, skin erosion, and necrosis (due to the size and weight of the generator) and premature battery depletion. Fortunately these problems are uncommon, occurring in less than 2% of patients. In addition, hematomas or seromas can form in the pulse generator pocket.

Twiddler's syndrome can also be included in the device-related complications, in which twisting or rotating the device in its pocket results in lead dislodgement and device malfunction, can occur in patients with an ICD. It is most likely to develop when the device is implanted in the abdomen of an obese patient who is able to rotate it within the abdominal pocket (Boyle NG et al. 1998). Patients most often present with an increase in bradycardic pacing threshold or lead impedance; however, there is a possibility that the device will fail to sense and treat an arrhythmia. Careful suturing of the device to the fascia and matching pocket and device size is important to avoid this complication.

Defibrillation-related problems represent a serious technical entity. A high defibrillation energy requirement (over 24 Joules) provides little margin for safety. However, in the absence of any changes in the clinical status of the patient, defibrillation energy requirements with a transvenous lead system are generally stable over a three month period (Newman D et al., 1997).

Inappropriate shocks most often occur due to supraventricular tachycardia, self-terminating VT, and sensing artifacts, e.g., myopotentials or T wave oversensing. It has been reported that inappropriate shocks for supraventricular tachyarrhythmias are more often in younger patients and in patients who have nonischemic dilated cardiomyopathy compared to patients with coronary artery disease (Alter P et al., 2005; Lin G et al., 2009; Lee DS et al., 2010). Potential induction of fatal ventricular fibrillation by inappropriate shocks is known from anecdotal reports (Messali A et al., 2004). Use of leads with true bipolar sensing can reduce sensing artifacts. The most important precipitating factor is myocardial ischemia, but other causes are electrolyte disturbances, and episodes of congestive heart failure resulting in an increase in sympathetic tone. However, newer atrial/dual chamber devices can effectively detect specific atrial and ventricular arrhythmias and can accurately discriminate between atrial tachycardia/atrial flutter and atrial fibrillation (Swerdlow CD et al., 2000). These devices can be programmed for mode switching to prevent inappropriate tracking of an atrial arrhythmia; to withhold inappropriate ventricular therapy; and to deliver appropriate therapy for the atrial tachyarrhythmia, such as pace termination of atrial flutter. Treatment with a sufficient dose of β-blockers may help to decrease the number of inappropriate shocks due to atrial flutter of fibrillation by slowing the ventricular rate (Pacifico A et al., 1999). In addition, prognostic benefits of β-blockers are well known in patients with coronary artery disease as well as in patients with heart failure (Packer M et al., 2001). Therefore, all patients with coronary heart disease and with non-ischemic dilated cardiomyopathy should receive β-blockers as standard therapy, unless there is a contraindication. Furthermore, it has been found a significantly lower incidence of inappropriate shocks due to supraventricular tachyarrhythmias in patients with versus without amiodarone therapy (Alter P et al., 2005). In addition, the rate cut-off for detecting ventricular tachyarrhythmias should not be programmed too low in order to decrease the overlap with supraventricular tachyarrhythmias. Since the latter is not possible in many patients with symptomatic slow ventricular tachyarrhythmias, state-of-the-art ICD discrimination algorithms should be used in order to distinguish supraventricular arrhythmias from VT.

Moreover, ICD related shocks to rescuers during CPR have been reported (Clements PA., 2003, Siniorakis E et al., 2009). In the case presented by Siniorakis E et al., CPR was performed in a patient bearing an ICD and presenting cardiac arrest with an initial rhythm of pulseless electrical activity. Ten minutes after starting CPR, the rescuer received an electric shock. This first shock of 21.9 J affecting the rescuer was triggered by chest compression-related muscular noise. This was mistaken by the ICD as ventricular fibrillation. In this context, there should be a warning from ICD manufacturers about the risks of shocks from ICDs during CPR.

An increase in the chronic defibrillation threshold may also occur (Martin DT et al., 1995). This problem may result from intense fibrosis and the cumulative acute damage produced by defibrillation discharges at the ICD electrode-myocardial interface (Epstein AE 1998 et al., 1998). However, the increase in defibrillation threshold may not be clinically significant with modern devices. In addition, changing the polarity of the leads may result in a reduction in the defibrillation threshold (Schauerte P et al., 1997).

6. Conclusions

The potential complications of ICDs are significant in terms of diversity and patient impact. For this reason, the decision to implant a device should be based on sound guidelines with definite expected patient benefit. Although it is a relatively simple procedure the potential complications may, at times, be life-threatening. Early recognition of these complications is the prerequisite for advances in ICD technology, in management strategies to avoid their recurrence and in improved patient quality of life. With a clear understanding of the accepted implant indications and possible complications and a meticulous approach to the implant and post-implant follow-up, the incidence of complications can be minimised.

7. References

[1] Anguera I, Del Río A, Miró JM, Matínez-Lacasa X, Marco F, Gumá JR, Quaglio G, Claramonte X, Moreno A, Mestres CA, Mauri E, Azqueta M, Benito N, García-de la María C, Almela M, Jiménez-Expósito MJ, Sued O, De Lazzari E, Gatell JM; Hospital Clinic Endocarditis Study Group. Staphylococcus lugdunensis infective endocarditis: description of 10 cases and analysis of native valve, prosthetic valve, and pacemaker lead endocarditis clinical profiles. Heart. 2005 Feb;91(2):e10.

[2] Bocker, D, Block, M, Isbruch, F, et al. Comparison of frequency of aggravation of ventricular tachyarrhythmias after implantation of automatic defibrillators using epicardial versus nonthoracotomy lead systems. Am J Cardiol 1993; 71:1064.

[3] Boyle, NG, Anselme, F, Monahan, KM, et al. Twiddler's syndrome variants in ICD patients. Pacing Clin Electrophysiol 1998; 21:2685.

[4] Brady, PA, Friedman, PA, Trusty, JM, et al. High failure rate for an epicardial implantable cardioverter-defibrillator lead: Implications for long-term follow-up of patients with an implantable cardioverter-defibrillator. J Am Coll Cardiol 1998; 31:616.

[5] Cacoub P, Leprince P, Nataf P, Hausfater P, Dorent R, Wechsler B, Bors V, Pavie A, Piette JC, Gandjbakhch I. Pacemaker infective endocarditis. Am J Cardiol. 1998 Aug 15;82(4):480-4.

[6] Clements PA. Hazards of performing chest compressions in collapsed patients with internal cardioverter defibrillators. Emerg Med J. 2003 Jul;20(4):379-80.

[7] Chevalier, P, Moncada, E, Canu, G, et al. Symptomatic pericardial disease associated with patch electrodes of the automatic implantable cardioverter defibrillator: An underestimated complication? Pacing Clin Electrophysiol 1996; 19:2150.

[8] Chopra A, Gulati D, Woldenberg N, Singh M. Intracardiac lead endocarditis due to Staphylococcus lugdunensis.Int J Infect Dis. 2010 Sep;14 Suppl 3:e291-3. Review.

[9] Cone LA, Sontz EM, Wilson JW, Mitruka SN. Staphylococcus capitis endocarditis due to a transvenous endocardial pacemaker infection: case report and review of Staphylococcus capitis endocarditis. Int J Infect Dis. 2005 Nov;9(6):335-9.

[10] Cook RJ, Orszulak TA, Nkomo VT, Shuford JA, Edwards WD, Ryu JH.Aspergillus infection of implantable cardioverter-defibrillator. Mayo Clin Proc. 2004 Apr;79(4):549-52.

[11] Curtis, AB, Bigger, JT, DiMarco, JP, et al, for the CABG Patch Trial Investigators. Epicardial; cardioverter-defibrillators do not cause postoperative arrhythmias. Am J Cardiol 1998; 82:1114.

[12] Epstein, AE, Kay, N, Plumb, VJ, et al. Gross and microscopic pathologic changes associated with nonthoracotomy implantable defibrillator leads. Circulation 1998; 98:1517.

[13] Friedman, PA, Foley, DA, Christian, TF. Stability of the defibrillation probability curve with the development of ventricular dysfunction in the canine rapid paced model. Pacing Clin Electrophysiol 1998; 21:339.

[14] Gold MR, Peters RW, Johnson JW, Shorofsky SR. Complications associated with pectoral cardioverter-defibrillator implantation: Comparison of subcutaneous and submuscular approaches. Worldwide Jewel Investigators. J Am Coll Cardiol 1996; 28: 12781282.

[15] Henrikson CA, Leng CT, Yuh DD, Brinker JAComputed tomography to assess possible cardiac lead perforation. Pacing Clin Electrophysiol. 2006 May;29(5):509-11.

[16] Huang RM, Naidich DP, Lubat E, Schinella R, Garay SM, McCauley DI. Septic pulmonary emboli: CT-radiographic correlation. AJR Am J Roentgenol. 1989;153:41-45.

[17] Ioannides MA, Christodoulides TA, Georgiou GM, Konis PA, Nicolaides EP. Recurrent Pneumonia Related To Pacemaker Lead Infection. The Internet Journal of Cardiology. 2006; 3(2)

[18] Joglar, JA, Kessler, DJ, Welch, PJ, et al. Effects of repeated electrical defibrillations on cardiac troponin I levels. Am J Cardiol 1999; 83:270.

[19] Kao N, Messersmith RN, Klich J.Hemoptysis complicating AICD patch placement controlled by temporary selective bronchial balloon occlusion.Chest. 1991 May;99(5):1301-3.

[20] Kenneth A. Ellenbogen MD, Mark A. Wood MD (2005). Cardiac pacing and ICDs. BlackWell Publishing

[21] Khan MN, Joseph G, Khaykin Y, Ziada KM, Wilkoff BL. Delayed lead perforation: A disturbing trend. Pacing Clin Electrophysiol 2005; 28:251–253.

[22] Kremers MS, Hastings JC 3rd, Herndon WM, Howe H. Delayed ICD patch migration after thoracoscopic placement with resultant hemothorax. Pacing Clin Electrophysiol. 1995 Jun;18(6):1335-7.

[23] Kron J, Herre J, Renfroe EG, et al. Lead- and device-related complications in the antiarrhythmics versus implantable defibrillators trial. Am Heart J 2001; 141: 9298.

[24] Kron J. Clinical significance of device-related complications in clinical trials and implications for future trials: insights from the Antiarrhytmics Versus Implantable Defibrillators (AVID) trial. Card Electrophysiol Rev 2003; 7: 473478

[25] Lee DS, Krahn AD, Healey JS, Birnie D, Crystal E, Dorian P, Simpson CS, Khaykin Y, Cameron D, Janmohamed A, Yee R, Austin PC, Chen Z, Hardy J, Tu JV; Investigators of the Ontario ICD Database. Evaluation of early complications related to De Novo cardioverter defibrillator implantation insights from the Ontario ICD database. J Am Coll Cardiol. 2010 Feb 23;55(8):774-82.

[26] Lick SD, Conti VR.Automatic internal cardioverter-defibrillator patch erosion into the upper airway presenting as a cavitary lesion. Chest. 1997 Oct;112(4):1144-6.

[27] Lin G, Nishimura RA, Gersh BJ, Phil D, Ommen SR, Ackerman MJ, Brady PA. Device complications and inappropriate implantable cardioverter defibrillator shocks in patients with hypertrophic cardiomyopathy. Heart 2009;95:709-714

[28] Liu PY, Huang YF, Tang CW, Chen YY, Hsieh KS, Ger LP, Chen YS, Liu YC. Staphylococcus lugdunensis infective endocarditis: a literature review and analysis of risk factors. J Microbiol Immunol Infect. 2010 Dec;43(6):478-84.

[29] Lurie AL, Udoff EJ, Reid PJ. Automatic implantable cardioverter-defibrillator: appearance and complications. AJR Am J Roentgenol. 1985 Oct;145(4):723-5.

[30] Mahapatra S, Bybee KA, Bunch TJ, et al. Incidence and predictors of cardiac perforation after permanent pacemaker placement. Heart Rhythm 2005; 2:907–911.

[31] Martin C, Auffray JP, Saux P, Albanese J, Gouin F. The axillary vein: an alternative approach for percutaneous pulmonary artery catheterization. Chest. 1986 Nov;90(5):694-7.

[32] Martin DT, John R, Venditti FJ. Increase in defibrillation threshold in non-thoracotomy implanted defibrillators using a biphasic waveform. Am J Cardiol 1995; 76:263.
[33] Mehta D, Nayak HM, Singson M, et al. Late complications in patients with pectoral defibrillator implants with transvenous defibrillator lead systems: High incidence of insulation breakdown. Pacing Clin Electrophysiol 1998; 21:1893.
[34] Messali A, Thomas O, Chauvin M, Coumel P, Leenhardt A. Death due to an implantable cardioverter defibrillator. J Cardiovasc Electrophysiol 2004; 15: 953956.
[35] Mewis C, Kuhlkamp V, Dornberger V, Mermi J, Seipel L. [High incidence of isolator fractures in transvenous implantation of cardioverter defibrillators]. Z Kardiol 1997; 86: 8594
[36] Mirowski M, Mower MM, Reid PR, Watkins L, Langer A. The automatic implantable defibrillator. New Modality for treatment of life-threatening ventricular arrhythmias. Pacing Clin Electrophysiol. 1982 May;5(3):384-401.
[37] Newman, D, Barr, A, Greene, M, et al. A population-based method for the estimation of defibrillation energy requirements in humans. Assessment of time-dependent effects with a transvenous defibrillation system. Circulation 1997; 96:267.
[38] Nolan RL, McAdams HP Bronchopericardial fistula after placement of an automatic implantable cardioverter defibrillator: radiographic and CT findings. AJR Am J Roentgenol. 1999 Feb;172(2):365-8.
[39] Pai RK, Pergam SA, Kedia A, Cadman CS, Osborn LA. Pacemaker lead infection secondary to Haemophilus parainfluenzae. Pacing Clin Electrophysiol. 2004 Jul;27(7):1008-10.
[40] Pacifico A, Hohnloser SH, Williams JH, et al. Prevention of implantable-defibrillator shocks by treatment with sotalol. d,l-Sotalol Implantable Cardioverter-Defibrillator Study Group. N Engl J Med 1999; 340: 18551862.
[41] Packer M, Coats AJ, Fowler MB, et al. Effect of carvedilol on survival in severe chronic heart failure. N Engl J Med 2001; 344: 16511658.
[42] Pai RK, Wall TS, Macgregor JF, Abedin M, Freedman RA. Klebsiella pneumoniae: a rare cause of device-associated endocarditis. Pacing Clin Electrophysiol. 2006 May;29(5):540-2.
[43] Pavia S, Wilkoff B.The management of surgical complications of pacemaker and implantable cardioverter-defibrillators. Curr Opin Cardiol. 2001 Jan;16(1):66-71. Review.
[44] Peterson PN, Daugherty SL, Wang Y, Vidaillet HJ, Heidenreich PA, Curtis JP, Masoudi FA; National Cardiovascular Data Registry. Gender differences in procedure-related adverse events in patients receiving implantable cardioverter-defibrillator therapy. Circulation. 2009 Mar 3;119(8):1078-84.
[45] Pfeiffer, D, Jung, W, Fehske, W, et al. Complications of pacemaker-defibrillator devices: Diagnosis and management. Am Heart J 1994; 127:1073.
[46] Quigley RL, Hamer ME, Swiryn S. Migration of an automatic implantable cardioverter-defibrillator patch causing massive hemothorax. Tex Heart Inst J. 1996; 23(1): 54–57
[47] Rosenqvist M, Beyer T, Block M, den Dulk K, Minten J, Lindemans F. Adverse events with transvenous implantable cardioverter-defibrillators: A prospective multicenter study. European 7219 Jewel ICD investigators. Circulation 1998; 98: 663670.

[48] Rossi SE, Goodman PC, Franquet T. Nonthrombotic pulmonary emboli. AJR Am J Roentgenol. 2000;174:1499-1508.

[49] Rusanov A, Spotnitz HM. A 15-year experience with permanent pacemaker and defibrillator lead and patch extractions. Ann Thorac Surg. 2010 Jan;89(1):44-50.

[50] Ryu JH, Swensen SJ. Cystic and cavitary lung diseases: focal and diffuse. Mayo Clin Proc. 2003;78:744-752.

[51] Schauerte, P, Stellbrink, C, Schondube, FA, et al. Polarity reversal improves defibrillation efficacy in patients undergoing transvenous cardioverter defibrillator implantation with biphasic shocks. Pacing Clin Electrophysiol 1997; 20:301.

[52] Siniorakis E, Hardavella G, Arvanitakis S, et al. Accidental shock to rescuer from an implantable cardioverter defibrillator. Resuscitation 2009 Mar;80(3):293-4.

[53] Schirmer, U, Hemmer, W, Lindner, KH, et al. Ultrastructural alterations in the right and left ventricular myocardium following multiple low energy endocardial countershocks in anesthetized dogs. Pacing Clin Electrophysiol 1997; 20:79.

[54] Swerdlow, CD, Schsls, W, Dijkman, B, et al, for the Worldwide Jewel AF Investigators. Detection of atrial fibrillation and flutter by dual-chamber implantable cardioverter-defibrillator. Circulation 2000; 101:878.

[55] Takahashi T, Bhandari AK, Watanuki M, Cannom DS, Sakurada H, Hiraoka M. High incidence of device-related and lead-related complications in the dual-chamber implantable cardioverter defibrillator compared with the single-chamber version. Circ J 2002; 66: 746750.

[56] Verheyden CN, Price L, Lynch DJ, Knight WL. Implantable cardioverter defibrillator patch erosion presenting as hemoptysis. J Cardiovasc Electrophysiol. 1994 Nov;5(11):961-3.

[57] Voigt A, Shalaby A, Saba S. Rising rates of cardiac rhythm management device infections in the United States: 1996 through 2003 J Am Coll Cardiol 2006;48: 590-591

[58] Wong KS, Lin TY, Huang YC, Hsia SH, Yang PH, Chu SM. Clinical and radiographic spectrum of septic pulmonary embolism. Arch Dis Child. 2002;87:312 315.

[59] Yap SC, Roos-Hesselink JW, Hoendermis ES, Budts W, Vliegen HW, Mulder BJ, van Dijk AP, Schalij MJ, Drenthen W. Outcome of implantable cardioverter defibrillators in adults with congenital heart disease: a multi-centre study. Eur Heart J. 2007 Aug;28(15):1854-61.

7

New Ways to Avoid Unnecessary and Inappropriate Shocks

Jorge Toquero, Victor Castro, Cristina Mitroi and Ignacio Fernández Lozano
Hospital Puerta de Hierro Majadahonda, Madrid, España

1. Introduction

Implantable cardioverter-defibrillators (ICDs) reduce mortality by terminating ventricular arrhythmias (VAs), and it has become widely accepted that this is done by delivering shocks. From the initials of ICD therapy it is known that ICD shocks are associated with reduced quality of life. Most importantly, recent accumulated evidence indicates a clear association among shocks (appropriate and inappropriate) and increased risks of heart failure (HF) and death (Poole et al, 2008). Knowing that, one of our major objectives when dealing with an ICD patient has to be reducing shocks while keeping the certainty that all the VAs are adequately terminated.

When trying to reduce shocks our focus should be dual, inappropriate and unnecessary therapies. Inappropriate shocks are generally defined as those not delivered for ventricular tachycardia (VT) or fibrillation (VF), and may be due to oversensing (double counting of right and left ventricular depolarization, T-wave oversensing, noise, etc) or to atrial arrhythmias with rapid ventricular conduction. Unnecessary shocks are those that could have been avoided using other means of terminating the VT, namely antitachycardia pacing, or allowing the VT to spontaneously finish, in case of non-sustained episodes, prolonging the number of intervals needed to detect and initiate therapy.

Depending on the trial, only 3–35% of shocked episodes were sustained VT/VF that absolutely require a shock for termination. When considering the number of shocks delivered for SVT, T-wave oversensing (TWOS) and lead noise, primary prevention patients may experience more inappropriate shocks than shocks for VT/VF. This highlights the need for improved shock reduction strategies.

During this chapter we will review the most recent developments and algorithms to avoid inappropriate and unnecessary shocks.

2. Where do we stand now?

2.1 The problem of inappropriate and unnecessary shocks

ICD therapy has clearly shown its benefit in reducing sudden death and is now an accepted therapy, with increasing number of patients receiving a device. One of the most serious problems with this therapy is the rate of unnecessary and inappropriate shocks, that ranges between 10 and 25% on different studies (Figure 1), with the added limitation of many trials not reporting this data.

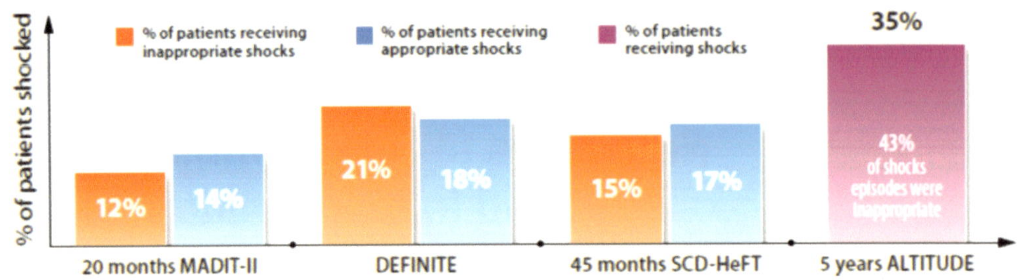

Fig. 1. Rate of inappropriate therapy (in orange) in some of the principal ICD trials.

Multiple studies have reported that ICD shocks are associated with several negative outcomes, both in the short term -such as increased troponin levels, decreased cardiac index or acutely reduced contractility-, as in the long term-increasing hospitalization rate or reducing quality of life. Inappropriate shocks might also be proarrhythmic in up to 10% of episodes and also reduce battery life.

Moreover, recent evidence indicates a clear association among appropriate shocks, inappropriate shocks, and increased risks of heart failure and death (Figure 2, reproduced from Poole et al, 2008). These data also demonstrates that the higher the number of shocks, the higher the death hazard ratio. An important corollary is that, even if it is impossible to completely avoid shocks, any reduction we obtain translates into lower hospitalization and death risk.

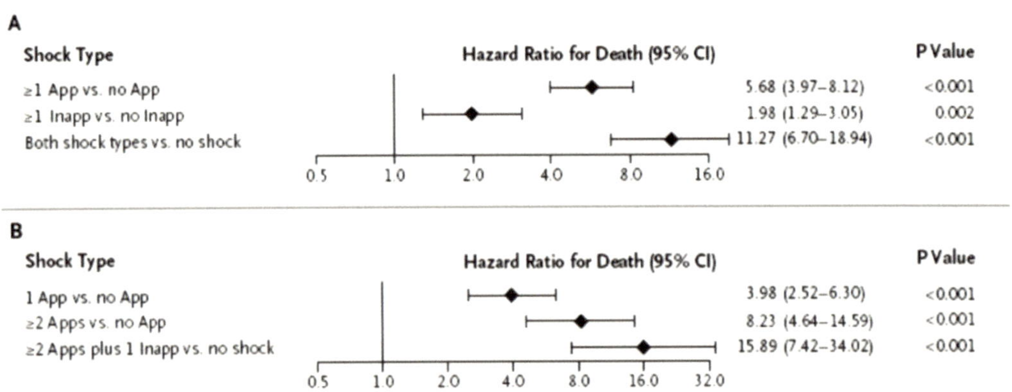

Fig. 2. Hazard Ratios for the association of ICD shock with the risk of death, according to shock type. Panel A shows the hazard ratios for the association of shock types (appropriate, inappropriate or both) with the risk of death. Panel B shows the adjusted hazard ratios for the risk of death according to the number of appropriate or inappropriate shocks.

From the SCD-HeFT we know that death from all causes was increased among patients who received an appropriate shock by a factor of nearly 6, with 30% of these deaths occurring within 24 hours after the first appropriate shock. After exclusion of these patients (in whom an appropriate shock was simply a harbinger of imminent death), appropriate shocks were still associated with a risk of death that was increased by a factor of 3. Data from MADIT II trial (Daubert et al, 2008) also clearly showed how shocks are associated with increased risk of all-cause mortality (by a factor of 3 after an appropriate ICD shock).

It is unclear whether this is due to the ventricular arrhythmia itself or to the shocks, but evidence is increasingly showing that ICD discharges are harmful per se. Pooled data from PainFREE I & II, EMPIRIC and PREPARE (Sweeney et al, 2010) has clearly shown the impact on survival depending on the type of therapy delivered by the ICD (Figure 3), demonstrating that antitachycardia pacing (ATP) termination of the VA can reduce the risk.

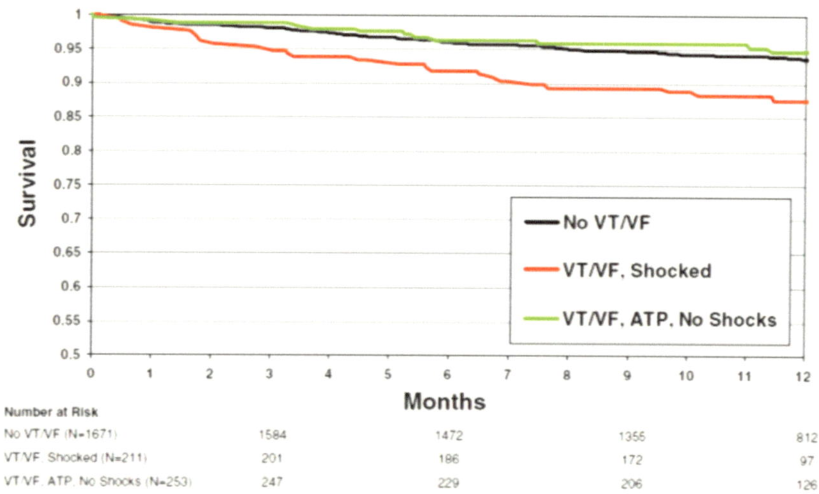

Fig. 3. Survival rates by rhythm and therapy type. Survival among patients treated only with ATP was identical to that in patients with no VT, whereas survival among patients who received shocks was significantly worse (reproduced from Sweeney et al, 2010).

An important issue to be considered is the high rate of inappropriate therapies in published studies, ranging from 10 to 25%. Benign events such as atrial fibrillation, supraventricular tachycardia (SVT), extra-cardiac noise, intracardiac oversensing, and nonsustained VT/VF are inappropriately treated with shocks by the ICD. Inappropriate therapy delivery remains the most frequent complication in patients with ICDs resulting in psychological distress, proarrhythmia, and battery life reduction. We could think that delivery of inappropriate shocks is something overcome in nowadays trials, but recent data from the MADIT II trial (Daubert et al, 2008) shows that one or more inappropriate shocks occurred in 83 (11.5%) of the 719 MADIT II ICD patients. Inappropriate shock episodes constituted 184 of the 590 total shock episodes (31.2%).

Atrial fibrillation was the most common trigger for inappropriate shock (44%), followed by supraventricular tachycardia (36%), and by abnormal sensing (20%). Due to the fact that the majority of inappropriate shocks are delivered because of a supraventricular rhythm incorrectly classified by the device (see Figure 4), nowadays most devices on the market contain some form of SVT discriminator.

Other causes of inappropriate therapy include oversensing of diaphragmatic potentials or myopotentials, T-wave oversensing, double or triple counting of intracardiac signals, lead fractures or header connection problems, lead chatter or noise, and electromagnetic interference. Strategies to reduce inappropriate therapy using device programming rely on the ability to distinguish supraventricular and atrial arrhythmias from ventricular tachycardia. Avoiding therapy for nonsustained ventricular arrhythmias and increasing the role of antitachycardia pacing to terminate ventricular tachycardia are key approaches to reducing shocks for ventricular arrhythmias.

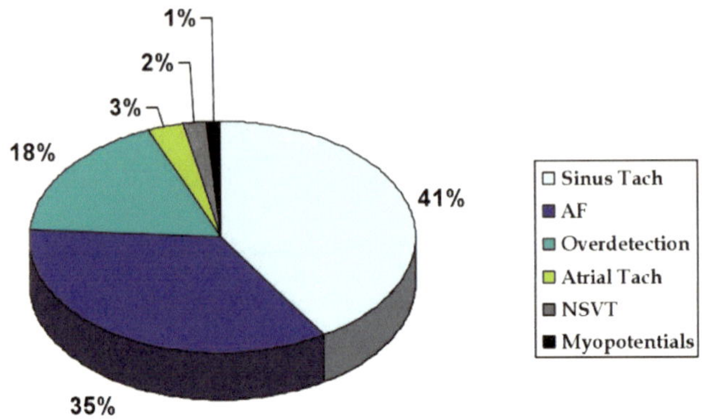

Fig. 4. Main causes of inappropriate shocks in ICD patients.

2.2 Algorithms to avoid inappropriate shocks

Although dual-chamber discrimination algorithms are frequently based on measurements of AV association, algorithms used in single-chamber ICDs focus on frequency-related tachycardia characteristics (beat-to-beat interval variability -rate stability- and abruptness of tachycardia initiation -onset-) and electrogram (EGM) morphology.

2.2.1 Sudden onset

Initially developed to avoid misclassification of sinus tachycardia as VT, the algorithm is based on the degree of prematurity of the first tachycardia cycle compared to the previous ones. If a tachycardia episode is declared, the device measures the RR intervals prior to the episode looking for the shortest RR interval. Then it compares this shortest RR interval with the RR interval initiating the episode. If the difference is above the programmed, the sudden onset criterion is satisfied. If the difference is below the programmed one, a non-sudden onset will be declared and therapy will be inhibited until the end of the sustained rate duration period if activated.

2.2.2 Stability

Measures the variability between RR intervals during tachycardia and was developed to avoid inappropriate shocks due to fast atrial fibrillation, a typically unstable rhythm. The device measures the stability during the programmed duration of the episode. If duration is satisfied, the mean difference in stability between consecutive RR intervals is compared to the programmed one. If stability is below the programmed one, the device declares the episode stable. If stability is above the programmed one, the device declares the episode unstable and therapy will be inhibited. Then it will continue to measure stability as long as the rate criterion is satisfied. If tachycardia becomes stable or the sustained rate duration period is satisfied, therapy will be initiated if the rate persists above the programmed cut-off rate.

Sudden onset carries a greater risk of error, since it analyses the rhythm only once upon initiation. In contrast, stability constantly reanalyzes the rhythm. These two algorithms have been traditionally underused due to concern of misclassification of a true VT as a non-shockable rhythm by the device, thereby continuously withholding a necessary therapy. However, several publications have demonstrated that programming sudden onset and stability detection criteria with a sustained rate duration safety net for triggering tachycardia

therapy results in appropriate device management in most patients with supraventricular and slow ventricular tachycardias (Brugada et al, 1998).
Recent data from the MADIT II trial (Daubert et al, 2008) showed that the stability detection algorithm was programmed less frequently in patients receiving inappropriate shocks (17% vs. 36%, p: 0.030), so we still have room to improve ICD programming by using consolidated algorithms.

2.2.3 Morphology algorithms

Morphology algorithms are the only single-chamber discriminators capable of distinguishing VT from abrupt-onset SVTs with regular V-V intervals, such as atrial flutter or atrial tachycardia. When integrated into dual-chamber algorithms, morphology algorithms may enhance discrimination of tachycardias with 1:1 AV relationships and detection of VT during atrial fibrillation (Swerdlow et al, 2002).
All morphology algorithms share general steps. (1) Create a template electrogram of baseline rhythm. (2) Construct a quantitative representation of this template. (3) Record electrograms from an unknown tachycardia. (4) Time align template and tachycardia electrograms. (5) Construct a quantitative representation of each tachycardia electrogram. (6) Compare the representation of each tachycardia electrogram with that of the template to determine the degree of morphologic similarity of the corresponding electrograms. (7) Classify each tachycardia electrogram as a morphology match or nonmatch with the template. (8) Classify the tachycardia as VT or SVT based on the fraction of tachycardia electrograms that match the template. The major differences among morphology algorithms are the electrogram source(s), methods of filtering and alignment, and waveform features used to compare tachycardia and template electrograms.

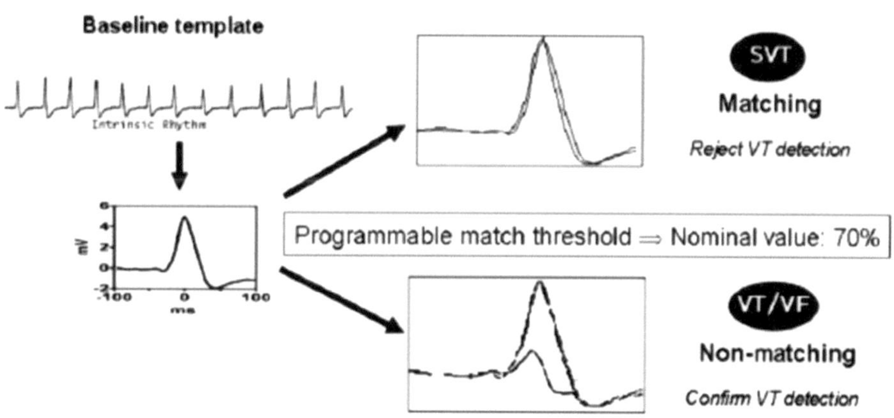

Fig. 5. Morphology analysis of tachycardia EGMs using the wavelet transform (Medtronic) The wavelet transform of the baseline rhythm template EGM is constructed and stored. When tachycardia is detected, each of the last eight tachycardia EGMs preceding detection is aligned with the template EGM. The wavelet transform of each EGM is performed and a match-percent score that describes the degree of morphological similarity to the template is calculated in real time. If the matching score is higher than the programmable threshold, VT is rejected. If the matching score is lower than the threshold, VT is confirmed and corresponding therapy initiated.

The Rhythm ID feature in Boston Scientific ICDs uses the vector timing and correlation algorithm -which incorporates both timing as well as morphological information- for supraventricular tachycardia discrimination. Clinical trials demonstrated high sensitivity and specificity of this feature in discriminating between ventricular tachycardia and supraventricular tachycardia. On detection of the unknown rhythm (when the ventricular tachycardia rate detection criteria is met), the vector timing and correlation algorithm compares the unknown rhythm beat-by-beat to a stored template of normal sinus rhythm. First, the algorithm aligns the signals coming from the near field and the far field EGMs. After that, the feature correlation coefficient computed over more than 8 points in the time-aligned signals is used for the comparison (see Figure 6).

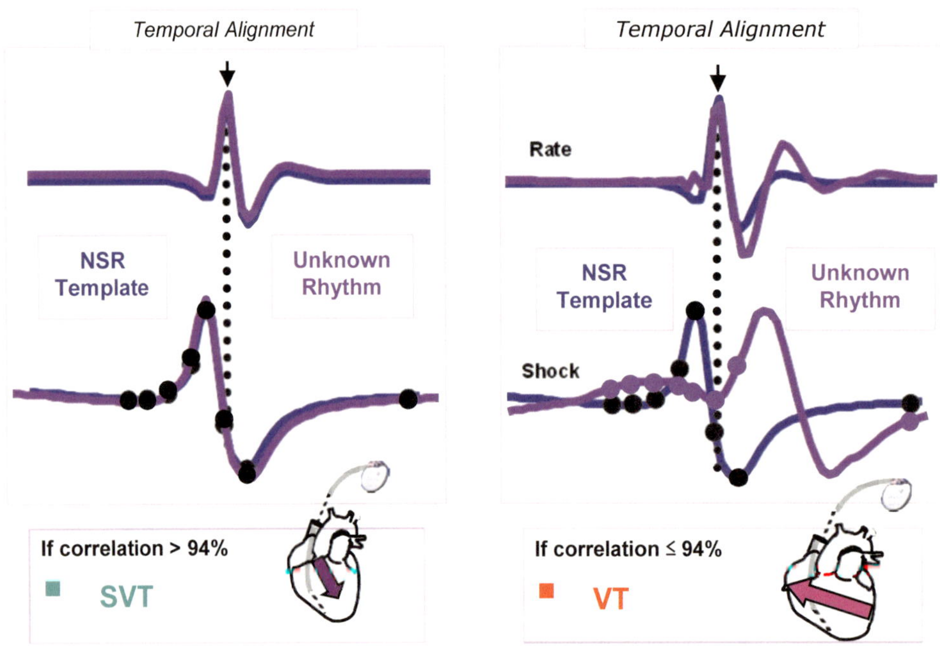

Fig. 6. Schematic representation of Rhythm ID algorithm functioning.

There are several limitations of morphology algorithms, such as:

- Truncation of EGMS that exceed the programmed range of the algorithm. Truncation both removed some electrogram features for analysis, and altered the timing of the highest peak used for alignment. It is, therefore, recommended to verify that recorded EGMs exceed 3 mV and are not clipped.
- Miopotential interference.
- Alignment errors: algorithm aligns electrograms in time based on their highest peaks. If an electrogram has two peaks of nearly equal amplitude, minor variation in their relative heights may result in an alignment error.
- Morphology algorithms may be applied in patients with baseline intraventricular conduction delays. However, rate-related aberrancy during rapidly conducted atrial fibrillation is likely to be misclassified.

As we stated in a recent publication (Toquero et al, 2009), probably morphology algorithms as an SVT discrimination criteria should be considered as an effective tool when used alone but, in order to maximize the benefits, a lower limit of 500 ms and the concomitant use of other discrimination criteria or combination with a high rate time-out feature should be considered. When programming several discriminators together, the more we use the better the specificity for SVT but carries a greater risk of underdetecting VT, so once again we have to individualize and tailor the programming to each patient.

2.2.4 Dual chamber detection

Dual chamber devices allow for ventricular and atrial rate analysis during tachyarrythmias, as well as establishing a relationship between them. As a concept, if the rhythm is faster in the ventricular chamber the device will deliver therapy. At the very beginning, it was expected a dramatic reduction of inappropriate shocks due to atrial tachyarrhythmias compared to single chamber devices, but finally it did not turn out to be that way due to atrial undersensing problems or difficulties programming the algorithm.

Evidence recently published (Ricci et al, 2009) shows that dual-chamber ICDs compared to single-chamber ICDs reduced the incidence of an endpoint composed by permanent AF, AF-related hospitalizations, and ICD shocks deemed inappropriate due to AF misclassification. So dual chamber detection helps to improve SVT discrimination but probably this is not enough to justify the implantation of a DDD device on this sole aim.

There are other algorithms intended to adequately discriminate SVT from true VT. Detailed description of PARAD+ from Sorin or SMART from Biotronik (using dual chamber discrimination) is beyond the aim of this chapter. Briefly, the PARAD+ combines several features of the tachyarrhythmia that are analyzed and inputted into a branching algorithm. It is the only algorithm that uses the chamber of acceleration to differentiate atrial from ventricular arrhythmias. It incorporates a feature termed VT long cycle, which monitors for longer intervals when the rhythm is classified as stable. Unlike VT, occasional longer RR intervals are common in rapid AF. SMART algorithm, like St Jude Devices, relies on a rate branch algorithm for discrimination. If the RR interval is shorter than the PP interval (V>A), the rhythm is considered VT.

For further description of different algorithms of several manufacturers, we strongly recommend the recent review by Mansour and Khairy, PACE 2011.

3. Ways to avoid shocks and new strategies

Even though it is plausible that shocks somehow have an adverse effect on myocardial function, this is unlikely to be a major factor. It is much more likely that the occurrence of a ventricular arrhythmia that causes a shock is signalling a meaningful change in the patient's clinical status. The important message is that the first occurrence of shocks is not a random event in an otherwise stable clinical course but a sign of clinical deterioration in the underlying disease process. Possible causes of shocks are to be considered, including a worsening of heart failure and myocardial ischemia.

There are several complementary ways to avoid both inappropriate and unnecessary shocks:

3.1 Optimize medical therapy, look for isquemia and other triggers, and early ablate clinical VTs

Antiarrhythmic medication is administered in patients with an ICD for a number of reasons. Most importantly, drug therapy can reduce or eliminate ICD shocks by suppressing ventricular arrhythmias, or by slowing VT to such a degree that it can be terminated with programmed ATP. In addition to the suppression of such "appropriate" shocks, antiarrhythmic therapy may suppress the "inappropriate" shocks precipitated by supraventricular arrhythmias (primarily atrial fibrillation). In routine practice, adjunctive antiarrhythmic therapy is administered to between 49% and 69% of patients who have an ICD.

The Optimal Pharmacological Therapy in Cardioverter Defibrillator Patients (OPTIC) trial was a randomized clinical trial evaluating the efficacy of amiodarone plus β-blocker and sotalol versus β-blocker alone for reduction of ICD shocks (Connelly et al, 2006). In 412 patients studied, mainly secondary prevention, with a median follow up of 359 days, the authors demonstrated that shocks occurred in 41 patients (38.5%) assigned to β-blocker alone, 26 (24.3%) assigned to sotalol, and 12 (10.3%) assigned to amiodarone plus β-blocker (Figure 7).

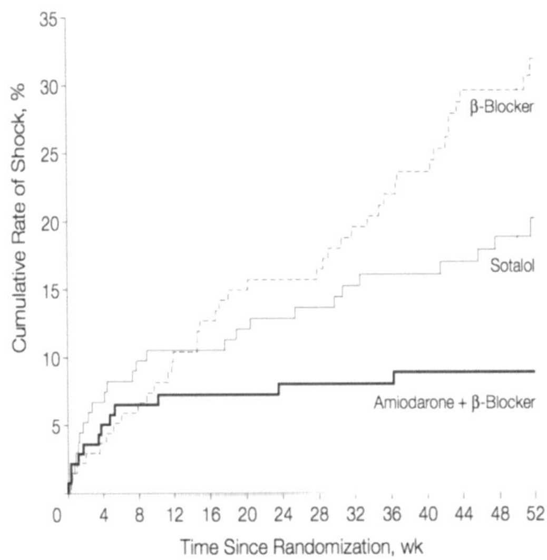

Fig. 7. Cumulative rate of shocks for the three treatment groups (β-blocker, Sotalol and Amiodarone+β-blocker) by time since randomization (Reproduced from Connolly et al, OPTIC trial).

The OPTIC study applies primarily to ICDs placed as secondary prevention, in which sustained ventricular arrhythmias have been clinically observed. There are less data to support the use of antiarrhythmic agents in patients with prophylactic or primary prevention ICD therapy and this group appears to have less frequent need for such therapy; thus, empirical antiarrhythmic therapy cannot be recommended for this setting. For patients who receive an ICD for secondary prevention, one could argue for empirical initiation of amiodarone or sotalol. However, such pharmacological intervention has important trade-offs. Adverse lung and thyroid effects were common among patients receiving amiodarone over just 1 year, and it can be expected that toxicity would be even more common over longer follow-up. In the OPTIC study, these and other adverse effects resulted in the discontinuation of 18% of those patients receiving amiodarone and 24% of those patients receiving sotalol. As noted by the authors, most patients taking β-blocker alone will not receive an ICD shock and

could avoid the inconvenience, cost, and risk of antiarrhythmic therapy. At present, all patients with an ICD who tolerate such therapy should receive a β-blocker.
Amiodarone is known to be effective in the prevention of ventricular arrhythmias; however, SCD-HeFT itself finally put to rest the notion that amiodarone could improve survival among patients with heart failure. Addition of amiodarone or substitution with sotalol cannot be advocated for all patients and should be considered on an individual basis.
Triggers of VT include electrolyte abnormalities (e.g., hypokalemia, hypocalcaemia, and hypomagnesaemia), ischemia, inflammation, and sleep apnea. It can also be triggered by drugs (sympathomimetic agents, digitalis toxicity, drugs prolonging the QT complex, etc.). Hypokalemia is the most important arrhythmia trigger clinically, followed by hypomagnesaemia. Hyperkalemia may also predispose to VT and VF, particularly in patients with structural heart disease. Electrolyte disturbances and ischemia are frequent VT triggers in ICD patients with reduced ejection fraction and heart failure. The greater prognostic significance of appropriate ICD shocks in patients with ischemic heart failure makes revascularization another possible intervention; however, there are currently no prospective data to suggest that this will improve prognosis. So, when facing a patient receiving a shock, we should be aware of all the possible triggers of VTs, actively look for them and make every effort needed to control these triggers.
The Ventricular Tachycardia Ablation in Coronary Heart Disease (VTACH) study (Kuck et al, 2010) assessed the potential benefit of catheter ablation before implantation of a cardioverter defibrillator in 110 patients that were randomized to receive catheter ablation and an ICD or ICD alone. They showed that time to recurrence of VT or VF was longer in the ablation group (median 18 months) than in the control group (5 months). At 2 years, estimates for survival free from VT or VF were 47% in the ablation group and 29% in the control group. The authors conclude that prophylactic VT ablation before defibrillator implantation seemed to prolong time to recurrence of VT in patients with stable VT, previous myocardial infarction, and reduced LVEF and should therefore be considered before implantation of an ICD in such patients.

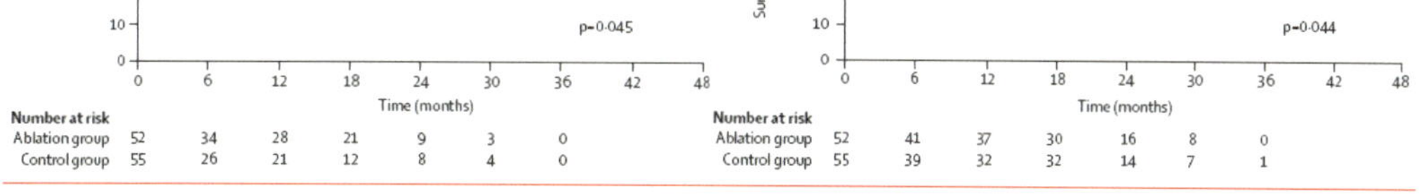

Fig. 8. Data from the VTACH trial. On the left, Kaplan Kaplan-Meier curves for survival free from VT or VF. On the right, estimates of survival free from hospital admission for cardiac reasons (Reproduced from V-TACH trial).

According to the latest guidelines of the American Heart Association, the American College of Cardiology, and the European Society of Cardiology, catheter ablation is indicated as adjunctive therapy in selected patients who have an ICD and who receive multiple shocks as a result of sustained ventricular tachycardia that is not manageable by reprogramming of the ICD or drug therapy.

Some evidence already exists on prophylactic ablation in ICD patients to prevent VTs and shocks. The SMASH-VT trial (Reddy et al, 2007) included 128 ischemic patients that were ICD implanted for spontaneous ventricular tachycardia or fibrillation. They were randomly assigned to defibrillator implantation alone or defibrillator implantation with adjunctive catheter ablation. Ablation was performed with the use of a substrate based approach in which the myocardial scar is mapped and ablated while the heart remains predominantly in sinus rhythm. During a mean follow-up of 22.5±5.5 months, twenty one patients assigned to defibrillator implantation alone (33%) and eight patients assigned to defibrillator implantation plus ablation (12%) received appropriate ICD therapy. So the authors conclude that prophylactic substrate-based catheter ablation reduced the incidence of ICD therapy in patients with a history of myocardial infarction who received ICDs for the secondary prevention of sudden death.

3.2 Optimize device programming

3.2.1 Tailored programming for each patient

The first way to avoid inappropriate shocks is to program the device considering patient characteristics such as age, underlying myocardiopathy, primary or secondary indication and concomitant arrhythmias or, at least, risk of future development. For instance, previous investigations have demonstrated substantial differences in frequency, rate, and mechanisms of tachycardia observed in patients with ICDs implanted for primary versus secondary prevention indications. The primary prevention patient population has been reported to have a lower incidence of ventricular arrhythmias compared with secondary prevention patients. Consequently, a higher proportion of ICD therapies in primary prevention patients could be due to inappropriate detections and therapies primarily due to arrhythmias such as sinus tachycardia and atrial fibrillation.

3.2.1.1 Cut-off rates

ICD recipients with primary compared to secondary prevention indications experience faster ventricular tachyarrhythmias, with average rates of 200 versus 153 beats per minute (bpm), respectively. In contrast, clinical supraventricular tachycardia (SVT) usually ranges between 160 and 180 bpm. Also patients under antiarrhythmic drug therapy experience slower tachycardias. For patients with secondary prevention indications, a safety margin of 30–60 ms between the slowest spontaneous or induced VT and the cut-off rate has been recommended (Mansour and Khairy, 2011).

If the VT rate is unknown or if a primary prevention patient is receiving antiarrhythmic therapy, an empirically programmed rate of 150–160 bpm appears reasonable. A higher rate of 170-175 bpm could be used in youngest patients, typically suffering from channelopathies. Modern devices allow us to program different detection zones (Ventricular Fibrillation-VF, Fast Ventricular Tachycardia-FVT and Ventricular Tachycardia-VT). Depending on ICD indication we can select one, two or the three of them, with different detection criteria and therapies on each one. In certain patients could be interesting to program a detection zone with no therapy, using the device to monitor the occurrence of slow tachycardias.

Limiting the use of SVT discriminators for tachycardias of 188 bpm or slower results in inappropriate ICD therapy since 22–44% of SVTs conduct faster than 188 bpm. Since the majority of SVTs leading to ICD shock have rates less than 230 bpm some authors (Volosin et al, 2011) have proposed the use of SVT discriminators for rates up to 230 bpm. Our usual policy is to program it up to 220 bpm.

3.2.1.2 Timers to override discriminators

Sustained rate duration (SRD; Boston Scientific, Natick, MA, USA), High rate time out (HRT; Medtronic, Minneapolis, MN, USA), SVT time out (St. Jude Medical, St. Paul, MN, USA), and sustained VT (Biotronik GmbH, Berlin, Germany) are timers used to override discriminators. Once the programmed timer elapses, therapy is delivered even if it had been appropriately withheld.

The literature suggests that this safety feature is of little value, especially for dual chamber devices. A reasonable option could be to activate the overriding timer while extending its nominal duration (in our opinion to, at least, 3 min).

3.2.1.3 Detection time/intervals

Classifying an arrhythmia as sustained is a somewhat arbitrary balance between overtreating otherwise self-terminating arrhythmias and delaying therapy for potentially unstable arrhythmias. The trend has been toward programming longer detection times, due to the fact that nominal detection settings are likely excessively conservative, erring on the side of overtreating nonsustained VT.

Recent publications (Wilkoff et al, 2008) have shown that adequately programming detection criteria, increasing the number of RR intervals needed to detect the arrhythmia and thus allowing for non-sustained VTs to spontaneously terminate (30 of 40 beats on this study), reduce number of shocks without increasing risk of syncope or serious adverse events.

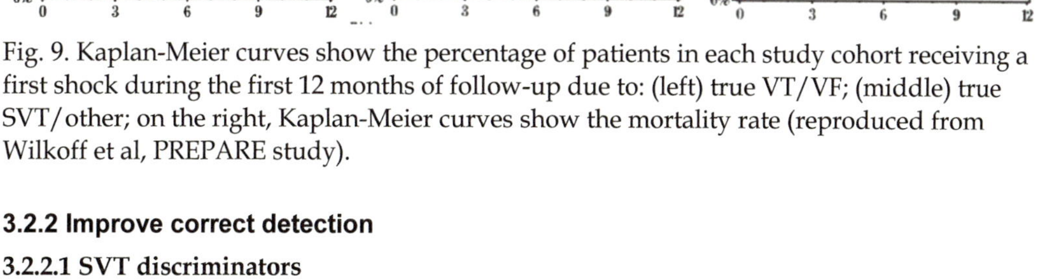

Fig. 9. Kaplan-Meier curves show the percentage of patients in each study cohort receiving a first shock during the first 12 months of follow-up due to: (left) true VT/VF; (middle) true SVT/other; on the right, Kaplan-Meier curves show the mortality rate (reproduced from Wilkoff et al, PREPARE study).

3.2.2 Improve correct detection

3.2.2.1 SVT discriminators

The main arguments against systematically enabling discriminators are their reliability and associated risks of underdetecting VT. With single chamber discriminators, underdetection occurs in 0–0.4% of VT episodes with stability, 0–2% with morphology, and 0.5–5% with onset criteria. For dual-chamber devices, VT underdetection has been reported in 0.6–1% of events.

Discriminators appear most useful in patients with secondary prevention ICDs or under antiarrhythmic drug therapy, since lower programmed cut-off rates expose them to a higher risk of inappropriate therapy for SVT. We currently program discriminators up to a rate of 220 bpm with a high-rate timer along with discriminators. In Medtronic's most recent ICD model (ProtectaTM), the SVT limit is nominally programmed to 230 bpm within the VT zone. For Boston and Sorin devices, discriminators apply to the entire VT zone.

In the event of inappropriate VT detection, reported values of onset, stability, AV association, and/or morphology should be examined, when available, to guide further programming to optimize cut-off values.

3.2.2.2 Algorithms to avoid shocks due to noise or T wave oversensing

New algorithms capable of increasing specificity without affecting sensitivity for VT detection have been developed by different ICD manufactures. Oversensing of T-waves and noise due to lead problems (loose set-screw or lead fractures) are among the leading causes of noise-driven VF detection.

One of these new algorithms recently introduced is intended to reduce inappropriate shocks caused by fractures of implantable cardioverter-defibrillator leads (Swerdlow et al, 2008). This lead-integrity algorithm (LIA), which can be downloaded into presently implanted Medtronic implantable cardioverter-defibrillators, alerts the patient and/or physician when triggered by either abnormally high impedance or sufficient evidence of nonphysiological, rapid oversensing. Once the LIA is triggered, it sets the programmed number of intervals to detect (NID) at 30 of 40 intervals to reduce inappropriate shocks, an audible alert sounds immediately and every 4 hours thereafter, and transmits a wireless, internet-based alert if enabled. The authors demonstrated on 15970 patients with Fidelis leads and 95 other fractured leads that increasing the NID reduced inappropriate shocks and the LIA provided at least a 3-day warning of inappropriate shocks in 76% of patients.

A new T-wave discrimination algorithm by Medtronic analyzes the sensing electrogram for alternating patterns of amplitude and frequency content by comparing the standard sensing signal to a first-order difference signal that attenuates low-frequency content dominating T-waves. Other functions like SenseAbility available in St Jude Medical ICDs allows avoidance of TWOS by means of four key parameters: Threshold start, decay delay, maximum sensitivity and refractory periods (see Figure 10 for explanation). The algorithm adjusts the sensitivity setting based on intrinsic signals and changes sensitivity on every beat so it adjusts as the patient's intrinsic activity changes.

The new lead noise oversensing algorithm available in Medtronic devices analyzes the far-field EGM (e.g., right ventricular (RV) coil-can) in an amplitude measurement window centered around each event sensed on the near-field EGM (e.g., RV tip-RV ring). The concept behind RV Lead Noise Discrimination algorithm is that lead noise oversensing is typically isolated to the near-field EGM (RVtip-RVring sense channel). Therefore, a far-field electrogram signal (Can to RV coil or RV coil to superior vena cava –SVC-) is used to confirm that VT/VF senses on the near-field electrogram are not present on the far-field signal in the case of lead noise (see Figure 11). Oversensing due to a lead or connection problem is identified when the peak to peak amplitudes seen on the far field signal have a large disparity, indicating that these amplitude measurement windows are sensing both R-wave as well as absence of R-waves (isoelectric potentials).

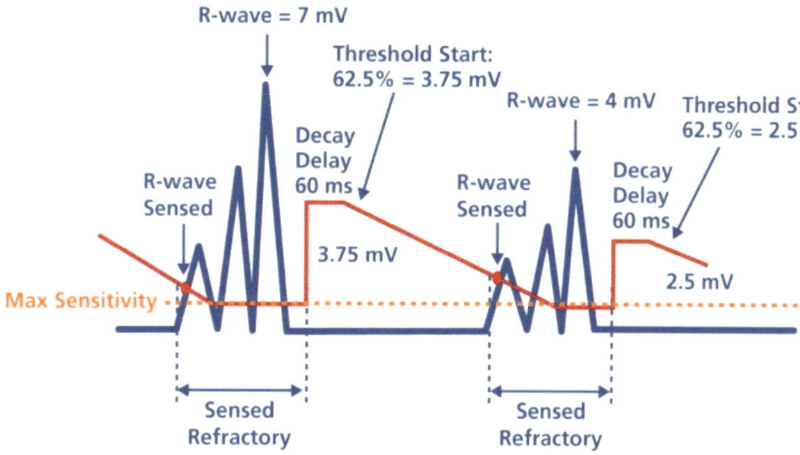

Fig. 10. SenseAbility algorithm: Threshold Start is a programmable percentage of the previous peak amplitude. Decay Delay "delays" the time before the linear decay occurs (60 ms on this example). Max Sensitivity defines the most sensitive level the ICD can reach.

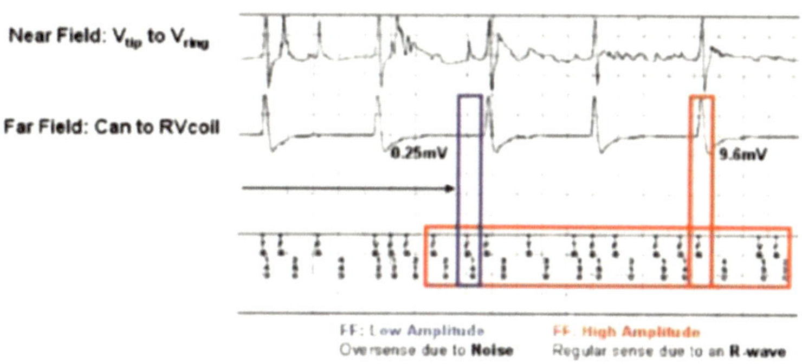

Fig. 11. Example of lead noise oversensing algorithm: Top line, near field EGM between tip to ring. Middle line, far field EGM between can to RV coil. Bottom line: marker channel. As the detection of noise continues, the algorithm withholds detection. Timeout is available to ensure that detection is not withheld for long periods of time.

3.2.3 Shock reduction strategies

Several recent publication have consistently demonstrated the usefulness of antitachycardia pacing and shock withholding for supraventricular rhythms, oversensing, and nonsustained ventricular tachycardia. During the following pages we will further discuss the evidence supporting this approach, as well as new developments incorporated in the newest devices to ensure correct VT diagnosis and delivery of shock only when needed.

3.2.3.1 Antitachycardia pacing

This function allows terminating VTs by pacing faster than the ventricular rate, thus blocking the re-entrant circuit sustaining the tachycardia. ATP is painless and much less associated with atrial tachycardia induction. Nevertheless, it may accelerate the VT or even transform it into VF.

There are several different types of ATP, basically referred to as burst and ramps. Burst means that all the stimulation pulses given during the ATP maintain the same interval whereas ramp means that the pacing interval decreases from one beat to the following one (Figure 12).

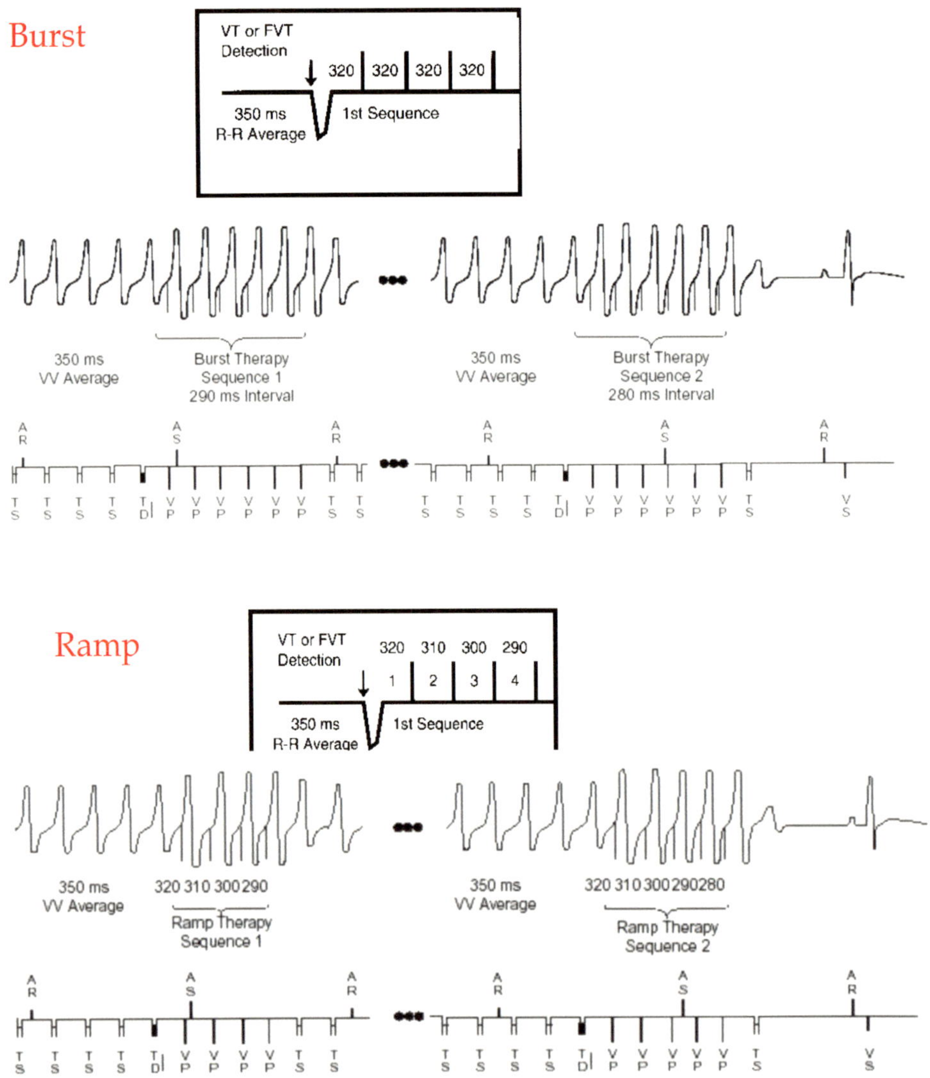

Fig. 12. Top. Burst pacing: after VT is detected, burst pacing is initiated. 2 sequences of 6 beats each are programmed, with a 91% coupling interval and 10 ms decrement between both. Bottom. Ramp pacing: only 2 sequences programmed, first one 4 beats, second one of 5. During ramp pacing, the 10 ms decrement programmed decreases each pacing interval in the same sequence.

ATP effectiveness is related to tachycardia cycle length, being higher in slower VTs and decreasing for VTs faster than 200 bpm (Ormaetxe-Merodio et al, 2008). Several publications have compared effectiveness and safety of both types of ATP, without finding statistically significant differences for slow VTs. Nevertheless, the PITAGORA ICD trial (Gulizia et al, 2009) randomized patients to one burst (eight stimuli, 88% of the cycle length) versus one ramp (eight stimuli, 91% cycle length) in the FVT zone (188–250 bpm). Bursts had a significantly higher success rate than ramps (72% vs 52%) for fast VTs, with a trend toward less acceleration (2.3% vs 7.4%).

There are some ICD models that memorize therapy effectiveness but it is known that failure of an ATP sequence does not predict subsequent failure. For Medtronic devices, in case it does not appear in four consecutive episodes, the device annulates it and, for the next episode, jumps directly to the next therapy programmed (Smart mode). Biotronik has a programmable option: ATP optimization. A successful ATP setting is memorized by the ICD and delivered as the first therapy for future events.

Concerning the number of pulses to use and stimulation rate, published data is scarce. Peinado et al, 1998, compared the efficacy and safety of different ATPs, namely 15 vs 7 pulses at rates of 91 vs 81% of tachycardia cycle length. They showed that for an isolated sequence of stimulation, burst pacing using 15 pulses was more effective than 7 pulses (78% vs 68%, p: 0,01) and stimulation rates of 91% of the tachycardia cycle length were better than 81% (80% vs 56%, $p<0{,}001$). So the authors conclude than ATP using 15 pulses at 91% of tachycardia cycle length was the most effective combination (87%, $p<0{,}001$ in comparison with the other ATP combinations).

Due to the scarce data we have concerning number of pulses to program, is our usual policy to program 10-12 pulses at 88-91% of tachycardia cycle length.

We can say that ATP in ICD recipients allows to successfully terminate 85-90% of VTs with cycle length higher than 320 ms, with a low acceleration rate (1-5%). Besides, these figures are applicable to different cardiomyopathies (ischemic and non-ischemic), confirming reentry as the most probable mechanism of these arrhythmias. 10 to 25% of ICD recipients present VTs with a CL lower than 320 ms. Even though effectiveness is lower than for slower VTs, there are published data supporting their use. In this way, Wathen et al 2001 (Pain-FREE trial), analyzed ATP results when using 2 burst of 8 pulses at 88% of tachycardia CL for VTs between 240 and 320 ms. Out of 442 studied episodes in 52 ischemic patients, 85% successfully terminated with the therapy, 90% with the first delivered burst. On top of that, a third therapy programmed in some patients by caring physician criteria successfully terminated 18 more VTs, rising global efficacy to 89%. With this stimulation protocol, VT acceleration rate was only 4%.

Several years later, Wathen et al published the Pain-FREE II trial (Wathen et al, 2004), comparing only one burst of 8 pulses at 88% with high energy shocks for VTs between 188 and 250 bpm. 1837 episodes were able for analysis, 73% of witch corresponded to monomorphic fast VTs. ATP efficacy for VTs faster than 188 bpm was 81%, with an acceleration rate of only 2%. On the population randomized to receive shocks, 34% of episodes ended spontaneously and 66% required the programmed therapy. So, shock reduction by using ATP for fast VTs was 70% in this study. Mean duration of episodes was shorter in the ATP group ($10{,}7\pm0{,}7$ vs $12{,}7\pm0{,}8$ ms; $p<0{,}001$). There were no differences between groups in sincopal episodes. Another important finding in this study was the fact that the number of intervals to detect the tachycardia was prolonged to 18, compared to 12 for the Pain-FREE I. That reduced significantly the number of episodes that required therapy, and settled the fundamentals for more recent studies investigating the results of prolonging the time to detect the tachyarrhythmia and start treatment.

Several smaller but more recent studies have also demonstrated that ATP is safe and effective for fast VTs termination. Following this evidence, most of the newest devices from different manufacturers offer the possibility of antitachycardia pacing delivery during ICD charging. The obvious advantage of ATP during charging is that, in case the VT terminates, the shock is avoided and, in case it does not, successful therapy is not delayed. One step forward is to deliver ATP even before initiating ICD charging. In case of success, not only shocks are avoided, but also battery depletion due to repeated charging thus prolonging ICD total life.

A less studied issue is the number of ATP attempts (burst or ramps) that are to be programmed. Published evidence shows that the majority of VTs ended with the first ATP, but is far from negligible the episodes terminated by the second or even the third attempt, not only for slow VTs but also for the fast ones. The main advantage of several ATPs programmed is avoiding shock delivery to terminate the episode. On the contrary, the risk is to prolong VT total duration, that could be dangerous depending on arrhythmia tolerance. So we have to tailor the therapy by programming different VT/FVT/VF zones and therapies on each, guided by cycle length and arrhythmia tolerability in each patient.

The PainFREE RX II (Pacing Fast VT REduces Shock ThErapies) and EMPIRIC (Comparison of Empiric to Physician-Tailored Programming of Implantable Cardioverter Defibrillators) trials demonstrated that specific VT and VF detection and therapy programming strategies reduced the frequency of shocked episodes. The use of detection algorithms designed to distinguish supraventricular and ventricular tachyarrhythmias and the use of ATP to terminate rapid VTs have been reported to be important components of programming strategies designed to optimize ICD programming and to reduce unnecessary shocks. Sweeny et al recently published that, combining the data of the studies PainFREE I & II, EMPIRIC and PREPARE, most ventricular episodes were potentially ATP-terminable VTs or FVTs, since ATP was able to terminate 92,4% of VT and 82,5% of FVT episodes attempted.

On the basis of this data, we think that programming the VT zone should include at least four ATPs, and for fast VTs, the weight of evidence suggests that at least one ATP sequence should be programmed for VTs between 188 and 250 bpm and that two sequences are superior to one.

3.2.3.2 Shock withholding for supraventricular rhythms, oversensing, and nonsustained ventricular tachycardia

The PREPARE (Programming of Detection and Therapy Parameters in ICDs Reduces Shock) trial was a prospective, cohort-controlled study that analyzed 700 patients with primary prevention indications for an ICD followed for 1 year. VT/VF was detected for rates ≥182 beats/min that were maintained for at least 30 of 40 beats. ATP was programmed as the first therapy for regular rhythms with rates of 182 to 250 bpm, and SVT discriminators were used for rhythms ≤200 bpm. The primary end point was a combined morbidity index, including incidence of device-delivered shocks, arrhythmic syncope, and untreated sustained symptomatic VT/VF. The authors demonstrated that programming strategies that prolong detection duration (30 of 40 ventricular beats), increase the heart rate threshold of tachycardia detection (182 beats/min), use supraventricular detection discrimination algorithms and ATP, and encourage first shock termination of tachyarrhythmias can safely and substantially reduce the number of tachyarrhythmias subjected to shock therapy.

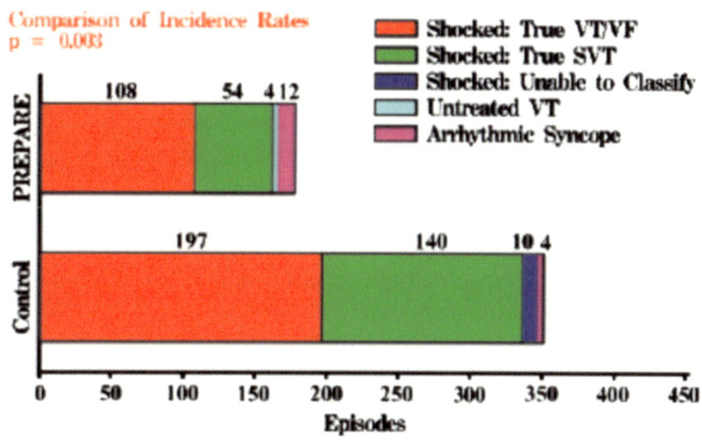

Fig. 13. Data from the PREPARE study. Both appropriate and inappropriate shocks were substantially reduced in the PREPARE study programmed patients. (Reproduced from Wilkoff et al, 2008).

The PREPARE study data clearly demonstrate that by waiting and permitting nonsustained and slower arrhythmias to self-terminate, there are fewer shocked and treated ventricular and SVTs.

New ways of further advancing our knowledge about how to avoid inappropriate and unnecessary shocks have been recently published (Volosin et al, 2011). The authors developed and validated a computer model using clinical data from other published ICD studies and nicely demonstrated how, by using the shock reduction strategies tested (see table 1), hypothetically were able to reduce the number of VT/VF shocked episodes in the SCD-HeFT ICD population by an estimated 59% (from 952 observed to 395 modelled shocks, probability of >0.999). The percentage of patients experiencing inappropriate shocks over 5 years was decreased by 15% (23.5–8.4%), and the number of shocks for non-VT/VF episodes was decreased from 423 to 77 (82% reduction).

Reducing Inappropriate Shocks
1. Using SVT discriminators to cycle lengths of 260 ms or greater. 2. Longer detection time to allow more episodes to terminate spontaneously. 3. Enhanced T wave oversensing algorithm avoids shocks due to oversensed T waves. 4. Lead noise algorithm avoids shocks due to noise oversensing. 5. Combination of atrial and ventricular timing/pattern analysis (PR Logic) with electrogram morphology analysis (Wavelet). 6. Tachycardia detection rate cutoff.
Reducing Unnecessary Shocks
1. ATP therapies to a cycle length of 240 ms. 2. Longer detection time to allow more episodes to terminate spontaneously. 3. New synchronization intervals to reduce shocks for nonsustained events. 4. Tachycardia detection rate cutoff.

Table 1. Strategies for reducing ICD Shocks tested by Volosin et al, 2011.

4. Conclusions

The number of unnecessary or inappropriate shocks is still not zero, which is the goal. ICD discharges have a negative impact on patient prognosis and quality of life, so every effort should be made by programming physicians and ICD manufacturers to reach this goal.
It has been suggested that the "out of box" settings for current ICD systems should be changed in light of the programming strategies shown in clinical trials to reduce shocks, and some manufacturers are already working on it. This may be worthwhile but, since there are so many patient specific issues to be considered, the important point is that the devices should be optimally programmed at implant, not how the devices are shipped.
The initial one-zone one-lead "shock box" approach has progressively become obsolete, as attention has increasingly turned toward avoidance of preventable shocks and inappropriate therapies for lead failure, SVT, and self-terminating tachyarrhythmias. ATP therapy should be systematically programmed, algorithms to discriminate from supraventricular rhythms are to be used and spontaneous episodes of VT have to be aggressively treated, with special consideration to ablation. Recently published evidence suggests that shock reduction strategies could and should be combined to reduce the incidence of unnecessary and inappropriate ICD shocks. New discrimination algorithms could significantly increase specificity without affecting sensitivity.
As in many other fields in Medicine and to the greatest extent possible, ICD programming should be guided by evidence based medicine and every effort should be made to translate this evidence to bedside by ICD programming physicians.

5. Reference

Brugada et al (1998). Enhanced Detection Criteria in Implantable Defibrillators. *J Cardiovasc Electrophysiol* 1998;9:261-268.

Connolly et al (2006). Comparison of β-Blockers, Amiodarone Plus β-Blockers, or Sotalol for Prevention of Shocks From Implantable Cardioverter Defibrillators. The OPTIC Study: A Randomized Trial. *JAMA* 2006;295:165-171.

Daubert et al (2008). Inappropriate Implantable Cardioverter-Defibrillator Shocks in MADIT II. Frequency, Mechanisms, Predictors, and Survival Impact. *J Am Coll Cardiol* 2008;51:1357–65.

Gulizia et al (2009). A randomized study to compare ramp versus burst antitachycardia pacing therapies to treat fast ventricular tachyarrhythmias in patients with implantable cardioverter defibrillators: The PITAGORA ICD trial. Circ Arrhythm Electrophysiol 2009; 2:146–153.

Kuck et al (2010). Catheter ablation of stable ventricular tachycardia before defibrillator implantation in patients with coronary heart disease (VTACH): a multicentre randomised controlled trial. *Lancet* 2010; 375: 31–40.

Mansour and Khairy (2011). Programming ICDs in the Modern Era beyond Out-of-the Box Settings. *PACE* 2011; 34:506–520.

Ormaetxe-Merodio et al (2008). Programación del desfibrilador automático implantable. *Rev Esp Cardiol* Supl. 2008;8:65A-75A.

Peinado R et al (1998). Randomized, prospective comparison of four burst pacing algorithms for spontaneous ventricular tachycardia. *Am J Cardiol.* 1998;82:1422-1425, A8-9.

Poole J et al (2008). Prognostic Importance of Defibrillator Shocks in Patients with Heart Failure. *N Engl J Med* 2008;359:1009-17.

Reddy et al (2007). Prophylactic Catheter Ablation for the Prevention of Defibrillator Therapy. *N Engl J Med* 2007;357:2657-65.

Ricci et al (2009). Dual-chamber implantable cardioverter defibrillators reduce clinical adverse events related to atrial fibrillation when compared with single-chamber defibrillators: a subanalysis of the DATAS trial. *Europace* 2009;11:587–593.

Sweeney et al (2010). Differences in effects of electrical therapy type for ventricular arrhythmias on mortality in implantable cardioverter-defibrillator patients. *Heart Rhythm* 2010;7:353–360.

Swerdlow et al (2002). Discrimination of Ventricular Tachycardia from Supraventricular Tachycardia by a Downloaded Wavelet- Transform Morphology Algorithm: A Paradigm for Development of Implantable Cardioverter Defibrillator Detection Algorithms. *J Cardiovasc Electrophysiol,* 2002;13:432-441.

Swerdlow et al (2008). Downloadable Algorithm to Reduce Inappropriate Shocks Caused by Fractures of Implantable Cardioverter-Defibrillator Leads. Circulation 2008; 118:2115-2116.

Toquero et al (2009). Morphology discrimination criterion wavelet improves rhythm discrimination in single chamber implantable cardioverter-defibrillators: Spanish Register of morphology discrimination criterion wavelet (REMEDIO). *Europace* 2009 ;11(6):727-733.

Volosin et al (2011). Combining Shock Reduction Strategies to Enhance ICD Therapy: A Role for Computer Modeling. *J Cardiovasc Electrophysiol,* 2011;22 (3): 280-289.

Wathen MS et al (2001). Shock reduction using antitachycardia pacing for spontaneous rapid ventricular tachycardia in patients with coronary artery disease. *Circulation* 2001;104:796-801.

Wathen MS et al (2004). Prospective randomized multicenter trial of empirical antitachycardia pacing versus shocks for spontaneous rapid ventricular tachycardia in patients with implantable cardioverter-defibrillators: Pacing Fast Ventricular Tachycardia Reduces Shock Therapies (PainFREE Rx II) trial results. *Circulation* 2004;110:2591-6.

Wilkoff et al (2008). Strategic Programming of Detection and Therapy Parameters in Implantable Cardioverter-Defibrillators Reduces Shocks in Primary Prevention Patients. Results From the PREPARE (Primary Prevention Parameters Evaluation) Study. *J Am Coll Cardiol* 2008;52:541–50.

Cardiovascular Implantable Cardioverter Defibrillator-Related Complications: From Implant to Removal or Replacement: A Review

Mariana Parahuleva
University Hospital of Giessen and Marburg/Location Giessen, Germany

1. Introduction

Implantable cardioverter defibrillators (ICDs) use has increased exponentially during the past decade. However, these devices are associated with complications related to the implantation procedure itself and morbidity caused by the adverse functioning of the components comprising the system. In 2003, 10.8% of patients undergoing cardioverter-defibrillator implantation experienced one or more early complications (Reynolds et al., 2006). Acute implantation complication rates range from 3% to 7%. For this reason a controlling in respect to the technology, indications for use, personnel involved in monitoring and the frequency and types of monitoring events is needed (Wilkoff et al., 2008).

The European Community (EN540, European Standard, 1993) and the International Standards Organization (ISO 14155, International Standard, 1996) have provided standards for adverse events observed during trials with implantable medical devices, defining an adverse event as any undesirable clinical occurrence in a subject whether it is considered to be device related or not. These standard criteria underwent sweeping changes in the past time. The first and most evident change is the standard's new title: "ISO 1415: Clinical investigations of medical devices in human subjects - good clinical practices", harmonized with the ICH E6 GCP guidelines (Stark et al., 2011). Few studies have systematically examined the predictors of complications in this population using multivariable analysis. These data suggest that complications are driven by the 3 major components that contribute to risk: device, physician, and patient factors. This may be most relevant for patients with complex device systems, particularly heart failure patients (Curtis et al., 2009; Al-Khatib et al., 2008). Even though prospective studies defining the risk associated with ICD implantation and optimal peri-, intra- and postoperative management to ICDs are needed. Therefore the aim of this review was to report the incidence of adverse events during the initial months after pectoral implantation or replacement of an ICD system with a transvenous lead system. The usual complication including implant procedure-related complications, ICD generator-related complications, as well as lead-related complications will be discussed. This review, however, limits discussion to surgical complications. In addition, it will be reviewed the relevant clinical trials as well as prescription guidelines, because the increasing clinical relevance of this topic is the reason for the future formulation of recommendations by an interdisciplinary working group.

2. Implant procedure-related complications

The early mortality effects of implant procedure-related complications may be the direct "mechanical" effect of the procedure, such as infection, pneumothorax, or perforation, that are not well tolerated. These risks probably are largely related to procedural complexity, reflected in system configuration risk in procedural volume, and operator expertise. The second contributor is the patient; the physiological duress of even minor surgery may exacerbate comorbidities, particularly heart failure, which contributes significantly to reduced survival.

2.1 Venous access related complications

Transvenous non-thoracotomy lead systems are available and are usually implanted safely and with a high success rate by an electrophysiologist and a surgeon. The axillary and subclavian vein puncture are the standard approach in ICD implantation. However, obtaining venous access for defibrillator implantation can be complicated by vascular injury, subclavian arteriovenous fistula and/or pneumothorax or hemothorax. No-puncture strategy using the cephalic cut-down technique obviates the complication in the majority of cases and improves the safety of device implantation. Thus, the subclavian route of insertion resulted in more complications than the cephalic vein route (Kron, 2003). In addition, conventional transvenous approaches for ICD lead placement are not possible in some patients with limited vascular access and/or tricuspid valve dysfunction. On the other site transvenous ICD lead failure rates are significant and their occurrence increases with time from implant. Therefore it was recently designed an entirely subcutaneous ICD system to eliminate the need for venous access and their complication (Bardy et al., 2010).

2.1.1 Subclavian arteriovenous fistula

Subclavian arteriovenous fistula is a rare and uncommon complication of ICD implantation and it could be successful closured using an Amplatzer vascular occlusion plug (Hess et al., 2010).

2.1.2 Pneumothorax

Pneumothorax is usually a complication of subclavian venous access and may be detected during the procedure or delayed until 48 h after implantation (Aggarwal at al., 1995). This complication is a problem in unexperienced operators and is directly related to the difficulty of the subclavian puncture. Often is the pneumothorax asymptomatic, but uncommonly occurs a tension pneumothorax with hemodynamic and clinical improvement, which needs immediately placement of chest tube. The diagnosis of pneumothorax was confirmed by chest x-ray. Pneumothorax due to perforation of the atrial lead through the wall of the atrial appendage has already been reported (Rosman et al., 2006). Perforation of the right ventricle with or without pericardial effusion is also well recognized (Gondi et al., 1981). However, isolated pneumopericardium reported as an exclusive complication of a cardiac resynchronisation therapy (CRT) implantation is very uncommon. We have previously reported pneumothorax recognised days after CRT implantation and concomitant pneumopericardium secondary as a late complication of a persisting connection between the pericardium and the pleura parietalis as consequence of the former aortal-coronary surgery, three years after coronary artery bypass graft surgery (CABG) (Fig.1, Parahuleva et al., 2009).

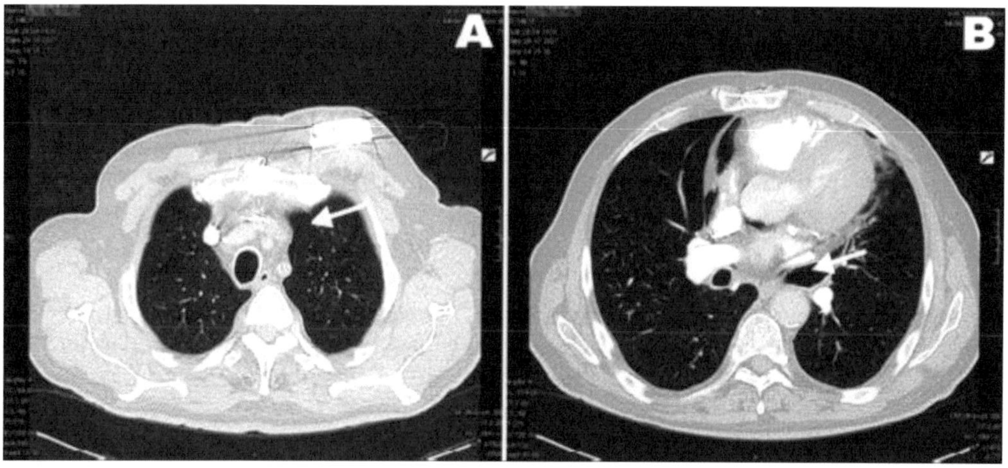

Fig. 1. Computed tomography (CT) scan of the thorax showing (A) left-sided pneumothorax with 30% reduction in lung volume and (B) moderate- sized pneumopericardium and pleuromediastinum (from Parahuleva et al., 2009).

2.1.3 Hemothorax

Hemothorax results most commonly from an arterial puncture and cannulate the artery with the intraducer, a situation that should indicate vascular surgical removal. This complication could also occur after right ventricular (RV) lead perforation beyond the cardiac border into the pleural space (Merla et al., 2007). The diagnosis of hemothorax and suspecting of RV perforation in patients with ICD implantation presenting with recurrent chest pain and/or pleural effusion is important, because it is potentially life threatening complication. Massive hemothorax may develop after placement of an ICD in patients who received postoperative anticoagulants (see also 2.2.1 ICD Hematoma). The perioperative management of anticoagulation in patients who are having implantation of a pacemaker or ICD is a common clinical problem in which best clinical practise is not established, but a strategy involving postoperative bridging with intravenous heparin confers a high risk for bleeding whereas perioperative continuation of a oral anticoagulation appears to reduce the risk for bleeding (see also 2.2.1 ICD Hematoma).

2.1.4 Venous thrombosis and superior vena cava syndrome (SVCS)

Significant vein occlusion was found in 25% of patients after placement of ICD (Lickfett et al., 2004) and in 27% of patients after pacemaker implantation (Antonelli et al., 1989). Subclavian venous obstruction or thrombosis following transvenous device implantation rarely cause clinical problems and become a significant challenge, when lead revision or device upgrade is indicated (Wilkoff et al., 2004, van Rooden et al., 2004). The reasons for these venous complications such as stenosis, occlusions, and superior vena cava syndrome have been discussed. The study has suggested that intravenous lead infection promotes local vein stenosis (Korkeila et al., 2009). Another found that the presence of a temporary wire before implantation is associated with an increased risk of stenosis (Haghjoo et al., 2007). Despite many years of experience with transcutaneous implanted intravenous pacing systems, it was unable to identify clear risk factors which lead to venous stenosis (Bar-Cohen et al., 2006). Neither the hardware (lead size, number and material) nor the access site choice (cephalic cut down, subclavian or axillary puncture) appears to affect rate of venous complications. A few factors were proposed as predictors of severe venous stenosis/occlusion: presence of multiple pacemaker leads (compared to a single lead), use of hormone therapy, personal history of venous thrombosis, new onset of atrial fibrillation, the presence of temporary wire before implantation, previous presence of a pacemaker (ICD as an upgrade) and the use of dual-coil leads (Bulur et al., 2010). A variety of different strategies to overcome the venous obstruction have been reported: controlateral LV lead placement (Fox, 2006), innominate vein as an alternative venous access (Aleksic et al., 2007), internal jugular vein approach (Bosa-Ojeda et al., 2007), opening an occluded subclavian vein and venoplasty (Worley et al., 2007), surgical approaches with the use of minimally invasive procedures (Jaroszewski et al., 2009), supraclavicular vein approach (Antonelli et al., 2010), use of a tunneling technique (Kim et al., 2010) or iliofemoral approach by patients with occluded superior venous access (Allred et al., 2008).

Anticoagulant therapy (for other reasons than pacemaker lead) seemed to have protective antithrombotic effect (Pavia et al., 2001), but the effect of prophylactic anticoagulant treatment after pacemaker implantation have not found positive results (Goto et al., 1998). Furthermore, it was found that oral anticoagulant treatment did not differ from antiplatelet treatment in respect to protection from venous obstruction occurrence (Haghjoo et al., 2007). The patients who are candidates for multiple pacemaker leads implantation have more risk factors for venous obstruction than other device patients. These patients should be evaluated with venography before lead revision and/or device upgrade procedures. In addition, large studies are needed to investigate whether anticoagulant or antiplatelet treatment could prevent venous obstruction.

2.2 ICD pocket related complications

2.2.1 ICD hematoma

Pocket hematoma is an acute, relatively common complication. The use of electrocautery and portable drainage device for 24 hours after implantation are useful to minimize pocket hematoma. The hematomas are managed usually conservatively. Expanding in size of hematoma, tense or painful in the ICD pocket are requiring re-operation to evacuate the hematoma (Belott et al., 2000). The risk of pocket hematoma is increased in anticoagulated patients. Dual antiplatelet therapy and periprocedural heparin appears to be associated with significantly increase risk of bleeding complications at the time of pacemaker or ICD implantation (Al-Khadra et al., 2003; Giudici et al., 2004). The study of Tompkins (Tompkins, 2010) evaluated patients (n=1388) undergoing permanent pacemaker and ICD implantation over a 3-year period to determine if patients with antiplatelet or anticoagulation therapy required normalization of coagulation factors in the periprocedural period. A significant bleeding complication was defined as need for pocket exploration or blood transfusion, hematoma requiring pressure dressing or change in anticoagulation therapy, or prolonged hospitalization. It has been shown that continuation of warfarin was associated with a trend toward increased bleeding complications when compared with controls, even when held to allow the international normalized ratio (INR) to decrease below 1.5 (Fig.2). There was no statistical difference in bleeding risk between patients continued on warfarin with an INR≥1.5 and patients who had warfarin withheld until the INR was normal. The use of periprocedural heparin (enoxaparin or unfractionated heparin) and dual antiplatelet therapy increase the risk of bleeding complication (Fig.2).

Appropriate periprocedural management requires a thorough understanding of indications for antiplatelet or anticoagulation medications and assessing the risks of thromboembolic versus bleeding complications (Douketis et al., 2008). Brake off of antiplatelet or anticoagulation medications before device implantation could be possible in patients at low risk for thromboembolic events. Patients at high risk for thromboembolic events should continue warfarin throughout the periprocedural phase and should need bridging anticoagulation with therapeutic dose heparin.

Operating with oral anticoagulation is the best alternative, because device implantation or replacement without withdrawing of oral anticoagulants and with an INR of about 2.0 is safe and was not associated with an increase of the hemorrhagic risk.

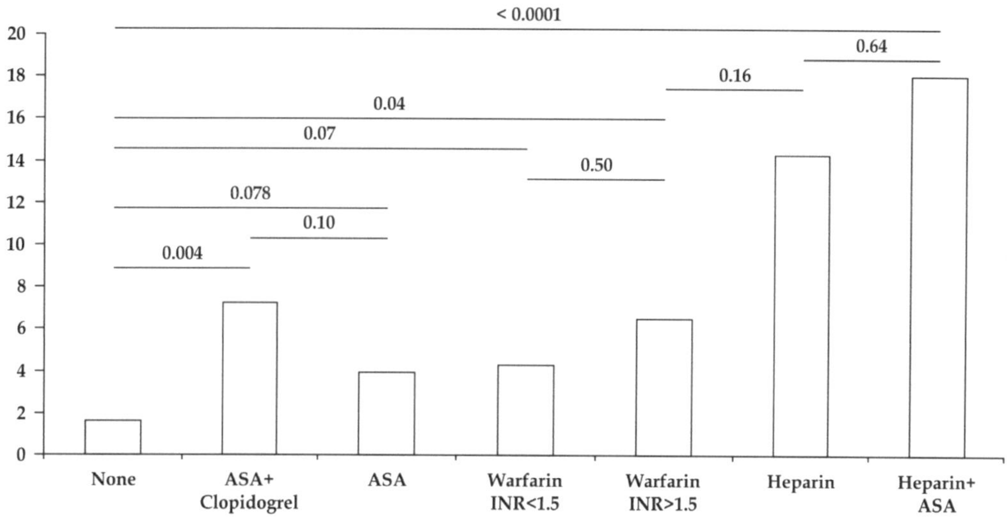

Fig. 2. Effect of antiplatelet and anticoagulation agents on bleeding complication in patients after device implantation (modified from Tompkins et al., 2010).

2.2.2 ICD infections

Device system infection is a serious complication and tended to occur within 1 year after implantation, or as late onset lead endocarditis (Mangram et al., 1999). The physical manifestations range from mild symptoms with local reaction to fulminant sepsis. Failure to use perioperative antibiotics is a predictor of system infection and ICD system infection ranges from 0.13 to 12.6% (Mela et al. 2001). Repeated operative procedures after the first device implantation were associated with increased risk of device infection (Margey et al., 2010). Female sex, older age, and preoperative antibiotics given at the first device implantation were associated with a lower risk of later device infection (Johansen et al., 2011). End-stage renal disease markedly increases bleeding and device-related infections (Tompkins, 2011).

When infection is present, complete device removal with transvenous lead extraction must be followed by antimicrobial therapy. Removal of the entire pacing system is crucial for the treatment of lead endocarditis (see also 3.2. Lead extraction-related complication). The development of laser-assisted extraction techniques for chronically implanted pacemaker and defibrillator leads has reduced the need for open surgical removal (Gaca et al., 2009).

2.2.3 ICD wound dehiscence and erosion

Wound healing is a major determent in the post-surgical course of patients after device implantation. Insufficient closure may lead to serious complications with pocket infections leading to the device's explantation. Therefore is the skin suture approach most important for the wound healing. The absorbable intracutaneous suture is frequently used to close surgical incisions and a form of skin adhesive surgical tape is commonly also placed over the wound. It was shown that early adverse events as insufficient closure, major and minor bleeding, pocket haematoma, erythema, incrustation, dehiscence, keloid, and explantation due to infection occurred significantly more often in the patients with skin adhesive in comparison to absorbable intracutaneous suture (Spencker et al., 2011).

Skin erosion is possible when the subcutaneous pocket at the time of initial implantation is too small or too superficial and the device makes undue tension on the overlying skin. The skin erosion is also associated with potential pocket infection and sub-pectoral placement after complete explantation of the device-lead system is usually advised (Gold et al., 1996).

2.2.4 Chronic pain

Chronic pain will usually manifest an obvious infection. An allergy to nickel/cobalt and chronic painful eczema could mimic a pocket infection (Citerne et al., 2011). Alternatively, mechanical trauma from the device location adjacent to chest wall may also be the reason for chronic pain. In this situation device relocation revision may be advised.

2.2.5 Twiddler's syndrome

Twiddler's syndrome is a rare complication well described in patients with subcutaneous permanent pacemakers, but is unusual in patients with CRT-D, which typically presents with device malfunction and inappropriate shocks. The condition occurs when the patient, either consciously or unconsciously, rotates the implanted pacemaker in its pocket, resulting in torsion, dislodgement, and often fracture of the pacing lead (Veltri et al., 1984). The placement of the pulse generator in a sub-pectoral position may help prevent Twiddler's syndrome.

2.3 Perioperative ICD implantation related-complications

2.3.1 Perioperative death

A serious complication such as perioperative death is rare in patients with transvenous device implantation. Elevated BNP level was significantly associated with increased risk of cardiac arrest periprocedural in patients received ICD implants (Wei et al., 2011) and studies are needed to investigate whether reducing preprocedural BNP could manage the procedural risk of cardiac arrest or in-hospital mortality. Although the benefit of ICD therapy in patients with hypertrophic cardiomyopathy (HCM) at risk for sudden cardiac arrest is well established, there may be a higher risk for device complications and inappropriate shocks (Lin et al., 2009).

2.3.2 Strokes

The most patients with perioperative strokes after device implantation had chronic atrial fibrillation without prior oral anticoagulation. Therefore, it would be routinely performed transesophageal echocardiography prior to device implantation in patients lacking maintained anticoagulation despite increased risk for cardiac thromboembolism, e.g., atrial fibrillation, severely reduced left ventricular function, ventricular aneurysms, and intracardiac thrombi. In the presence of intracardiac thrombi is not recommended to perform intraoperative defibrillation threshold testing (Healey et al., 2010).

2.4 Defibrillation testing-related complications

Defibrillation threshold (DFT) testing has traditionally been an integral part of ICD implantation. However, recent publications question the necessity of DFT testing during implantation, because of compelling evidence that it predicts or improves outcomes (Strickberger et al., 2004; Russo et al., 2005; Gula et al., 2008). DFT testing may now be the highest acute risk component of ICD implantation, quoting the effectiveness of the current generation of devices and the rate of complications associated with testing. The recently published experience revealed some serious testing-related complications: sudden cardiac death (SCD), spontaneous episodes of ventricular arrhythmia (sustained ventricular tachycardia, VT, and strokes (Birnie et al., 2008). Physicians favored performance of defibrillation testing in patients who are at lower risk of defibrillation testing-related complications and in those receiving amiodarone (Ruso et al., 2005). Lower left ventricular ejection fraction (LVEF) had a borderline predictive value for high DFT. The association between left ventricular function and failure of defibrillation was examined in the Post Implant Testing Study (PITS). As systolic function declined, there was a trend to a higher failure rate, which was not statistically significant (Brodsky et al., 1999). Other studies suggest that left ventricular mass or volumes are more predictive than ejection fraction to predict DFTs (Hodgson et al., 2002). The rate of complications associated with intraoperativ DFT testing appears small, even allowing for the underestimation of its true rate with the current study methodology (Birnie et al., 2008; Healey et al., 2010). These slight but measurable risks must be considered when assessing the risk-benefit ratio of the procedure. The serum markers NSE, PS1B rise significantly by the ICD-test as an expression of neuronal damage in patients with poor LVEF also significantly more (Prull et al., 2011). In the primary prophylaxis ICD indication ICD-test must be therefore a critical indication. Additional data from ongoing prospective ICD registries and/or clinical trials are required to clarify whether routine DFT testing may be safely abandoned leading to a revision of current guidelines.

3. Lead-related complications

3.1 Lead Implantation-related complications

3.1.1 Lead dislocation/malposition

Device leads are placed routinely with few notable complications. The lead dislocation occurs very early postoperative (usually 24–48 hours) but may occur up to 3 months after implantation. Adverse changes in sensing and pacing thresholds compared to implant values should prompt consideration of this complication and lead repositioning or replacement is required. Further management to avoid recurrence of this complication is essential and the follow-up of devices early postoperative will help to minimize her incidence.

The lead malposition is diagnosed by unacceptable pacing, sensing, and/or defibrillation thresholds. The placement of leads into the left ventricle is a rare complication of transvenous device implantation and may be occur by intracardiac abnormality such as a ventricular septal defect. This malpositioning places the patients at risk for thromboembolic events, including cerebrovascular insults (37% based on the reported cases of left ventricular leads, Van Gelder et al., 2000) and anticoagulation with warfarin is recommended. The median sternotomy or thoracotomy are the usual operative technique for the extraction of left ventricular lead. It was also reported a successful percutaneous removal of a left ventricular lead in patients who had been anticoagulated and had no evidence of thrombus on the lead (Trohman et al., 1991) or a minimally invasive technique for left ventricular lead extraction (Stouffer et al., 2010).

Diaphragmatic stimulation is another possible manifestation of lead malposition. It is usually due to direct phrenic nerve stimulation from the right or left ventricular lead.

Location of the left ventricular pacing lead is one of the determinants for success of cardiac resynchronization therapy (CRT). The implantation procedure includes several challenging technical issues and strongly depends on the highly variable anatomy of the coronary sinus. The optimal position of the LV pacing lead is the site of latest activation in the left ventricle, which enables effective resynchronization. Furthermore, phrenic nerve stimulation (PNS) occurs in 37% of CRT patients at implant or follow-up. To address this common problem, the manufacturers of CRT devices offer a range of configurations aimed at preventing PNS. A quadripolar LV lead has recently been designed which provides more programming configurations and may help to overcome high thresholds and PNS (Forleo GB et al., 2010; Shetty AK et al., 2011). There are several publications concerning quadripolar electrode implantation which show elimination of PNS, but the optimal LV pacing configuration should be determined on the basis of individual patient testing. We report a case in which the use of the quadripolar left ventricular lead pacing depended on the highly variable anatomy of the coronary sinus and resulted in the occurrence of stable PNS at 3- and 6-months follow-up. In this case report, even 10/10 configurations could not prevent occurrence of PNS (Parahuleva et al., 2011)

3.1.2 Lead fractures

Most dislodgements tended to occur in the 3 months following implantation, whereas lead fractures continued to occur throughout follow-up. Fractures of ICD leads may occur 5 years after the implantation and coaxial polyurethane leads have a particularly high incidence of failure. However, there are no parameters that can be used to predict lead failure during follow-up (Kitamura et al., 2006). Although implantation techniques and generator technology continue to evolve, the occurrence of lead fractures and the need for premature system revision supports the practice of close routine ICD system surveillance.

3.1.3 Lead perforation and cardiac tamponade

The device lead may perforate the atria, ventricle or coronary sinus during the implant procedure. Atrial leads perforated more frequently than ventricular leads, and ventricular ICD leads perforated more frequently than ventricular pacemaker leads. This complication almost always occurs after active fixation of pacing and ICD leads and may be associated with delayed right ventricular perforation and bleeding in to the pericardial space. Asymptomatic perforation is a common phenomenon with subacute or delayed perforation and without clinical signs (inappropriate shock, syncope, abdominal pain, mammary hematoma, diaphragm stimulation, and chest pain) of lead perforation at the time of the procedure or perforation of the right ventricle diagnosed more then 5 days (sometimes more then 6 months) after implantation. However, dyspnea with pericardial effusion may occur requiring emergency pericardial drainage by cardiac tamponade. The risk of cardiac tamponade is increased in anticoagulated patients. Subacute ventricular perforation is a rare but potentially life threatening complication of lead implantation and the diagnosis could be emergency confirmed by chest x-ray, echocardiography, or computed tomography. A lead perforation rate is low and there were no statistically significant differences in perforation or dislodgement rates between manufacturers or lead models (Turakhia et al., 2009).

3.2 Lead extraction-related complication

Transvenous lead extraction is an essential component of management of infections and other device-related complications (Smith et al., 2008). Despite the development of more efficient and safer tools, the procedure continues to be associated with risk of major complications such as venous or myocardial damage, tamponade, and even death (Field et al. 2007). It has also been recognized that chronic leads (more than 1 year) occasionally break during the process of extraction and extraction of a fractured lead from the right ventricle is sometimes difficulty.

Thus, implantation of an additional device lead versus extraction of the defective lead and implantation of a new one is one possible therapeutic approach in cases of a defective lead. Implantation of an additional or replacement of the lead in case of high-voltage pace/sense lead failure is statistically not different concerning mortality and morbidity (Wollmann et al., 2007). There are no predictors for further lead defects. Implantation of an additional lead should not be recommended in young patients. Predictors for death were an age over 70 years and renal insufficiency.

4. Pacing/sensing-related complications

Pacing/sensing-related and ICD-specific complications (oversensing, undersensing, exit block, pacemaker-mediated tachycardia, ineffective and inappropriate therapy) detected during routine follow-up visits are relatively rare. Recommended routine follow-up intervals for ICD patients are range from 3 to 6 months and 6 month follow-up interval appear to be the safest (Senges-Becker et al., 2005). In addition, inappropriate pacing/sensing parameters of right ventricular lead implanted at the right ventricular apex could occur in the perioperative period. An alternate location for implantation in these situations is the right ventricular outflow tract. However, active-fixation of right ventricular leads should be considered to limit the risk of electrode dislodgment (Lubinski et al. 2000).

5. Complications after ICD replacement and/or upgrade procedures

Device replacement is generally technically less challenging than a new implant but is associated with complications that may place the patient at substantial risk, including system infection requiring complete extraction (Gould et al., 2008; Moore et al., 2009). Patients who undergo ICD replacement or upgrade procedures often have significant cardiac conditions and noncardiac comorbidities and may therefore be at higher risk of developing complications from the procedure than has been demonstrated in randomized trials (Poole et al., 2010; Santini et al., 2006). The Canadian Heart Rhythm Society has previously reported on a retrospective series that involved 533 ICDs that were replaced because of an advisory, which demonstrated an overall complication rate of 8.1% (Gould et al., 2006). This unexpectedly high complication rate was associated with major complications in 2.0% of patients, including death in 2 patients. A voluntary German ICD registry focusing on new implants reported rates of specific complications and found that pocket hematoma, chronic pain, and lead and device dislodgments leading to operative revisions were the most common events, with reoperation in 3.0% (Gradaus et al., 2003). Recently, the REPLACE registry reported a 4.0% complication rate in 1031 patients undergoing generator replacement and 15.3% in 713 patients with replacement and a lead addition (Poole et al., 2010). This prospective registry reported that ICDs and particularly CRT ICDs were associated with a greater risk of complications, consistent with the current study that found a higher complication in upgrade and CRT patients. However, identifying factors contributing to complications may permit identification of high-risk individuals that warrant incremental monitoring and therapy to attenuate risk. Recently, a prospective, multicenter, population-based registry of all ICD patients at 18 centers in Ontario, Canada showed, that risk factors associated with complications after ICD replacement, include the presence of angina, antiarrhythmic therapy, increased number of previous procedures, and low implanter volume (Krahn et al., 2011). Generator change is a higher risk procedure than new implants. This suggests that clinicians and researchers should consider strategies to minimize the need for device replacement, particularly because most devices are implanted for primary prevention.

6. Conclusion

Cardiovascular implantable cardioverter defibrillator-related complications are rare in patients with transvenous device implantation. The cardioverter-defibrillator can be life saving, but its potential complications could be significant and enormous. For this reason, the recognition of potential cardiovascular implantable cardioverter defibrillator-related complications is essential for advances in ICD technology and management strategies to avoid their recurrence and will assist and educate clinicians who care for an increasing number of patients with cardiovascular devices to minimize the incidence of this complication.

7. Acknowledgment

Very special thanks to Mr Svetozar Borislavov, for his loving support and understanding during my scientific and medical researches in past few years. His encouragement was the reason to complete this book chapter and I want to dedicate it to him.

8. References

Aggarwal RK, Connelly DT, Ray SG, Ball J, Charles RG. Early complications of permanent pacemaker implantation: no difference between dual and single chamber systems. *Br Heart J*, 1995, 73: 571–5.

Aleksic I, Kottenberg-Assenmacher E, Kienbaum P, Szabo AK, Sommer SP, Wieneke H et al. The innominate vein as an alternative venous access for complicated implantable cardioverter defibrillator revisions. *PACE*, 2007, 30:957–60.

Al-Khadra AS. Implantation of pacemakers and implantable cardioverter defibrillators in orally anticoagulated patients. *Pacing Clin Electrophysiol*, 2003, 26:511– 4.

Al-Khatib SM, Greiner MA, Peterson ED, Hernandez AF, Schulman KA, Curtis LH. Patient and implanting physician factors associated with mortality and complications after implantable cardioverter-defibrillator implantation, 2002–2005. *Circ Arrhythm Electrophysiol*, 2008, 1:240–249.

Allred JD, McElderry HT, Doppalapudi H, Yamada T, Kay GN. Biventricular ICD implantation using the iliofemoral approach: providing CRT to patients with occluded superior venous access. *Pacing Clin Electrophysiol*, 2008 Oct;31(10):1351-4.

Antonelli D, Turgeman Y, Kaveh Z, Artoul S, Rosenfeld T. Short term thrombosis after transvenous permanent pacemaker insertion. *PACE*, 1989, 12:280–2.

Antonelli D, Freedberg NA, Turgeman Y. Supraclavicular vein approach to overcoming ipsilateral chronic subclavian vein obstruction during pacemaker-ICD lead revision or upgrading. *Europace*, 2010 Nov, 12(11):1596-9.

Bar-Cohen Y, Berul CI, Alexander ME, Fortescue EB, Walsh EP, Triedman JK, Cecchin F. Age, size, and lead factors alone do not predict venous obstruction in children and young adults with transvenous lead systems. *J Cardiovasc Electrophysiol.* 2006 Jul, 17(7):754-9.

Bardy GH, Smith WM, Hood MA, Crozier IG, Melton IC, Jordaens L, Theuns D, Park RE, Wright DJ, Connelly DT, Fynn SP, Murgatroyd FD, Sperzel J, Neuzner J, Spitzer SG, Ardashev AV, Oduro A, Boersma L, Maass AH, Van Gelder IC, Wilde AA, van Dessel PF, Knops RE, Barr CS, Lupo P, Cappato R, Grace AA. An entirely subcutaneous implantable cardioverter-defibrillator. *N Engl J Med*, 2010 Jul 1, 363(1):36-44.

Belott P, Reynolds D. Permanent pacemaker and implantable cardioverterdefibrillator implantation. In Ellenboggen K, Kay G, Wilkoff B (Eds): Clinical cardiac pacing and defibrillation. *WB Saunders*, Philadelphia: Saunders; 2000, 573–644.

Birnie D, Tung S, Simpson C, Crystal E, Exner D, Ayala Paredes FA, et al. Complications associated with defibrillation threshold testing: the Canadian experience. *Heart Rhythm*, 2008, 5:387-90.

Bosa-Ojeda F, Bethencourt-Munoz M, Vergara-Torres M, Lara-Paoron A, Rodriguez-Gonzales A, Marrero-Rodriguez F. Upgrade of a pacemaker defibrillator to a biventricular device: the internal jugular vein approach in a case of bilateral subclavian veins occlusion. *J Interv Card Electrophysiol*, 2007, 19:209–11.

Brodsky CM, Chang F, Vlay SC. Multicenter evaluation of implantable cardioverter defibrillator testing after implant: the Post Implant Testing Study (PITS). *Pacing Clin Electrophysiol*, 1999, 22:1769-76.

Bulur S, Vural A, Yazıcı M, Ertaş G, Özhan H, Ural D. Incidence and predictors of subclavian vein obstruction following biventricular device implantation. *J Interv Card Electrophysiol*, 2010 Dec, 29(3):199-202, Epub 2010 Oct 2.

Citerne O, Gomes S, Scanu P, Milliez P. Painful Eczema mimicking pocket infection in a patient with an ICD: a rare cause of skin allergy to nickel/cobalt alloy. *Circulation*, 2011 Mar 22, 123(11):1241-2.

Curtis JP, Luebbert JJ, Wang Y, Rathore SS, Chen J, Heidenreich PA, Hammill SC, Lampert RI, Krumholz HM. Association of physician certification and outcomes among patients receiving an implantable cardioverter-defibrillator. *JAMA*, 2009, 301:1661–1670

Douketis JD, Berger PB, Dunn AS, Jaffer AK, Spyropoulos AC, Becker RC, Ansell J; American College of Chest Physicians. The perioperative management of antithrombotic therapy: American College of Chest Physicians Evidence-Based Clinical Practice Guidelines (8th Edition). *Chest*, 2008 Jun, 133(6 Suppl):299S-339S.

EN540, European Standard. *Clinical Investigation of Medical Devices for Human Subjects*, 1993, Brussels, Belgium: European Committee for Standardization.

Field ME, Jones SO, Epstein LM. How to select patients for lead extraction. *Heart Rhythm* 2007;4:978-85.

Forleo GB, Della Rocca DG, Papavasileiou LP, Di Molfetta A, Santini L, Romeo F. Left ventricular pacing with a new quadripolar transvenous lead for CRT: early results of a prospective comparison with conventional implant outcomes. *Heart Rhythm*, 2010, Sep 28.

Fox DJ, Petkar S, Davidson NC, Fitzpatrick AP. Upgrading patients with chronic defibrillator leads to a biventricular system and reducing patient risk: controlateral LV lead placement. *PACE*, 2006, 29:1025–7.

Gaca JG, Lima B, Milano CA, Lin SS, Davis RD, Lowe JE, Smith PK. Laser-assisted extraction of pacemaker and defibrillator leads: the role of the cardiac surgeon. *Ann Thorac Surg*. 2009 May;87(5):1446-50; discussion 1450-1.

Giudici MC, Barold SS, Paul DL, Bontu P. Pacemaker and implantable cardioverter defibrillator implantation without reversal of warfarin therapy. *Pacing Clin Electrophysiol*, 2004, 27:358–60.

Gold MR, Peters RW, Johnson JW, Shorofsky SR. Complications associated with pectoral cardioverter-defibrillator implantation: comparison of subcutaneous and submuscular approaches. Worldwide Jewel Investigators. *J Am Coll Cardiol*, 1996 Nov 1, 28(5):1278-82.

Gondi B, Nanda NC. Real-time, two-dimensional echocardiographic features of pacemaker perforation. *Circulation*, 1981, 64: 97–106.

Goto, Y., Abe, T., Sekine, S., & Sakurada, T. (1998). Long-term thrombosis after transvenous permanent pacemaker implantation. *Pacing and Clinical Electrophysiology*, 21(6), 1192–1195.

Gould PA, Gula LJ, Champagne J, Healey JS, Cameron D, Simpson C, Thibault B, Pinter A, Tung S, Sterns L, Birnie D, Exner D, Parkash R, Skanes AC, Yee R, Klein GJ, Krahn AD. Outcome of advisory implantable cardioverter-defibrillator replacement: one-year follow-up. *Heart Rhythm*, 2008, 5:1675–1681.

Gould PA, Krahn AD. Complications associated with implantable cardioverter-defibrillator replacement in response to device advisories. *JAMA*, 2006, 295:1907–1911

Gradaus R, Block M, Brachmann J, Breithardt G, Huber HG, Jung W, Kranig W, Mletzko RU, Schoels W, Seidl K, Senges J, Siebels J, Steinbeck G, Stellbrink C, Andresen D. Mortality, morbidity, and complications in 3344 patients with implantable cardioverter defibrillators: results from the German ICD Registry EURID. *Pacing Clin Electrophysiol*, 2003, 26:1511–1518.

Gula LJ, Massel D, Krahn AD, Yee R, Skanes AC, Klein GJ. Is defibrillation testing still necessary? A decision analysis and Markov model. *J Cardiovasc Electrophysiol*, 2008, 19:400-5.

Haghjoo, M., Nikoo, M. H., Fazelifar, A. F., Alizadeh, A., Emkanjoo, Z., & Sadr-Ameli, M. A. Predictors of venous obstruction following pacemaker or implantable cardioverterdefibrillator implantation: a contrast venographic study on 100 patients admitted for generator change, lead revision, or device upgrade. *Europace*, (2007), 9(5), 328–332.

Healey JS, Birnie DH, Lee DS, Krahn AD, Crystal E, Simpson CS, Dorian P, Chen Z, Cameron D, Verma A, Connolly SJ, Gula LJ, Lockwood E, Nair G, Tu JV; Ontario ICD Database Investigators. Defibrillation Testing at the Time of ICD Insertion: An Analysis From the Ontario ICD Registry. *J Cardiovasc Electrophysiol*, 2010 Dec, 21(12):1344-8.

Hess CN, Ohman EM, Patel MR.Amplatzer vascular plug closure of a subclavian arteriovenous fistula associated with implantable cardioverter-defibrillator implantation. *Catheter Cardiovasc Interv*, 2010 Sep 17.

Hodgson DM, Olsovsky MR, Shorofsky SR, Daly B, Gold MR. Clinical predictors of defibrillation thresholds with an active pectoral pulse generator lead system. *Pacing Clin Electrophysiol*, 2002, 25:408-13.

ISO 14155, *International Standard for Clinical Investigation of Medical Devices*, Geneva, Switzerland: International Organisation for Standardization, 1996.

Jaroszewski DE, Altemose GT, Scott LR, Srivasthan K, Devaleria PA, Lackey J et al. Non traditional surgical approaches for implantation of pacemaker and cardioverter defibrillator systems in patients with limited venous access. *Ann Thorac Surg*, 2009, 88:112–6.

Johansen JB, Jørgensen OD, Møller M, Arnsbo P, Mortensen PT, Nielsen JC. Infection after pacemaker implantation: infection rates and risk factors associated with infection in a population-based cohort study of 46299 consecutive patients. *Eur Heart J*. 2011 Apr;32(8):991-8. Epub 2011 Jan 20.

Kim JB, Joung B, Lee MH, Kim SS. Use of a tunneling technique to achieve a lower defibrillation threshold during implantable cardioverter defibrillator implantation via the right subclavian vein. *J Korean Med Sci*, 2010 Oct, 25(10):1526-8.

Kitamura S, Satomi K, Kurita T, Shimizu W, Suyama K, Aihara N, Niwaya K, Kobayashi J, Kamakura S. Long-term follow-up of transvenous defibrillation leads: high incidence of fracture in coaxial polyurethane lead. *Circ J*, 2006 Mar, 70(3):273-7.

Korkeila P, Ylitalo A, Koistinen J, Airaksinen KE. Progression of venous pathology after pacemaker and cardioverter-defibrillator implantation: A prospective serial venographic study. *Ann Med*, 2009, 41(3):216-23.

Krahn AD, Lee DS, Birnie D, Healey JS, Crystal E, Dorian P, Simpson CS, Khaykin Y, Cameron D, Janmohamed A, Yee R, Austin PC, Chen Z, Hardy J, Tu JV; for the Ontario ICD Database Investigators. Predictors of Short-Term Complications After Implantable Cardioverter-Defibrillator Replacement: Results From the Ontario ICD Database. *Arrhythm Electrophysiol*, 2011 Apr 1, 4(2):136-142.

Kron J. Clinical significance of device-related complications in clinical trials and implications for future trials: insights from the Antiarrhytmics Versus Implantable Defibrillators (AVID) trial. Card Electrophysiol Rev. 2003 Dec;7(4):473-8.

Laborderie J, Barandon L, Ploux S, Deplagne A, Mokrani B, Reuter S, Le Gal F, Jais P, Haissaguerre M, Clementy J, Bordachar P. Management of subacute and delayed right ventricular perforation with a pacing or an implantable cardioverter-defibrillator lead. *Am J Cardiol*, 2008 Nov 15, 102(10):1352-5.

Lickfett L, Bitzen A, Arepally A, Nasir K, Wolpert C, Jeong KM et al. Incidence of venous obstruction following insertion of an implantable cardioverter defibrillator. A study of systematic contrast venography on patients presenting for their first elective ICD generator replacement. *Europace*, 2004, 6:25–31.

Lin G, Nishimura RA, Gersh BJ, Phil D, Ommen SR, Ackerman MJ, Brady PA. Device complications and inappropriate implantable cardioverter defibrillator shocks in patients with hypertrophic cardiomyopathy. *Heart*, 2009 May, 95(9):709-14.

Lubinski A, Lewicka-Nowak E, Królak T, Kempa M, Bielawska B, Wilczek R, Swiatecka G. Implantation and follow-up of ICD leads implanted in the right ventricular outflow tract. *Pacing Clin Electrophysiol.* 2000 Nov;23(11 Pt 2):1996-8.

Mangram AJ, Horan TC, Pearson ML, Silver LC, Jarvis WR. Guideline for prevention of surgical site infection, 1999. Hospital Infection Control Practices Advisory Committee. *Infect Control Hosp Epidemiol.* 1999 Apr;20(4):250-78.

Margey R, McCann H, Blake G, Keelan E, Galvin J, Lynch M, Mahon N, Sugrue D, O'Neill J. Contemporary management of and outcomes from cardiac device related infections. Europace. 2010 Jan;12(1):64-70.

Mela T, McGovern BA, Garan H, Vlahakes GJ, Torchiana DF, Ruskin J, Galvin JM. Long-term infection rates associated with the pectoral versus abdominal approach to cardioverter- defibrillator implants. *Am J Cardiol.* 2001 Oct 1;88(7):750-3.

Merla R, Reddy NK, Kunapuli S, Schwarz E, Vitarelli A, Rosanio S. Late right ventricular perforation and hemothorax after transvenous defibrillator lead implantation. *Am J Med Sci*, 2007 Sep, 334(3):209-11.

Moore JW III., Barrington W, Bazaz R, Jain S, Nemec J, Ngwu O, Schwartzman D, Shalaby A, Saba S. Complications of replacing implantable devices in response to advisories: a single center experience. *Int J Cardiol*, 2009, 134:42–46.

Parahuleva M, Chasan R, Soydan N, Abdallah Y, Neuhof Ch, Tillmanns H, Erdogan A. Quadripolar left ventricular lead in a patient with CRT-D does not overcome phrenic nerve stimulation. *Clin Med Insights Cardiology*, 2011:5 45–47.

Parahuleva M, Schifferings P, Neuhof Ch, Tillmanns H, Erdogan A. Pneumopericardium and Pneumomediastinum as a Late Complication of Defibrillator Implantation after Coronary Artery Bypass Graft Surgery. *Thorac Cardiov Surg*, 2009, 57:489–495.

Pavia S, Wilkoff B. The management of surgical complications of pacemaker and implantable cardioverter-defibrillators. *Curr Opin Cardiol*, 2001 Jan, 16(1):66-71.

Poole JE, Gleva MJ, Mela T, Chung MK, Uslan DZ, Borge R, Gottipaty V, Shinn T, Dan D, Feldman LA, Seide H, Winston SA, Gallagher JJ, Langberg JJ, Mitchell K, Holcomb R. Complication rates associated with pacemaker or implantable cardioverter-defibrillator generator replacements and upgrade procedures: results from the REPLACE registry. *Circulation*, 2010, 122:1553–1561.

Reynolds MR, Cohen DJ, Kugelmass AD, Brown PP, Becker ER, Culler SD, Simon AW. The frequency and incremental cost of major complications among medicare beneficiaries receiving implantable cardioverter-defibrillators. *J Am Coll Cardiol*, 2006 Jun 20, 47(12):2493-7.

Prull M. W, Unverricht S, Bittlinsky A, Sasko B, Wirdemann H, Gkiouras G, Butz T, Trappe H.-J. Der ICD-Test führt zu einem zerebralen Schaden und verschlechtert die kognitive Funktion. *Clin Res Cardiol*, 100, Suppl 1, April 2011

Rosman J, Shapiro MD, Hanon S. Pneumomediastinum and right sided pneumothorax following dual chamber-ICD implantation. *J Interv Card Electrophysiol*, 2006 Nov, 17(2):157-8.

Russo AM, Sauer W, Gerstenfeld EP, Hsia HH, Lin D, Cooper JM, et al. Defibrillation threshold testing: is it really necessary at the time of implantable cardioverter-defibrillator insertion? *Heart Rhythm*, 2005, 2:456-61.

Santini M, Brachmann J, Cappato R, Davies W, Farre J, Levy S, Quesada A, Ricci RP, Rowland E, Sulke N. Recommendations of the European Cardiac Arrhythmia Society Committee on device failures and complications. *Pacing Clin Electrophysiol*, 2006, 29:653–669.

Senges-Becker JC, Klostermann M, Becker R, Bauer A, Siegler KE, Katus HA, Schoels W. What is the "optimal" follow-up schedule for ICD patients? Europace. 2005 Jul;7(4):319-26.

Shetty AK, Duckett SG, Bostock J, Roy D, Ginks M, Hamid S, Rosenthal E, Razavi R, Rinaldi CA. Initial Single-Center Experience of a Quadripolar Pacing Lead for Cardiac Resynchronization Therapy. *Pacing Clin Electrophysiol*, 2011 Jan 5.

Smith MC, Love CJ. Extraction of transvenous pacing and ICD leads. *Pacing Clin Electrophysiol* 2008;31:736-52.

Spencker S, Coban N, Koch L, Schirdewan A, Mueller D. Comparison of skin adhesive and absorbable intracutaneous suture for the implantation of cardiac rhythm devices. *Europace*, 2011 Mar, 13(3):416-20, Epub 2010 Nov 11.

Stark, J.N. (2011). A New Standard for Medical Device Investigations. *Journal of ClinicalResearch Best Practices*, Vol. 7, No. 2, (February 2011)

Stouffer CW, Shillingford MS, Miles WM, Conti JB, Beaver TM. Lead astray: minimally invasive removal of a pacing lead in the left ventricle. *Clin Cardiol*, 2010 Jun, 33(6):E109-10.

Strickberger SA, Klein GJ. Is defibrillation testing required for defibrillator implantation? *J Am Coll Cardiol*, 2004, 44:88-91.

Tompkins C, Cheng A, Dalal D, Brinker JA, Leng CT, Marine JE, Nazarian S, Spragg DD, Sinha S, Halperin H, Tomaselli GF, Berger RD, Calkins H, Henrikson CA. Dual antiplatelet therapy and heparin "bridging" significantly increase the risk of bleeding complications after pacemaker or implantable cardioverter-defibrillator device implantation. *J Am Coll Cardiol*, 2010 May 25, 55(21):2376-82.

Trohman RG, Wilkoff BL, Byrne T, et al. Successful percutaneous extraction of a chronic left ventricular pacing lead. *Pacing Clin Electrophysiol*, 1991, 14:1448–1451.

Turakhia M, Prasad M, Olgin J, Badhwar N, Tseng ZH, Lee R, Marcus GM, Lee BK. Rates and severity of perforation from implantable cardioverter-defibrillator leads: a 4-year study. *J Interv Card Electrophysiol.* 2009 Jan;24(1):47-52.

Van Gelder BM, Bracke FA, Oto A, et al. Diagnosis and management of inadvertently placed pacing and ICD leads in the left ventricle: a multicenter experience and review of the literature. *Pacing Clin Electrophysiol*, 2000, 23:877–883.

Van Rooden CJ, Molhoek SG, Rosendaal FR, Schalij MJ, Meinders AE, Huisman MV. Incidence and risk factors of early venous thrombosis associated with permanent pacemaker leads. *J Cardiovasc Electrophysiol*, 2004 Nov, 15(11):1258-62.

Veltri EP, Mower MM, Reid PR. Twiddler's syndrome: a new twist. *PACE*, 1984, 7:1004-09

Wilkoff BL. Lead-induced venous thrombosis:consequences? *J Cardiovasc Electrophysiol,* 2004 Nov, 15(11):1263-4.

Wilkoff BL, Auricchio A, Brugada J, Cowie M, Ellenbogen KA, Gillis AM, Hayes DL, Howlett JG, Kautzner J, Love CJ, Morgan JM, Priori SG, Reynolds DW, Schoenfeld MH, Vardas PE; (HRS; EHRA; ACC; AHA); European Society of Cardiology (ESC); Heart Failure Association of ESC (HFA); Heart Failure Society of America (HFSA). HRS/EHRA Expert Consensus on the Monitoring of Cardiovascular Implantable Electronic Devices (CIEDs): Description of Techniques, Indications, Personnel, Frequency and Ethical Considerations. *Europace,* 2008 Jun, 10(6):707-25.

Wollmann CG, Böcker D, Löher A, Paul M, Scheld HH, Breithardt G, Gradaus R.Two different therapeutic strategies in ICD lead defects: additional combined lead versus replacement of the lead. *J Cardiovasc Electrophysiol,* 2007 Nov, 18(11):1172-7.

Worley SJ, Ghon DC, Pulliam RW. Opening an occluded subclavian vein with a screw-like flexible hollow guide-wire and venoplasty. *PACE,* 2007, 30:1290–3.

9

Expanding Applications of Defibrillators and Cardiac Resynchronization Therapy to Include Adult Congenital Heart Disease

K Michael[1], B Mayosi[2], J Morgan[3] and G Veldtman[4]
[1]*Queen`s University Heart Rhythm Service, Kingston, Ontario*
[2]*University of Cape Town, Department of Medicine*
[3]*Wessex Cardiothoracic Unit and*
[4]*Grown Up Congenital Heart Disease Unit, Southampton University`s Hospital,*
[1]*Canada*
[2]*South Africa*
[3,4]*UK*

1. Introduction

Atrial redirection surgery, brought into common use by Mustard's modification of the Senning procedure, transformed the natural history of dextro-transposition of the great arteries (d-TGA) from a 90% one year mortality to a 90% 1 year survival(1). Although rendering the infant acyanotic with excellent functional capacity, the morphological right ventricle(sRV) is required to support the systemic circulation. The sRV faces substantial pressure overload resulting in a high incidence of late ventricular failure(2). This prompted an evolution to a more physiologically acceptable correction in the form of the arterial switch or Jatene operation(3). The arrhythmias and heart failure that usually manifest by the second decade of life in patients after atrial redirection surgery pose a challenge to management.

Apart from the progressive sRV dysfunction and heart failure, sinus bradycardia commonly arises because of surgical disruption to the sino-atrial node blood supply warranting early pacemaker implantation (4). The incidence of tachyarrythmias, most notably atrial flutter and fibrillation, may be related to ventricular dysfunction or as a consequence of atrial scarring following surgery. Ventricular tachycardia (VT) and fibrillation (VF) have been documented on holter monitoring in various long term studies and the incidence of sudden cardiac death (SCD) ranges between 2-11%(5). Cardiac resynchronization with a biventricular implantable cardioverter-defibrillator (ICD) therefore poses an attractive option particularly as a bridge to transplantation in this group of patients. We examine the challenges in terms of the anatomical constraints in a group of consecutive patients with surgically corrected TGA(6;7).

1.1 Relevant anatomical issues

Placement of intracardiac leads may compromise the haemodynamic status of the patient. Mechanical obstruction from an intra-baffle stenosis or thrombotic obstruction may be encountered or concomitant known associations such as severe tricuspid regurgitation, valvar and sub-valvar pulmonary stenosis must be borne in mind.

Intra-baffle leaks raise the possibility of systemic embolization and inadvertent lead positioning within the sRV.

The coronary sinus (CS) in d-TGA, as in the normal human heart, lies in the atrio-ventricular groove between the left atrium and sub-pulmonic left ventricle (pLV). In the case of surgically altered d-TGA, the resultant sRV, is therefore not encircled by the CS. This limits transvenous access to the lateral wall of the sRV, for lead placement. A large aberrant coronary vein arising from the sRV may drain into the CS or directly into the right atrium (RA) **figure 1**. This may present an option for lead placement. An anterolateral cardiac vein may be regarded as a poor pacing site for a failing systemic LV but may be entirely suitable for pacing the sRV. In an anatomical study by Uemura et al, in hearts with congenitally corrected transposition (atrio-ventricular and ventriculo-arterial discordance), the CS drained the sRV in the majority (87%) of specimens with 5 having partial or complete drainage directly into the atrium (8).

Electrical stimulation of the failing systemic ventricle is usually achieved transvenously via CS cannulation, utilising specially designed left venticular pacing leads. If this is unsuccessful (eg. lack of a suitable ventricular vein) a trans-sternal, surgical approach may be used. The latter, however, may be preferable if conducted at the time of cardiac surgery or with surgically or congenitally altered anatomy that makes transvenous CS access difficult or unachievable.

Access to the coronary venous vasculature post Mustard surgery in d-TGA is also dependent on whether the surgeon leaves the CS os open to the systemic-atrial side of the baffle or to the pulmonary-venous portion. The next challenge is percutaneous cannulation of the CS given the altered atrial structure. Pre-procedural imaging using cardiac magnetic resonance, computerized tomography, intracardiac or transoesophageal echocardiograpy improves identification of coronary venous anatomy (9-11).

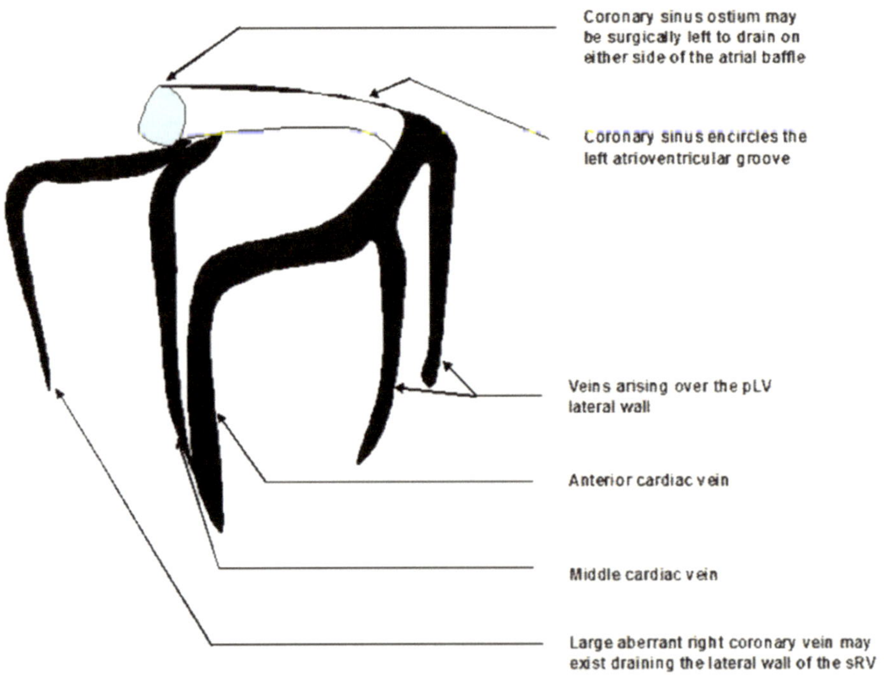

Fig. 1. The anticipated coronary venous structure in dTGA.

1.2 Evolving concepts of cardiac resynchronization therapy

Cardiac resychronization therapy (CRT) has become an integral part of the management of patients with ischaemic and non-ischaemic cardiomyopathies presenting with advanced heart failure. This device based strategy has also been successfully applied in patients with adult congenital heart disease and ventricular dysfunction (12).

Cardiac asynchrony has been traditionally defined in patients in terms of electrical (QRS width >120ms) and doppler echocardiography (conventional/ tissue doppler). The CRT non-responder population however remains between 20-30% warranting evaluation of additional or alternative measurements. Experience is however limited in patients with morphological sRVs and these selection criteria may not be relevant in this peculiar population (13;14;15).

1.3 Patients

All patients were derived from a a jointly managed group of patients at a tertiary referral centre for clinical electrophysiology and adult congenital heart disease. All patients had NYHA grade II-III heart failure symptoms with a perceived risk of SCD. Conventional management would have entailed inevitable cardiac transplantation, with its associated complications. The decision to resort to device therapy was therefore taken out of clinical and life-saving necessity and was conducted in terms of our current understanding of best clinical practice. Where innovative strategies were employed, this was used primarily to increase patient benefit from a more refined and patient specific technique.

1.4 Statistical analysis

Demographic data and simple statistical analysis was performed using SPSS and represented at mean±std dev. Where relevant a test of significance was performed using a t-test.

2. Application of cardiac defibrillator therapy for at risk patients with failing systemic right ventricles

Technical considerations implant details, and follow-up on 5 patients with d-TGA and a Mustard procedure receiving an ICD ± concomitant CRT are addressed below. Right ventricular function was assessed by a combining echocardiographic visual appraisal and planimetry as well as RV angiography. An individualized approach to implantation was undertaken, taking into consideration existing transvenous electrodes and post surgical cardiac anatomy. After implantation, patients were followed-up at 4-6 weeks and then 6-monthly intervals. Data at follow-up including functional assessment, device interrogation, ECG and transthoracic echocardiograms (TTEs) were reviewed.

The baseline characteristics of the 5 patients (4 male, age 18-35 years) studied are shown in **table 1**. All had significantly impaired sRV function (mean sRV EF=30%) and impaired functional class (NYHA class II-III). Two patients had sustained VT, 3 non-sustained VT, and 4 had atrial arrhythmias. Four patients had previously implanted pacemakers. Pre-implant electrophysiological studies were not performed.

2.1 Implant considerations

Implanting a transvenous electrode into the pLV requires that the lead navigates through the surgical baffle. Baffle stenosis impeding flow from the superior vena cava (SVC) to the pLV is common post Mustard modification(1). Defibrillator electrode placement will potentially further impede venous drainage and pLV filling. A strategic decision was therefore made not to implant multiple leads via anatomically narrow baffles and to treat any baffle stenosis prior to the implant. An entirely transthoracic defibrillation strategy was therefore employed in the first patient using a high energy defibrillator (maximum output of 41J) with subcutaneous, single finger arrays (Model 6996. 25cm coil, 500cm² surface. Medtronic, USA). Despite this defibrillation was ineffective figure 2.

	Patient 1	**Patient 2**	**Patient 3**	**Patient 4**	**Patient 5**
Age (years) at implantation	24	22	35	18	25
Documented arrhythmias	Sinus bradycardia, atrial flutter, *NSVT	Sinus bradycardia, ‡VT, *NSVT	Sinus bradycardia, atrial flutter, *NSVT	†SVT, *NSVT	Sinus bradycardia, †SVT, *NSVT, ‡VT
RVEF (%)	25	25	30	35	35
Pre-existing device	Yes	Yes	Yes	No	Yes
Weight (kg)	110.2	106.1	77	67.4	54
Implant	Surgical	Surgical	Transvenous	Transvenous	Transvenous

*NSVT=non sustained ventricular tachycardia, †SVT=supra-ventricular tachycardia, ‡VT=ventricular tachycardia

Table 1. Salient baseline clinical characteristics of patients receiving defibrillators.

Of the 4 patients with pre-existing pacemakers, 2 were demonstrated to have functional baffle stenosis and therefore underwent lead extraction and stent angioplasty at separate procedures at least 48 hours prior to transvenous insertion of a defibrillator lead. Those patients who had lead extractions and the patient with no pre-existing pacemaker underwent standard transvenous implantation with endocardial defibrillator coils placed via the subclavian vein into the pLV. Two patients with existing pacemakers and no evidence of baffle stenosis on cardiac catheterisation had their existing endocardial (pLV)

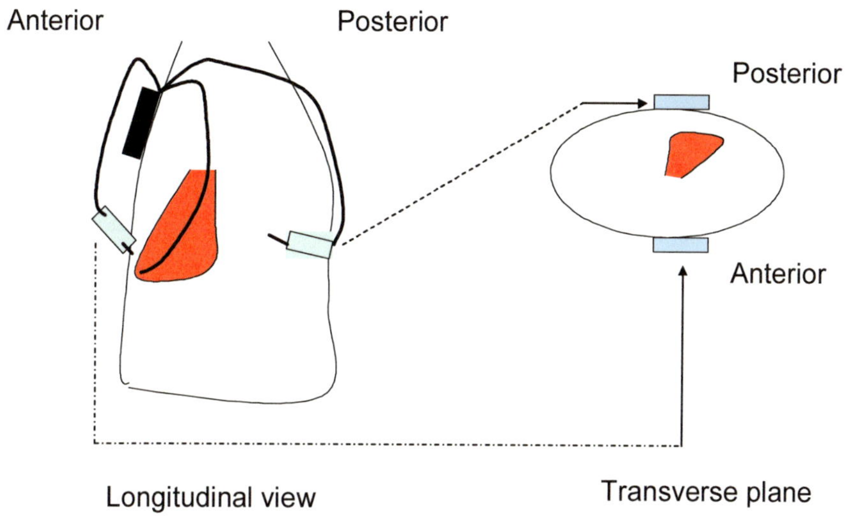

Fig. 2. Diagrammatic view of the placement of the subcutaneous arrays (arrowed) around the chest wall in patient 1 with a sensing lead in the pLV.

pace/sense electrodes conserved; 1 then had epicardial patch electrodes and 1 had subcutaneous arrays implanted at the time of trans-sternal, epicardial pacing lead placement for CRT.

2.2 Defibrillation circuits and testing

The patient with subcutaneous arrays, had the electrodes placed in an antero-posterior configuration around the left chest wall with a left sub-pectoral Can implantation (**figure2**).
Ventricular fibrillation was induced via the chronic pLV endocardial pace/sense lead and therapies were delivered between the anterior and posterior subcutaneous arrays. A series of 6 inductions were performed with therapies of 25 to 41J but none were successful in terminating VF and external rescue shocks were required. Inclusion of the active Can in the circuit did not improve defibrillation outcome.
One patient underwent epicardial patch electrode placement in the anterolateral and inferior positions over the systemic ventricle. This strategy was successful in defibrillating VF at 25J on the first induction (a 10J safety margin).
The remaining 3 patients underwent standard transvenous system implants. An active Can was placed in the left sub-pectoral region and a defibrillation coil advanced under fluoroscopy to the pLV via the subclavian vein. The first 2 transvenous implants received dual coil leads (as is our standard practice when high DFTs are anticipated) but both had failed initial defibrillation, requiring exclusion of the SVC coil from the circuit. In 1 of these patients, a pLV to Can vector provided effective defibrillation at 25J, and in the other it was also necessary to reverse the polarity of the circuit to achieve this safety margin. This patient underwent 4 VF inductions and subsequently developed pulmonary oedema during the procedure.

2.3 Follow up

The median follow-up in all 5 patients was 20 months (range 15-24). A total of 4083 non-sustained tachycardias were documented in the cohort over this period. One patient has had VT with pre-syncope which was correctly diagnosed and treated by a discharge by the ICD.

2.4 Discussion

Mustard patients are at increased risk of SCD defined by sRV dysfunction, heart failure functional status, non-sustained VT and atrial arrhythmias (5). Only 1 patient in the cohort had a preceding out-of-hospital arrest but all patients had documented multiple ventricular ectopics on 24-hour holter analysis. None of the patients received formal electrophysiological studies as we felt that a negative study should not disqualify them. The patients were < 40 years of age and lived productive lives up to the point of referral. The absence of therapies in the majority of the patients (4/5) over 2 years of follow-up does not mean that the decision to implant them was incorrect. The time to the first appropriate therapy in other patient groups with ICDs often exceeds 2 years (16).

It has also not previously been demonstrated that the gold standard treatment for prevention of SCD, namely ICDs, are effective in this population, and given the variation from normal anatomy, efficacy should not be assumed. Appropriate vectors of defibrillation, as determined by electrode placement, are the key determinants of defibrillation success (17). The SVC cavity to pLV vector in particular appears to exclude much of the sRV and septum **figure 3** whilst severe chamber dilatation, common in Mustard patients, is recognised from other populations to be associated with less effective defibrillation (18).

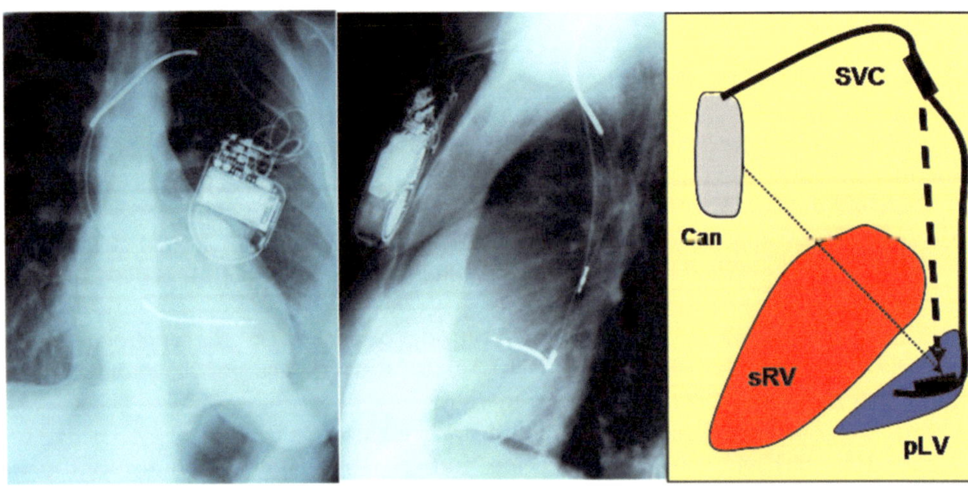

Fig. 3. Electrode positions and defibrillation pathways of a dual coil lead system in a patient post Mustard correction. A dual coil defibrillator lead implanted into the pLV tends to be located more superiorly than when it is in an apical position in the right ventricle. The result is that the proximal electrode rests within the SVC/left subclavian vein. The defibrillation vector between the SVC and pLV thus excludes the major myocardial mass, reducing defibrillation efficacy.

The role of polarity reversal is less well established. Data from randomised trials provides some evidence but no rational explanation, that by inverting vectors, efficacy may be improved in patients (19). However, with a limited number of inductions in any given individual, apparent differences in efficacy may be no more than a reflection of the probabilistic nature of defibrillation success and we need to be cautious in making finite decisions as regards what will and will not work in individual patients.

The single patient experience with subcutaneous defibrillation was plainly suboptimal with no successful defibrillation achieved. This may be a reflection of the Mustard anatomy or other independent factors that potentially may affect defibrillation efficacy. This patient had a body mass index of 33 and gross cardiomegaly.

Our experience demonstrates that transvenous implantation is feasible but may require interventions such as lead extraction and angioplasty of the atrial baffle to avoid venous pathway obstruction. The optimal defibrillation vector with a transvenous implant appears to be pLV to active Can and as such, single coil leads are preferred. Our experience with subcutaneous arrays alone was unsatisfactory. Efficacy may be improved by selecting patients with a smaller body habitus and by incorporating intra-thoracic electrodes. Epicardial patches require an open chest procedure and may be placed at the time of concomitant epicardial CRT if indicated in the individual patient.

The findings mandate the use of high output devices, regardless of the configuration, in anticipation of compromised defibrillation efficacy in similar patients which ultimately may prove more cost effective than undertaking revision procedures.

2.5 Conclusion

Defibrillator implantation in Mustard patients is feasible though challenging. Clinicians planning to implant such patients must be prepared to optimise the systemic venous access of the baffle prior to implantation and then to have strategies in place to tackle high defibrillation thresholds and the decompensation that may result from multiple VF inductions. Endocardial pLV to active Can and epicardial patches are effective defibrillation strategies in this group.

3. Cardiac resynchronisation therapy

Although the atrial switch was abandoned in the 1980s for the Jatene (arterial switch) procedure, a considerable number of patients have survived into their third decade of life (20). The right ventricle is not capable of supporting the systemic circulation for this extended period. Patients post Senning or Mustard operations, invariably experience right ventricular failure by the second and third decades of life (4;21). If cardiac transplantation is their only option, these patients face a post operative average life expectancy of just 10 years (22). Coupled with the limited availability of donors, this management plan is suboptimal for these, generally young patients. We present here 3 consecutive cases who had pre-existing dual chamber pacemakers upgraded to CRT/D. Two required a hybrid approach using epicardial leads implanted by surgical thoracotomy while a 3rd successfully had an endocardial sRV pace/sense lead implanted. Although the results varied for these cases, they demonstrate plausible alternatives to management.

3.1 Case presentations

3.1.1 Case 1

Patient 1 was 110 kg and 22 years old at time of implantation of his CRT/D system (**table2**). The underlying congenital anomaly of simple transposition was initially temporised by an atrial septostomy soon after birth and then with a Mustard operation at 7 months of age. At 18 years of age he presented with sino-atrial node dysfunction (a common complication

	Patient 1	Patient 2
Age (years) at implantation	22	24
Wight (kg)	110	106
Onset of symptoms	15	16
Initial symptoms	Effort intolerance	Breathlessness & chest pain
Gender	M	M
NYHA	III	III
Drug therapy		
ACE inhibitor	Lisinopril	Lisinopril
Beta Blocker	Bisoprolol	Bisoprolol
Cardiac glycoside	Y	Y
Frusemide	Y	Y
Spironolactone	N	Y
Amiodarone	Y	N
Echo features		
sRV	Dilated. Severely impaired	Dilated, severely impaired
pLV	Moderately impaired	"Normal"
TR	Mild	Mild
MR	Trivial	-
ECG features		
BBB	RBBB	RBBB
AVB	First degree	First degree
QRS duration	120ms	160 ms
CXR Cardiothoracic ratio	0.6	0.7
SAN dysfunction	Sinus bradycardia	Sinus bradycardia
NSVT	Y	Y
VT	N	Y
VF	N	N
SVT	Atrial Flutter (ablated)	N

*N-No Y-Yes mRV- morphological right ventricle mLV- morphological left ventricle TR-tricuspid regurgitation MR-mitral regurgitation BBB-Bundle branch block AVB-atrioventricular block SAN-sino-atrial node NSVT-non sustained VT VT-ventricular tachycardia VF-ventricular fibrillation SVT-supraventricular

Table 2. Baseline clinical characteristics of 2 patients with Mustard corrections and prexisting pacemakers receiving an upgrade to CRT.

following Mustard surgery) and therefore received a dual chamber pacemaker (Medtronic THERA DR 7968i. Medtronic. Inc., MA). Transthoracic echocardiogram revealed a dilated and myopathic sRV with an EF of 25% and a dp/dt ratio = 438.3 with evidence of asychronous ventricular contraction. The systemic ventricle (sRV) myocardial performance index was 0.53. An exercise treadmill test showed a suboptimal response with a cardiac output of 3.9 l/min pre-exercise to 9.0 l/min at maximal exercise. He had an underlying right bundle branch block QRS morphology. Recent evidence from other series also suggest an increase risk of VT/VF and SCD in patients following Mustard procedures presenting with sRV dysfunction and atrial tachyarrhythmias (1). Cardiac resynchronization and defibrillator therapy offered a plausible alternative to delaying cardiac transplantation. The implant was performed via a mini-thoracotomy through the lower part of the previous sternal incision. The chronic atrial and pLV leads were conserved and a steroid eluting pace/sense electrode was sutured to the inferior epicardial surface of the right ventricle (Medtronic 4968). Two single-finger subcutaneous defibrillator arrays (Medtronic 6996) were implanted in an antero-posterior configuration and connected to the defibrillator ports of a Contak RENEWAL 4HE defibrillator (Guidant Inc.). Attempts at biventricular pacing (BVP) were also of limited benefit. A TTE guided optimization of CRT resulted in the sRV being paced 40ms before the pLV. The paced QRS remained predominantly right bundle branch block in morphology but had increased to 200ms from a baseline width of 120ms. Apart from not experiencing a subjective improvement in symptoms, the patient presented with episodes of recurrent paroxysmal atrial flutter documented on holter analysis.

A successful flutter ablation was performed using non-contact mapping (Ensite™. St. Jude Medical). Two lines of block were created extending from the inferior vena cava to the inferior limb of the baffle and also from the tricuspid valve to the pulmonary venous side of the baffle. Despite further adjustment to the paced atrioventricular delay (AVD) and ventricular off-set, there was no improvement in symptoms. At his most recent follow-up doppler parameters suggested atrial pacing provided the optimal configuration (AAIR).

His effort tolerance was quantified objectively on the treadmill using the Bruce protocol and he exercised for 6.58 minutes.

3.1.2 Case 2

The second patient (24 years) weighed 106kg, was born with simple d-TGA and a large patent ductus arteriosus which had spontaneously closed by the time of atrial baffle construction at 6 months of age. Thereafter periodic surveillance with TTE revealed a mild stenosis of the inferior limb of the atrial baffle. Onset of dyspnoea and effort related chest pain with diaphoresis occurred at 17 years and was assumed to be due to sRV dysfunction and demand ischaemia after demonstration of unobstructed coronary arteries. Like the previous patient, profound sinus bradycardia was documented on holter monitoring which resulted in pacemaker implantation at the age of 22. Two years later, his effort tolerance deteriorated from NYHA grade II to III/IV with an episode of VT and accompanying syncope. The decision was made to upgrade to a CRT/D. Preceding angiography demonstrated a stenosis in the inferior limb of the atrial baffle for which balloon angioplasty was successfully performed.

The upgrade was performed by surgical thoracotomy, conserving the chronic atrial and ventricular pacing leads (Medtronic 5076). An epicardial steroid eluting electrode (Medtronic 4968) was attached to the inferior epicardial surface of the sRV. The pacing threshold of the sRV epicardial lead at implantation was 5.5v @ 0.5ms, with an R wave measuring 4.6mV and an impedance of 1100 ohms. The epicardial system showed a great variability in pacing parameters over a 9 month follow-up period post procedure **(table3)**.

Once again, the atrioventricular delay (AVD) and ventricular pacing off-set was guided by echocardiography and the sRV was paced 40ms ahead of the pLV in the final programming. The patient symptomatically improved to NYHA grade II status.

	sRV epicardial lead		pLV endocardial lead		RA endocardial lead	
	Threshold	Resistance (ohms)	Threshold	Resistance (ohms)	Threshold	Resistance (ohms)
Implant	0.5ms@5.5v	1100	0.2ms@1.5v	448	0.3ms@1.5v	480
1 month*	0.5ms@6.0v	576	0.2ms@1.0v	432	0.4ms@1.0v	496
6 month	0.3ms@5.0v	624	0.4ms@1.2v	464	0.4ms@1.0v	624
9 month	0.3ms@5.0v	648	0.2ms@1.5v	448	0.3ms@1.5v	480

* follow-up

Table 3. Comparison of pacing parameters of epicardial and endocardial leads at sequential follow-up in patient 2 implanted post Mustard surgery with a hybrid CRT system.

Cardiac resynchronization therapy has dramatically improved the quality of life in patients presenting with grade III and IV NYHA symptoms of heart failure (23). We have demonstrated here its application in two patients with sRV dysfunction using surgically positioned epicardial leads.

It may be argued that preceding angioplasty of significant baffle related stenoses in both patients may have contributed to functional improvement. The baffle angioplasties were performed in both patients as a separate procedure at least 48 hours before device implantation. This was done primarily to reduce the duration of the device implantation procedure but neither patient demonstrated appreciable clinical or echocardiographic benefit from relief of the stenoses on myocardial function in the period leading up to the actual implant.

The RV in a normal heart is a thinner walled and crescent shaped structure, that is not a suitable long term substitute for the left ventricle. The concave intrusion of the septum into the cavity of the RV also provides the optimal geometry for overall RV function (24). If left to chronically support the systemic circulation, the RV hypertrophies and dilates with subsequent flattening of the interventricular septum. The resultant dyskinetic septal motion further worsens the functional impairment of the dysfunctional RV. Resynchronization therapy should therefore serve not only to pace the RV free wall but co-ordinate this with septal motion. This complex anatomical and functional interaction suggests that we need to take greater care in positioning pacing leads over the sRV, to ensure adequate septal and free wall recruitment during biventricular pacing.

From this discussion we can infer why CRT failed in the first patient. The epicardial lead was placed on the sRV at the discretion of the surgeon over its inferior border with no formal guidance. It was only limited by the pacing threshold at the respective site. This arbitrary placement may have been responsible for the non-response. Perhaps a more guided approach such as that suggested by Dekker et al using intra-procedural pressure-volume loop monitoring may have altered the outcome (25).

Epicardial pacing systems have been more frequently associated, than transvenous systems, with higher pacing thresholds, diaphragmatic stimulation, lead fracture and insulation breaks (26).The use of steroid eluting leads, does alleviate some of the deterioration in pacing parameters but this unfortunately did not offer an advantage in the second patient (27). Due to previous surgery, the location of viable myocardium for pacing is difficult and placement of electrodes on the inferior aspect of both the sRVs was because of limited access to the sRV free wall.

Transvenous attempts at coronary sinus cannulation may also result in failure to deliver a appropriately positioned lead. Mair et al in a comparative study, also demonstrated a higher complication rate with transvenous CS lead placement than with epicardial implantation via a mini-thoracotomy procedure (26). A video-assisted thoroscopy creating a minimally invasive percutaneous approach may be a solution but the option requires expertise and is dependent on centre availability (28). This prompted us to consider endocardial delivery of the pace/sense lead to the sRV in the next case study.

The feasibility and safety of endocardial pacing of the systemic ventricle using a transseptal route to the left ventricle in normally "transposed" hearts was shown by Jais et al in a small series of 11 patients (29). In patients post Mustard correction, this would mean perforation through the atrial baffle or passage through a baffle leak to implant the lead onto the endocardial surface of the sRV followed by life long anticoagulation because of the potential for paradoxical and systemic embolization. Disruption to the atrial structures and interference with the atrioventricular valve may become issues in the long term follow-up of these patients but this remains an option with the benefit of more stable endocardial pacing thresholds.

3.1.3 Case 3

A 27 year old female with a Mustard procedure for d-TGA, and subsequent DDDR pacemaker implantation for sinus node dysfunction at age 17years, presented with progressive effort intolerance. Transthoracic echocardiogram and angiography revealed a dilated sRV with systolic dysfunction (EF=23%) and predominant lateral free wall hypokinesia.

Holter monitoring revealed episodes of non-sustained ventricular tachycardia. The 12-lead electrocardiogram (ECG) revealed atrial and ventricular sequential pacing with fused sinus/paced QRS complexes measuring 130ms. She achieved just 4.8 minutes on treadmill testing (Bruce protocol) compared to just 8.4 minutes documented 10 years earlier.

Preceding diagnostic cardiac catheterization revealed severe stenosis of the inferior baffle and a minor leak in the superior baffle communicating with the pulmonary venous atrium. Stent angioplasty of the inferior baffle was performed to relieve the obstruction (**figure 4**).

A multi-electrode (MEA) catheter (Ensite 3000. St. Jude Medical. USA) was then inserted retrogradely across the aortic valve into the sRV and isopotential (voltage) maps were created of the sRV during AAI, DDD pacing (RA+pLV then RA+sRV). Biventricular pacing (BVP) was simulated by pacing from a roving ablation catheter (7F Stinger. Bard. Minneapolis.USA) within the sRV and by triggering sRV pacing after the sensed pLV impulse (**figure 5**). Because of this there was an inherent delay of 20ms after pLV chamber pacing. Atrial pacing (AAI) achieved diffuse and rapid activation of the sRV however Wenckebach's phenomenon of the atrioventricular node was noted at just 70 beats per minute making constant ventricular pacing necessary. Voltage mapping during pLV apical pacing showed inhomogenous activation of the sRV in that the peak voltage activation waveform failed to involve considerable areas of the sRV free wall. Direct pacing of the endocardial surface of the sRV resulted in diffuse and rapid activation This was achieved from multiple sites on the sRV free-wall endocardium extending from the apex to the base.

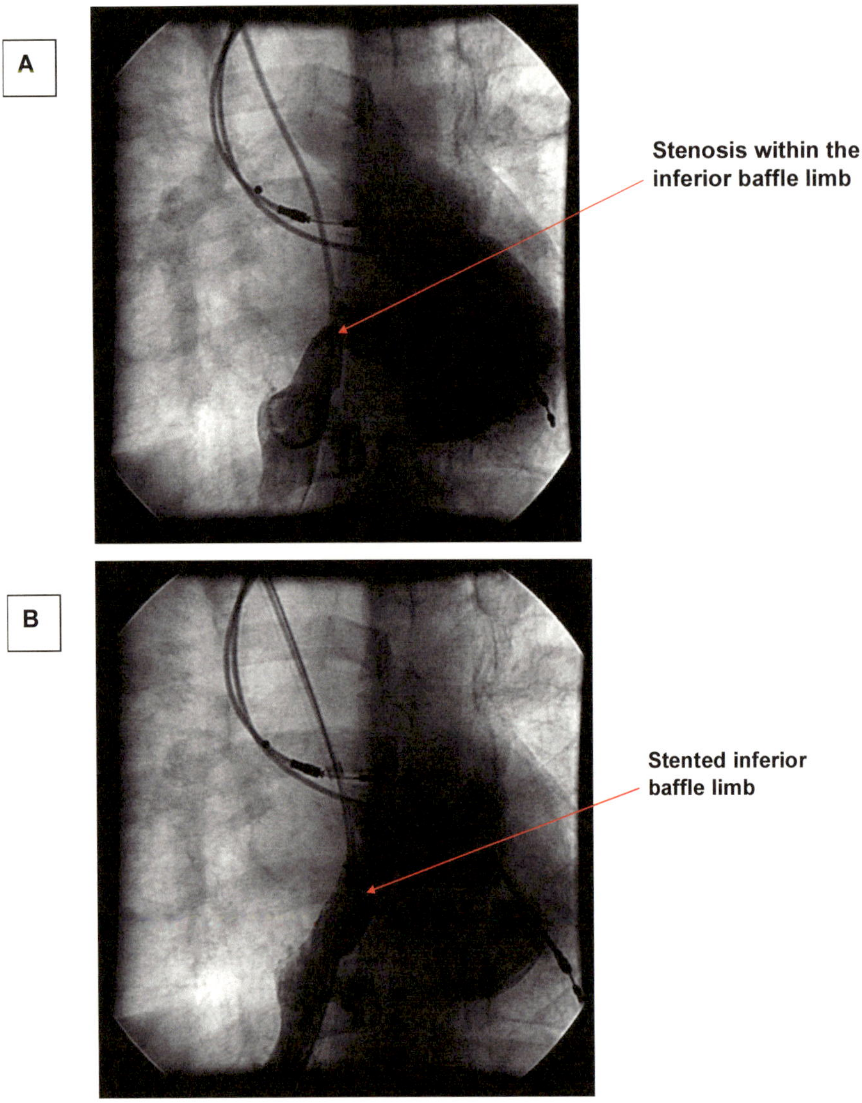

Fig. 4. A. Shows the RA and pLV leads of the existing DDD pacemaker. Contrast injection into the IVC demonstrates a stenosis within the inferior baffle limb but was adequate to allow passage of the pigtail catheter. B. Shows the satisfactory post stent result.

Baffle angioplasty and was initially performed thereafter a 4F lumenless pace/sense active fixation lead (model 6996, SelectSecure™. Medtronic Inc.) was deployed using a steerable delivery sheath via a standard left subclavian vein approach with anticoagulation (heparin 1000units/kg maintaining an activated clotting time of ± 300seconds). The superior limb of the systemic baffle was crossed through the baffle leak and positioned in the antero-basal segment of the sRV (**figure 6**).

Instantaneous intra-arterial blood pressure response was assessed during AAI, DDD (RA+pLV and RA+sRV) and simulated biventricular pacing (BVP) (pLV+ sRV)(2). An arbitrary paced AVD of 110 ms was selected for DDD configurations (**table 5**).

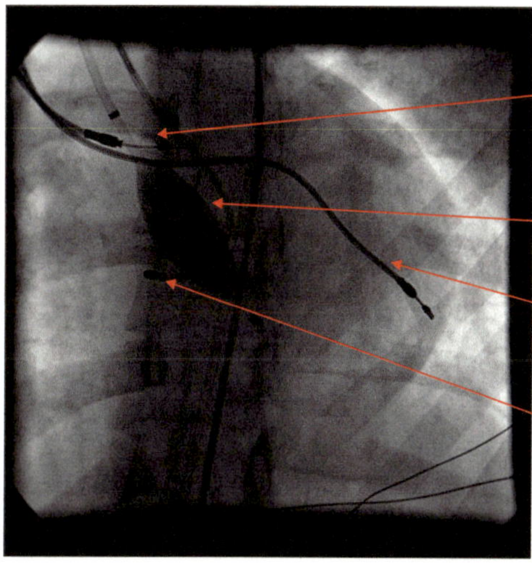

Fig. 5. The MEA catheter is deployed in the sRV. Isopotential maps of the sRV are created from pacing off the RA & pLV leads and from a roving ablation catheter within the sRV.

Despite the shortest activation time of 90ms occurring with AAI pacing, the maximal acute, blood pressure response of 73mmHg(average 60±9 mmHg) occurred during BVP (Table 5). An early (1week TTE) and sustained (after 6 months) 43% improvement in EF was also noted (23% to 33%). Effort tolerance improved from NYHA III to II accompanied by a decrease in QRS width from 130 to 120ms during consistent synchronous BVP in DDDR mode. No antitachycardia therapies have thus far been documented.

Blood pressure response during pacing		
	Blood pressure (mmHg)	Mean Blood pressure
AAI	75/43	53
DDD (RA/pLV)*	76/41	55
DDD (RA/sRV)*	78/48	58
BVP (sRV+pLV)	100/58	73
		60±9 mmHg
**AVD=110 ms.*		

Table 5. Tabulation of the maximal, acute, intra-procedural arterial blood pressure response obtained with each pacing modality. The AVD was arbitrarily set at 110ms.

We have presented here a novel strategy using ventricular activation maps to direct endocardial lead placement in an effort to achieve successful BVP in patients with a Mustard procedure and a failing sRV. The application of CRT has been extrapolated to the adult congenital heart disease population following success in treating patients with cardiomyopathies. Although no randomised controlled data exists for these patients, there has been documentation in the form of small case series (30). What is apparent is that conventional selection criteria may not apply and that there is variation in technical approaches sometimes requiring a combined endocardial and epicardial system.

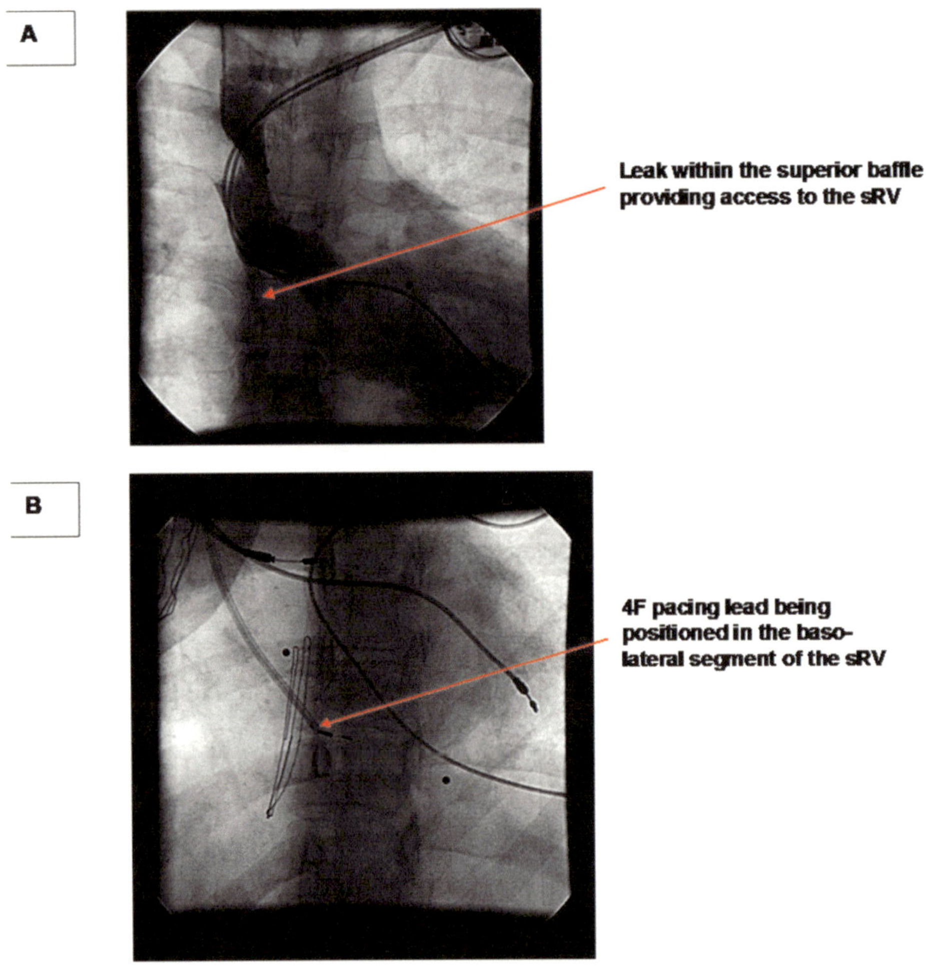

Fig. 6. A. Illustrates a small baffle leak in the superior limb allowing access for a sheath to deliver the 4F pacing lead into the sRV pictures in B.

3.2 Conclusion

The advent of atrial redirection surgery heralded potential survival to adulthood for patients with d-TGA who would have otherwise faced inevitable childhood death. However, the late complications arising from this surgery, particularly progressive heart failure and the increase risk of SCD remain challenges for management. The indications and best methods to effect successful CRT/D therapy however remain unknown apart from combined anecdotal evidence. In this patient cohort, we have demonstrated that the pLV to active defibrillator Can was the most successful as was the use of epicardial patches. An exclusively transthoracic system utilizing subcutaneous electrodes proved unreliable because of the influence of weight in adult patients. A combination of intracardiac, intrathoracic and subcutaneous electrodes is however sometimes necessary to enhance defibrillation efficacy.

The initial experience with CRT using a combined endocardial and epicardial lead system proved inconsistent and may have been because of poor patient selection but also because of suboptimal epicardial lead placement. The use of non contact mapping in addition to echocardiographic criteria was used to define asynchrony and guide endocardial placement of a pacing lead within the sRV. This warranted anticoagulation, but was performed with relative ease.

4. References

[1] Helbing WA, Hansen B, Ottenkamp J et al. Long-term results of atrial correction for transposition of the great arteries. Comparison of Mustard and Senning operations. J Thorac Cardiovasc Surg 1994;108:363-72.

[2] Poirier NC, Yu JH, Brizard CP, Mee RB. Long-term results of left ventricular reconditioning and anatomic correction for systemic right ventricular dysfunction after atrial switch procedures. J Thorac Cardiovasc Surg 2004;127:975-81.

[3] Konstantinov IE, Alexi-Meskishvili VV, Williams WG, Freedom RM, Van Praagh R. Atrial switch operation: past, present, and future. Ann Thorac Surg 2004;77:2250-8.

[4] Dos L, Teruel L, Ferreira IJ et al. Late outcome of Senning and Mustard procedures for correction of transposition of the great arteries. Heart 2005;91:652-6.

[5] Kammeraad JA, van Deurzen CH, Sreeram N et al. Predictors of sudden cardiac death after Mustard or Senning repair for transposition of the great arteries. J Am Coll Cardiol 2004;44:1095-102.

[6] Warnes CA. Transposition of the great arteries. Circulation 2006;114:2699-709.

[7] Feder E, Meisner H, Buhlmeyer K, Struck E, Sebening F. Operative treatment of TGA: comparison of Senning's and Mustard's operation in patients under 2 years. Thorac Cardiovasc Surg 1980;28:7-12.

[8] Uemura H, Ho SY, Anderson RH et al. Surgical anatomy of the coronary circulation in hearts with discordant atrioventricular connections. Eur J Cardiothorac Surg 1996;10:194-200.

[9] Bashir JG, Frank G, Tyers O, Lampa M, Yamaoka R. Combined use of transesophageal ECHO and fluoroscopy for the placement of left ventricular pacing leads via the coronary sinus. Pacing Clin Electrophysiol 2003;26:1951-4.

[10] Shalaby AA. Utilization of intracardiac echocardiography to access the coronary sinus for left ventricular lead placement. Pacing Clin Electrophysiol 2005;28:493-7.

[11] Roberts PR, Paisey JR, Betts TR et al. Comparison of coronary venous defibrillation with conventional transvenous internal defibrillation in man. J Interv Card Electrophysiol 2003;8:65-70.

[12] Dubin AM, Janousek J, Rhee E et al. Resynchronization therapy in pediatric and congenital heart disease patients: an international multicenter study. J Am Coll Cardiol 2005;%20;46:2277-83.

[13] Diller GP, Okonko D, Uebing A, Ho SY, Gatzoulis MA. Cardiac resynchronization therapy for adult congenital heart disease patients with a systemic right ventricle: analysis of feasibility and review of early experience. Europace 2006;8:267-72.

[14] Mital S, Addonizio LJ, Lamour JM, Hsu DT. Outcome of children with end-stage congenital heart disease waiting for cardiac transplantation. J Heart Lung Transplant 2003;22:147-53.
[15] Bristow MR, Feldman AM, Saxon LA. Heart failure management using implantable devices for ventricular resynchronization: Comparison of Medical Therapy, Pacing, and Defibrillation in Chronic Heart Failure (COMPANION) trial. COMPANION Steering Committee and COMPANION Clinical Investigators. J Card Fail 2000;6:276-85.
[16] Ermis C, Zhu AX, Vanheel L et al. Comparison of ventricular arrhythmia frequency in patients with ischemic cardiomyopathy versus nonischemic cardiomyopathy treated with implantable cardioverter defibrillators. Am J Cardiol 2005;96:233-8.
[17] Stajduhar KC, Ott GY, Kron J et al. Optimal electrode position for transvenous defibrillation: a prospective randomized study. J Am Coll Cardiol 1996;27:90-4.
[18] Gold MR, Khalighi K, Kavesh NG, Daly B, Peters RW, Shorofsky SR. Clinical predictors of transvenous biphasic defibrillation thresholds. Am J Cardiol 1997;79:1623-7.
[19] Schauerte P, Stellbrink C, Schondube FA et al. Polarity reversal improves defibrillation efficacy in patients undergoing transvenous cardioverter defibrillator implantation with biphasic shocks. Pacing Clin Electrophysiol 1997;20:301-6.
[20] Alva C, Horowitz E, Ho SY, Rigby ML, Anderson RH. The feasibility of complete anatomical correction in the setting of discordant atrioventricular connections. Heart 1999;81:539-45.
[21] Roos-Hesselink JW, Meijboom FJ, Spitaels SE et al. Decline in ventricular function and clinical condition after Mustard repair for transposition of the great arteries (a prospective study of 22-29 years). Eur Heart J 2004;25:1264-70.
[22] Politi P, Piccinelli M, Poli PF et al. Ten years of "extended" life: quality of life among heart transplantation survivors. Transplantation 2004;78:257-63.
[23] Bristow MR, Saxon LA, Boehmer J et al. Cardiac-resynchronization therapy with or without an implantable defibrillator in advanced chronic heart failure. N Engl J Med 2004;350:2140-50.
[24] Guarracino F, Cariello C, Danella A et al. Right ventricular failure: physiology and assessment. Minerva Anestesiol 2005;71:307-12.
[25] Dekker AL, Phelps B, Dijkman B et al. Epicardial left ventricular lead placement for cardiac resynchronization therapy: optimal pace site selection with pressure-volume loops. J Thorac Cardiovasc Surg 2004;127:1641-7.
[26] Mair H, Sachweh J, Meuris B et al. Surgical epicardial left ventricular lead versus coronary sinus lead placement in biventricular pacing. Eur J Cardiothorac Surg 2005;27:235-42.
[27] Horenstein MS, Walters H, III, Karpawich PP. Chronic performance of steroid-eluting epicardial leads in a growing pediatric population: a 10-year comparison. Pacing Clin Electrophysiol 2003;26:1467-71.
[28] Furrer M, Fuhrer J, Altermatt HJ et al. VATS-guided epicardial pacemaker implantation. Hand-sutured fixation of atrioventricular leads in an experimental setting. Surg Endosc 1997;11:1167-70.
[29] Jais P, Douard H, Shah DC, Barold S, Barat JL, Clementy J. Endocardial biventricular pacing. Pacing Clin Electrophysiol 1998;21:2128-31.
[30] Janousek J, Tomek V, Chaloupecky VA et al. Cardiac resynchronization therapy: a novel adjunct to the treatment and prevention of systemic right ventricular failure. J Am Coll Cardiol 2004;44:1927-31.

10

Role of Automated External Defibrillators (AED) in Sports

Saqib Ghani and Sanjay Sharma
St. George's University of London,
United Kingdom

1. Introduction

Sudden cardiac death (SCD) in young athletes is a tragic event with devastating effects on the family, athletic team, and the local community. Unfortunately sudden cardiac arrest (SCA) due to ventricular fibrillation (VF) is often the first manifestation of underlying cardiovascular disorders and is associated with high mortality. Sudden death in sport is rare and is usually due to congenital or hereditary structural and electrical cardiovascular disorders in young athletes (< 35 years), and atherosclerotic coronary artery disease (CAD) in older athletes. There is debate over the most appropriate screening strategy to identify athletes at risk of SCD. Since some cardiac disorders cannot be identified without elaborate and cost-prohibitive pre-participation cardiovascular screening (PPS) programmes, additional strategies such as an effective programming using automated external defibrillators (AED) may be crucial in minimising cardiovascular deaths in athletes. Furthermore PPS would not prevent acquired cases of cardiovascular fatality in sports such as myocarditis, commotio cordis, and heatstroke or electrolyte disturbances. This chapter provides an overview of the magnitude of the problem, causes of SCD in athletes, the efficacy of automated external defibrillator (AED) in managing SCA, and the importance of emergency response planning to ensure effective management of SCA in athletes.

2. Sudden cardiac death & Sudden Arrhythmic Death Syndrome (SADS)

Sudden cardiac death (SCD) is defined as an unexpected, non-traumatic, non-violent event resulting from sudden cardiac arrest (SCA) within six hours of previously witnessed normal health. A sudden cardiac death where no cause of death is found despite detailed examination of the heart by an expert cardiac pathologist is referred to as Sudden Arrhythmic Death Syndrome (SADS).

2.1 Causes of sudden cardiac death in athletes

Cardiovascular disorders remain the most common cause of death in western world. The commonest cause of sudden cardiac death in individuals aged over 35 years is coronary artery disease. In young athletes aged less than 35 years, hypertrophic cardiomyopathy (HCM) is the most common cause of SCD (Maron BJ, 2003). Other causes of SCD that affect heart structurally include arrhythmogenic right ventricular cardiomyopathy (ARVC), dilated cardiomypathy (DCM), coronary artery anomalies, aortic root rupture (can be

associated with Marfan's syndrome) and valvular heart disease (Figure 1). According to the Italian data, ARVC accounts for approximately 25% of all cases of SCD in athletes (Corrado et al., 2005). This discrepancy in the prevalence of ARVC between the US and Italy could be attributed to several factors, notably the existence of a legal and mandatory PPS programme in Italy that has proven effective in the early diagnosis of HCM with subsequent disqualification from sport. Most data on SCD in Italy is derived from the Veneto region which is internationally renowned for pathological expertise in the diagnosis of ARVC.
In approximately 4% of all cases of SCD in sport the heart may appear structurally normal. The most commonly implicated conditions in such circumstances include the hereditary ion channelopathies and congenital accessory pathways e.g. long QT syndrome (LQTS), Brugada syndrome, Wolff-Parkinson-White Syndrome (WPW), catecholaminergic polymorphic ventricular tachycardia (CPVT) and Lenegre's disease. Other acquired causes of SCD include electrolyte disturbances, drugs, myocarditis and Commotio Cordis (blunt trauma to chest leading to ventricular arrhythmia).

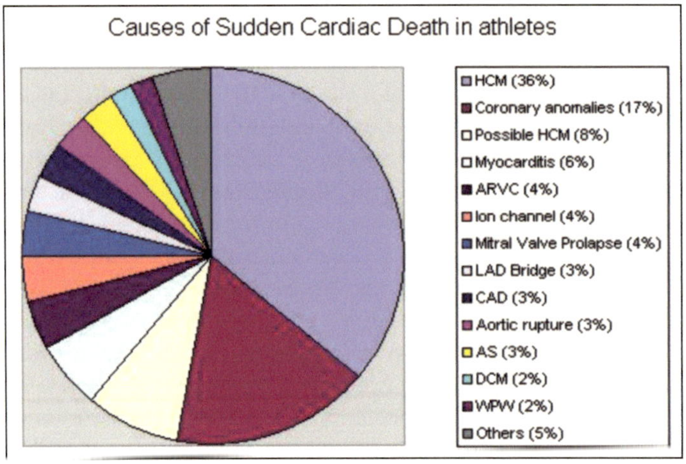

Fig. 1. Causes of sudden cardiac death in young athletes (adapted from Maron *et al.*, 2009). HCM, hypertrophic cardiomyopathy; ARVC, arrythmogenic right ventricular cardiomyopathy; LAD, left anterior descending artery; CAD, coronary artery disease; AS, aortic stenosis; DCM, dilated cardiomyopathy; WPW, Wolff-Parkinson-White syndrome.

2.2 Prevalence of SCD / SCA in athletes

The precise frequency of SCA in athletes remains disputed, but there is general agreement that vigorous exercise is a trigger for SCA in athletes with underlying cardiac disease (Drezner, 2009). The incidence of SCD in young competitive athletes (age 12-35 years) from Veneto region of Italy, was found to be 3.6/100,000 prior to implementation of national screening program (Corrado et al., 2006). In a comparative population study, the relative risk of SCD in young competitive athletes was found to be 2.8 times greater than age-matched non-athletes (Corrado et al., 2003). In general, athletes are perceived as healthier group of individuals compared to non-athletes; however the risk of SCD is higher in this group if they harbour a quiescent cardiovascular disorder. Fortunately these tragic events are rare. Sudden death occurs mostly during or soon after exercise, and has shown to affects males more commonly.
The incidence of SCA in high school student athletes was found to be 4.4/100,000 in a survey of US high schools with AED (Drezner et al., 2009), and was reported as 3.75/100,000

for children and young adults (age 14-24 years) in a prospective, population-based study in US and Canada (Atkins et al., 2009).

3. Role of pre-participation cardiovascular screening (PPS)

A majority of cardiac conditions implicated in SCD may not cause any symptoms prior to cardiac arrest; therefore the only way to detect these abnormalities is by testing or screening healthy individuals. This makes the role of pre-participation cardiovascular screening (PPS) important in young healthy individuals particularly those participating in sporting activities. Identification of high risk individuals based purely on health questionnaire focusing on cardiovascular symptoms has a low yield. The addition of 12-lead ECG as a screening tool to identify young apparently healthy individuals at risk of sudden death increases the diagnostic yield of such screening programmes but increases the false positive rates. There is also considerable resistance to implementation of widespread cardiovascular screening of athletes due to low incidence of SCD in athletes and low prevalence rates of implicated cardiac disorders thus challenging cost effectiveness of such programmes. There is also an overlap between physiological adaptation to exercise and cardiac disorders which may result in false positive results causing unnecessary anxiety and the need for further evaluation and the potential for unfair disqualification from competitive sports.

PPS is not mandatory in UK and most western countries. In USA and Italy, PPS programmes are in existence to minimise risk of SCD in athletes. The US screening protocol comprises of a health questionnaire about cardiac symptoms and family history, and physical examination. Italian screening model includes 12 lead ECG in addition to the health questionnaire and physical examination. A state-sponsored cardiac screening programme has been in place in Italy since 1970s. Recent experience from Veneto region of Italy has shown a significant reduction in SCD in athletes (Figure 2) from cardiomyopathies and heart rhythm disorders since the implementation of nationwide pre-participation screening programme (Corrado et al., 2006).

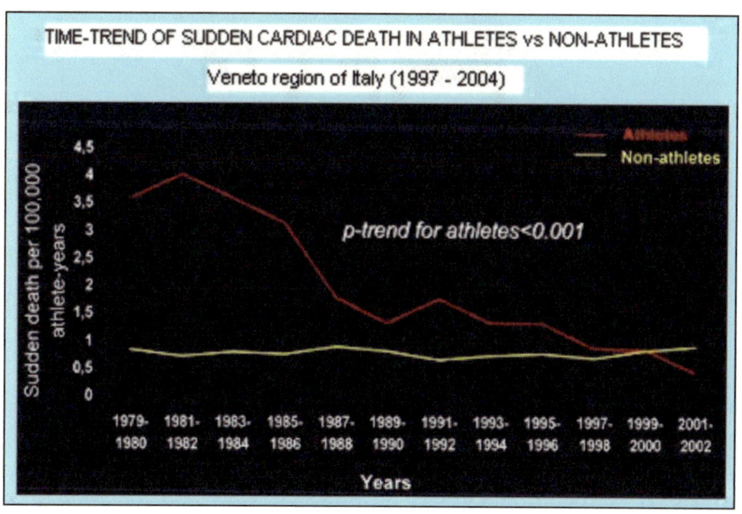

Fig. 2. Annual incidence rates of SCD in screened competitive athletes and unscreened non-athletes aged 12 to 35 years in Veneto region of Italy after introduction of nationwide PPS programme. *(Adapted from Corrado et al., 2006)*

4. The role of automated external defibrillators (AED)

The majority of out-of-hospital cardiac arrests occur by the initial mechanism of ventricular fibrillation (VF) and in some occasions ventricular tachycardia (VT) with loss of cardiac output (pulseless VT); therefore community based portable defibrillators, since becoming first available in late 1960s, have emerged as one approach to this problem. As discussed previously, pre-participation cardiovascular screening (PPS) using ECG may not identify certain cardiac disorders e.g. premature coronary artery disease, anomalous coronary arteries and valvular heart disease, and certain acquired conditions are also implicated in SCD in athletes e.g. myocarditis, commotio cordis and electrolyte imbalance. Therefore it is important to have alternative strategy for secondary prevention of SCD. Automated external defibrillators (AED) have thus become an important part of overall management of victims of cardiac arrest particularly in public places and in sports and fitness centres.

AEDs are sophisticated, reliable and computerised devices capable of delivering electric shocks to victims of cardiac arrest when ECG shows a shock-able rhythm (VF or pulseless VT). A key feature of AED is the simplicity of its operation; controls are kept to a minimum, and voice and visual prompts are used to guide rescuers. Modern AEDs are suitable to be used by both lay rescuers and healthcare professionals (Resuscitation Council UK, 2010).

AEDs can be semi-automatic or fully automatic (example shown in Figure 3). All AEDs can determine victim's ECG and determine the need for shock. A semi-automatic AED indicates the need for a shock which is then delivered by the operator. The automatic AED administers shock without the need for intervention by the operator. Some semi-automatic AEDs have the facility to enable the operator to override the device and deliver a shock manually (Perkins & Colquhoun, 2010).

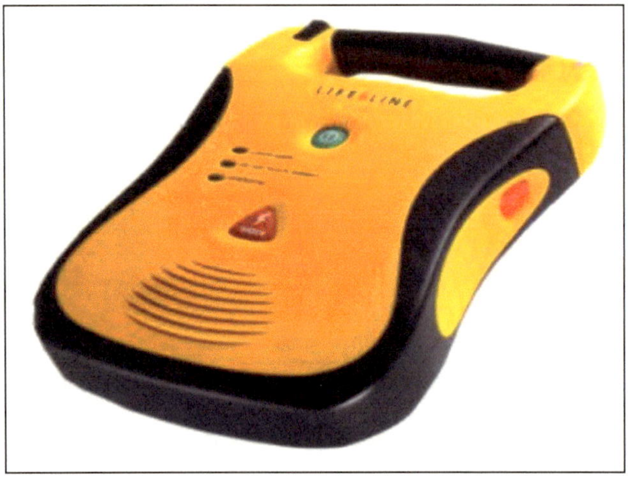

Fig. 3. Defibtech Lifeline Automated External Defibrillator.

4.1 Time chain of survival

The American Heart Association (AHA) emphasises the time-sensitive intervention for victims of SCA and has outlined four critical steps in a "Chain of Survival" to save lives in the event of cardiovascular emergency (Figure 4). The chain of survival includes a series of actions designed to reduce mortality associated with cardiac arrest. The important links in this sequence include (1) early recognition of cardiorespiratory arrest, (2) early CPR, (3) early defibrillation when indicated, and (4) early advanced cardiac life support.

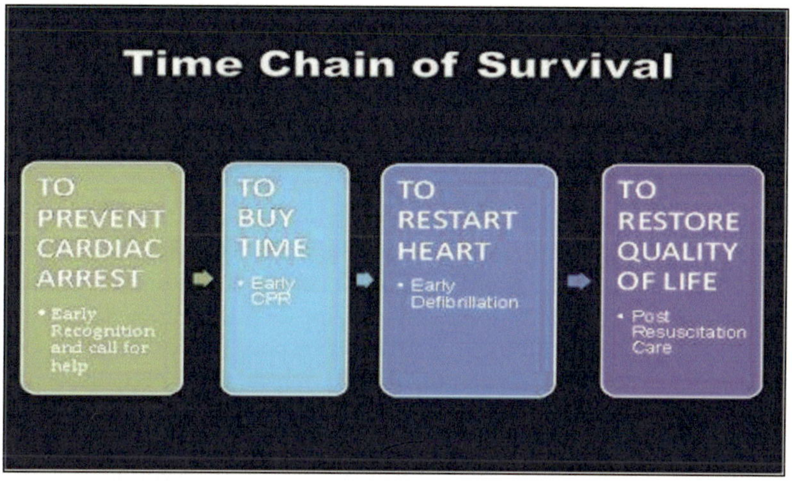

Fig. 4. Important links in the "chain of survival".

The single greatest factor affecting survival from SCA is the time interval from cardiac arrest to defibrillation (Balady et al., 2002; Drezner et al., 2007). Survival rates from out-of-hospital cardiac arrests have improved since the introduction of public access AED programs which have allowed lay rescuers to deliver early defibrillation (Hallstrom et al., 2004).

The ability to recognise cardiac arrest plays a key role in initiation of a successful chain of survival. This can be achieved by basic life support (BLS) training and general awareness amongst general population. A delay in recognition of cardiac arrest in a collapsed athlete or individual can lead to loss of crucial moments that may then translate into a poor outcome. Brief seizure like activity or involuntary myoclonic jerks have been reported in approximately 50% of young athletes with SCA, and thus SCA can be mistaken for a seizure (Drezner et al., 2006). Another challenge includes inaccurate assessment of pulse and respiration. Occasional or agonal gasping can occur in first minutes after SCA and is often misinterpreted. In athletes with SCA, on-going respiration and pulse was reported in approximately 50% cases (Drezner et al., 2006). Therefore careful and prompt assessment and recognition of SCA plays a crucial part in management of cardiac arrest in any situation but particularly in athletes. Early and effective CPR is the best treatment for cardiac arrest until the arrival of AED or advanced life support. It can prevent ventricular fibrillation from deteriorating to asystole, may increase the chance of successful defibrillation, contributes to preservation of heart and brain function, and significantly improves survival (AHA and International Liaison Committee on Resuscitation, 2000 as cited in Balady et al., 2002).

Public access AEDs play an important role in chain of survival by reducing the time delay from cardiac arrest to delivery of shock. A survival rate of up to 90% has been reported in victims of VF cardiac arrest when defibrillation is achieved within first minute (Franklin et al., 1998 as cited in Balady et al., 2002). Survival rates decline 7-10% with every minute delay in defibrillation; beyond 12 minutes the survival may be as low as 2-5% (AHA, 2000 as cited in Balady et al., 2002). The importance of early defibrillation in "chain of survival" by using AED is further emphasised by evidence of high survival rates with use of public access

AEDs in casinos (Valenzuale et al., 2000) and airplanes (Page et al., 2000) in USA, and in public places nationwide in Japan (Kitamura et al., 2010).

4.2 Efficacy of AED in preventing SCD in athletes

As mentioned previously sudden death of a young athlete is a tragic event and attracts media coverage. Pre-participations screening has shown to reduce incidence of SCD in athletes, but it is not widely mandated and certain cardiac conditions cannot be identified on routine ECG. Hence the need for alternative secondary prevention measures; AED plays an important role in preventing SCD in athletes.

Resuscitation in nine intercollegiate athletes with SCA reported a survival rate of only 11% despite witnessed collapse and timely cardio-pulmonary resuscitation (CPR). This study showed a relatively low survival rate despite use of AED. Mean time to defibrillation was 3.1 minutes (range 1 to 7.5 minutes). All arrests happened during or just after exercise. A detailed scrutiny in this series revealed a delay in response times in 44% of cases, and 5 victims had hypertrophic cardiomyopathy (HCM) which may have influenced the low survival rate (Drezner & Rogers, 2006).

Recent evidence from a cohort of 1710 US high schools with an on-site AED program showed an improved survival rate when early defibrillation in young athletes with SCA (Drezner et al., 2009). Letters were sent out to 18,974 schools; of these 2084 replied (11%); 1710 schools had at least 1 AED on site. A survey relating to SCA was conducted in these 1710 schools between January 2006 and July 2007. A total of 36 cases of SCA were reported. Of these 14 victims were high school student athletes with a mean age of 16 years; 22 were older non-students with mean age of 57 years. 35 (97%) cases were witnessed, 34 (94%) received bystander CPR, and 30 (83%) received an AED shock. Mean time from collapse-to-CPR was 1.5 minutes; mean time from SCA-to-shock was 3.6 minutes. Overall 64% survival to hospital discharge was achieved, which made this study the first to suggest an apparent survival benefit from early defibrillation in young athletes with SCA.

In this study a significant proportion of victims of SCA were non-students and represented an older age range. This group comprised of school staff and spectators. This highlights the importance of AED in managing SCA in general population in addition to athletes. As one would expect a large number of spectators at any major sporting event, the availability of public access AED can also improve survival from SCA in such non-athletic population. Hence AEDs should be made readily available at all sporting clubs and facilities. Likewise, AEDs should be present in public places where lay rescuers could use this device to deliver shock in cases of SCA. This is further elaborated in the following section.

Sudden cardiac death may occur as a result of being struck with a blunt projectile object over the anterior left hemi-thorax. This phenomenon is referred to as Commotio Cordis (Latin word meaning 'agitated heart'). Such blunt trauma can trigger VF or VT and lead to subsequent cardiac arrest. Unfortunately the general survival rate in commotio cordis is approximately 16%, and with early CPR rates of 25% have been seen. In animal models AED had 98% sensitivity for detecting VF and produced 100% termination of arrhythmia in swine struck with baseball. Based on swine model of commotio cordis, the practice of making AED available on-site may have an advantageous effect on outcome.

4.3 Use of AED in public places by healthcare professionals and lay rescuers

Historically the survival rates from out-of-hospital cardiac arrests using standard emergency medical services have been less than 5% in the USA. A majority of out-of-hospital cardiac arrests occur by the initial mechanism of ventricular fibrillation (VF) therefore it would seem reasonable that early public access to defibrillation would result in better survival rates. Since becoming first available in 1960s, AEDs have emerged as one approach towards the issue of out-of-hospital cardiac arrests.

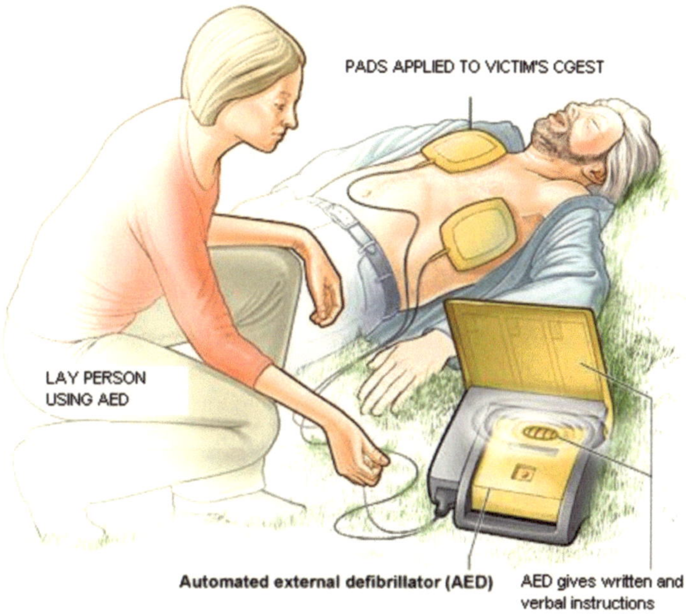

Fig. 5. Demonstration of AED use by lay rescuer.

A high discharge survival rate after out-of-hospital VF with rapid defibrillation by police and paramedics was reported in retrospective observational study in 1990s (White et al., 1996). It was noted that when shock resulted in return of spontaneous circulation (ROSC) without the need for advanced life support (ALS), 96% victims survived. Overall survival rate was 49% (41 out of 84 victims survived); 58% survival rate in police group with mean call-to-shock time of 5.6 minutes and 43% survival rate in paramedic group with mean call-to-shock time of 6.3 minutes. The results of this study showed that early defibrillation not only increases survival from out-of-hospital VF cardiac arrests but increases the likelihood that initial shocks will result in ROSC with the need for costly time-consuming ALS care.

Successful use of public access AEDs by lay rescuers with impressive survival rates has been reported in public places like planes, airports and casinos. These studies not only show that public use of AED is safe but also emphasises the need to encourage use of AED by lay rescuers. The survival rates were similar when AED was used by trained health professionals or by lay people. The single most important factor defining high survival rate was time interval between cardiac arrest to delivery of first shock.

In 1997 a major US airline started equipping its planes with AEDs. From 1997 to 1999, AED was used on 200 occasions; ECGs from all these events were analysed for appropriateness of use; the results suggested that use of AED aboard commercial aircrafts is effective with good survival rate of 40% (Page et al., 2000). During this study AED was also used as a cardiac monitor in conscious patients; no complications or inappropriate shocks were observed in these cases. A 2 year prospective study at 3 Chicago airports showed 56% one year survival rate with effective use of AED by random bystanders (Caffrey et al., 2002). AED use by casino security guards also demonstrated good survival to discharge from hospital rates of 53% (Valenzuela et al., 2000). In cases of witnessed arrest, mean collapse to shock time was 4.4 minutes. A high survival rate of up to 74% was observed when AED shock was delivered in less than 3 minutes from collapse; 49% survival rate when collapse to shock time was more than 3 minutes.

In a recent study involving over 12,000 victims of out-of-hospital VF cardiac arrest in Japan, nationwide dissemination of AED has shown to increase 1-month survival rates with minimal neurological impairment with early defibrillation by lay rescuers using public access AED (Kitamura et al., 2010). In cases where public access AED was used, 31.6% patients were alive at 1 month with minimal neurological impairment. Mean time to shock decreased with AED being more readily available.

4.4 Emergency Response Planning (ERP)

Emergency response planning (ERP) is required to ensure an efficient and structured response to SCA. It is recommended that every school, club and organisation sponsoring sporting activities should have an emergency response plan for SCA with written policies and procedures (Anderson et al., 2002). The core elements of an emergency response plan (ERP) for SCA include development of a written ERP for SCA, establishment of an efficient communication system, identification and training of likely responders in CPR and AED use, access to early defibrillation by on-site AED, registering AED with local emergency medical services, and annual review of the response plan (Drezner, 2007, 2009). The key elements of ERP are tabulated below.

Key elements of emergency response planning (ERP)
• Develop a written emergency response plan
• Establish an effective and efficient communication system
• Identify and train likely first responders in CPR and AED use
• Access to early defibrillation through on-site AED
• Practice and review EPR at least annually

Table 1. Key elements of Emergency Response Planning (ERP).

The first responder to a medical emergency may widely vary, and may include a coach, official, student, teammate, teacher, school nurse, lay bystander, or a health professional like team physiotherapist, sports medicine professional, trained ALS provider, paramedic or a doctor. All such potential rescuers should be familiar with ERP and should ideally be trained. Coaches and physiotherapists are more likely to be present near the sporting and training activities, therefore they receive training in CRR and use of AED. In high schools, coaches were found to be first responders to SCA in 34% of cases (Drezner et al., 2009). The personnel should particularly be trained to detect and identify SCA in a collapsed athlete. Seizure like activity and occasional agonal respirations have been reported in up to 50% athletes with SCA, therefore a high suspicion of SCA should be maintained in any collapsed individual or athlete (Drezner et al., 2006).

An efficient and easily accessible communication system is important to prevent critical delays in the chain of survival. All parts of school or athletic facility should be developed to enable effective communication for first responder so that an emergency medical service (EMS) can be activated, and on-site emergency response team alerted (Drezner, 2009). Public access AEDs should be located such that collapse-to-shock target of 3 to 5 minutes can be achieved (Drezner et al., 2007). A central location should be chosen with consideration given to most populated areas; multiple AEDs may be needed for large facilities. AED should be highly visible, easily accessible and preferably near a telephone to ensure efficient communication. The equipment should be maintained as per manufacturer recommendations. For large events like distance running, triathlons etc. the location of AED is important; use of bicycles or mobile rescue teams can be helpful (Drezner, 2009).

An ERP should be reviewed at least annually with all potential first responders. Any modifications to the response plan based on drills should be documented. Finally, the ERP should be coordinated with local emergency medical services (EMS), including awareness of types and locations of AED. The latter may be useful for receiving information from EMS about AEDs if an unfamiliar person happens to be the first responder to SCA.

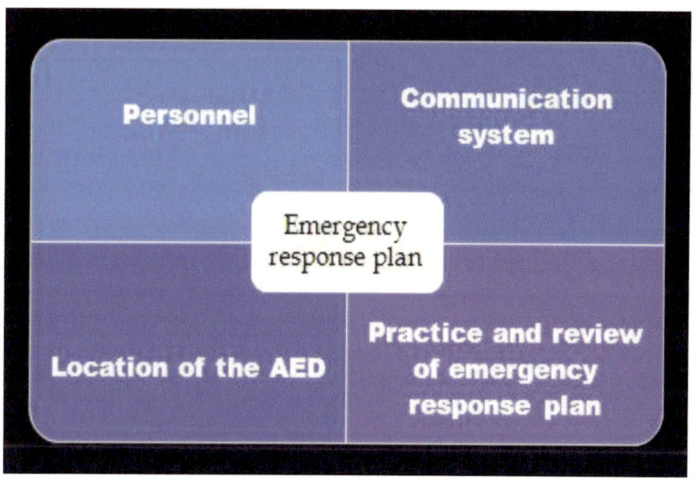

Fig. 6. Emergency Response Planning (ERP).

The European Society of Cardiology (ESC) and European Resuscitation Council (ERC) have been supporting various AED programmes as per ESC-ERC recommendations (Priori et al., 2004). A recent study (Arena study) investigated the cardiovascular safety procedures of major sports arenas in Europe with special attention to the availability of AEDs (Borjesson et al., 2010). A total of 190 football clubs in 10 European countries were included in the study. AED was present in 72% of the venues and 64% clubs reported the existence of a written emergency response plan; only 65% clubs had basic CPR training programme with advanced CPR training programme practiced in only 26% of the clubs. A vast majority (97%) of the clubs had some form of communication system in existence. Furthermore the mean distance from sporting arena to hospital was 4.2km with mean time for transportation of ≤5min achievable in 59% of clubs. Surprisingly, of the 79 clubs with >5min transportation time to hospital, 25% did not have AED on site. The study therefore highlighted the inadequacies in major European sporting clubs in relation to prevention of SCD; 28% of clubs did not have an AED, 36% did not have a written ERP, 41% clubs had transportation time of over 5min and 25% of these clubs did not have an AED.

Major sporting events attract thousands of spectators including adult and senior individuals with risk factors for cardiac events; these spectators are exposed to intense emotions, and such circumstances have been demonstrated to trigger cardiac events (Chi, 2004 and Wilbert-Lampen, 2008 as cited in Borjesson et al., 2010). During the Arena study, a total of 39.4 million spectators were estimated for 190 clubs. A total 77 sudden cardiac arrests were reported in one season, making estimated adjusted incidence of SCA to be 1 in 589,000 spectators. No cardiac arrests occurred in football players or officials. Therefore the availability of AED as a part of ERP in sporting arenas is crucial for minimising the risk of SCD in both players and members of general public. Efforts are therefore required to further promote AED programmes across Europe and enable sporting venues to implement efficient emergency response planning.

4.5 Recommendations regarding AED use and emergency response planning

There is need for comprehensive emergency planning to ensure an efficient response to SCS in schools, sports clubs and arenas, and public places in general. In US several national recommendations have emerged over time with regards to use of AED and developing an emergency response plan. In 2002 National Athletic Trainers' Association released a position statement recommending any organisation or institution sponsoring athletic activities to develop and implement a written emergency plan for SCA including acquisition of necessary equipment and training of involved personnel in CPR and AED use (Anderson et al., 2002, as cited in Drezner et al., 2009). The American Heart Association (AHA) issued consensus recommendations in 2004 for Medical Emergency Response Plan in schools, emphasising that an AED programme should be in place in every school that cannot reliably achieve call-to-shock time of less than 5 minutes using emergency medical services (Hazinski et al, 2004, as cited in Drezner et al., 2009). American College of Cardiology (ACC) 36th Bethesda Conference suggested that every school providing sports activities should have access to defibrillation within 5 minutes of collapse (Myenburg et al., 2005). In 2007, an inter-association task force strongly recommended access to AEDs with a target collapse-to-shock time of less than 3 to 5 minutes, in a consensus recommendation for emergency preparedness for SCA in high school and college athletic programs (Drezner et al., 2007).

In 2004 the European Society of Cardiology (ESC) and European Resuscitation Council (ERC) joined forces to develop European recommendations for legislation on defibrillation, for training in AED use and for the development of AED community programmes (Priory et al., 2004). Priorities and needs for the prevention of SCD were identified; it was recommended that AED programmes should stem from emergency medical services and hospitals and then progressively move to community programmes; common standards for defibrillation should be set for European countries; legislation regarding public use of AED to be introduced; training requirements for CPR and AED use should be defined for individuals participating in public access AED programmes; the need for systematic data collection and analysis to enable sharing information between various programmes to facilitate research and development; the ESC and ERC should support AED programmes by promoting education in the community. The panel advocated support from ESC and ERC to involve Ministers of Health and the European Parliament in the promotion of a "European Cardiac Arrest Survival Directive".

5. Conclusion

Sudden cardiac death is often the first presentation in an athlete harbouring a potentially sinister cardiac disorder. Prompt identification and disqualification by trained coach or physician can reduce fatality rate significantly. In the current financial climate where resources for pre-participation screening are limited in most countries, consideration should be given to implementation of an on-site AED programme with an adequate emergency response plan. Automated external defibrillators improve survival from sudden cardiac arrest in young athletes and also when used by ley persons and healthcare professionals in public places. The availability of AEDs during competitive sporting events also provides the potential for life-saving support to spectators and other bystanders.

6. References

Anderson J, Courson RW, Kleiner DM, et al. (2002). National Athletic Trainers' Association Position Statement: Emergency Planning in Athletes. *Journal of Athletic Training,* Vol. 37, No. 1, (Jan 2002), pp. 99–104.

Atkins DL, Everson-Stewart S, Sears GK. et al. (2009). Epidemiology and outcomes from out-of-hospital cardiac arrest in children: The Resuscitation Outcomes Consortium Epistry–Cardiac Arrest. *Circulation,* Vol. 119, No. 11, (Mar 2009), pp. 1484-491.

Balady GJ, Chaitman B, Foster C. et al., (2002). Automated external defibrillators in health/fitness facilities: Supplement to the AHA/ACSM recommendations for cardiovascular screening, staffing, and emergency policies at health/fitness facilities. *Circulation,* Vol. 105, No. 9, (Mar 2002), pp. 1147–1150.

Borjesson M, Dugmore D, Mellwig KP. et al., (2010). Time for action regarding cardiovascular emergency care at sports arenas: a lesson from the Arena study. *European Heart Journal,* Vol. 31, No. 12, (Jun 2010), pp. 1438–1441.

Caffrey SL, Willoughby PJ. et al (2002). Public use of automated external defibrillators. *New England Journal of Medicine,* Vol. 347, No. 16, (Oct 2002), pp. 1242–1247.

Corrado D, Basso C, Pavei A. et al. (2006). Trends in sudden cardiovascular death in young competitive athletes after implementation of a preparticipation screening program. *The Journal of the American Medical Association,* Vol. 296, No. 13 (Oct 2006), pp. 1593-1601.

Corrado D, Pellicia A, Bjornstad HH. et al. (2005). Cardiovascular preparticipation screening of young competitive athletes for prevention of sudden death: proposal for a common European protocol. *European Heart Journal,* Vol. 26, No. 5, (Mar 2005), pp. 516-524.

Corrado D, Basso C, Rizzoli G. et al. (2003). Does sports activity enhance the risk of sudden death in adolescents and young adults? *Journal of American College of Cardiology,* Vol. 42, No. 11 (Dec 2003), pp. 1959–1963.

Drezner JA. (2009). Preparing for sudden cardiac arrest - the essential role of automated external defibrillators in athletic medicine: a critical review. *British Journal of Sports Medicine,* Vol. 43, No. 9, (Sept 2009), pp. 702–707.

Drezner JA, Courson RW, Roberts WO. et al. (2007). Inter-association task force recommendations on emergency preparedness and management of sudden cardiac arrest in high school and college athletic programs: a consensus statement. *Clinical Journal of Sports Medicine,* Vol. 17, No. 2, (Mar 2007), pp. 87-103.

Drezner JA, Rao AL, Heistand J. et al. (2009). Effectiveness of emergency response planning for sudden cardiac arrest in United States high schools with automated external defibrillators. *Circulation*, Vol. 120, No. 6, (Aug 2009), pp. 518–525.

Drezner JA, Rogers KJ. (2006). Sudden cardiac arrest in intercollegiate athletes: detailed analysis and outcomes of resuscitation in nine cases. *Heart Rhythm*, Vol. 3, No. 7, (Jul 2006), pp. 755–759.

Hallstrom AP, Ornato JP, Weisfeldt M. et al. (2004). Public-access defibrillation and survival after out-of-hospital cardiac arrest. *New England Journal of Medicine*, Vol. 351, No. 7, (Aug 2004), pp. 637-646.

Kitamura T, Iwami T, Kawamura T. et al. (2010). Nationwide public-access defibrillation in Japan. *New England Journal of Medicine*, Vol. 362, No. 11, (Mar 2010), pp. 994-1004.

Maron BJ. (2003). Sudden death in young athletes. *New England Journal of Medicine*, Vol. 349, No. 11, (Sep 2003), pp. 1064-1075.

Maron BJ. (2009). Distinguishing hypertrophic cardiomyopathy from athlete's heart physiological remodelling: clinical significance, diagnostic strategies and implications of preparticipation screening. *British Journal of Sports Medicine*, Vol. 43, No. 9, (Sep 2009), pp. 649-656.

Myenburg RJ, Estes NA III, Fontaine JM. et al. (2005). Task force 10: Automated external defibrillators. *Journal of American College of Cardiology*, Vol. 45, No. 8, (Apr 2005), pp. 1369-1371.

Page RL Joglar JA, Kowal RC. et al. (2000). Use of automated external defibrillators by US airlines. *New England Journal of Medicine*, Vol. 343, No. 17, (Oct 2000), pp. 1210-1216.

Perkins G, Colquhoun M. (2010). The use of automated external defibrillators, In: *Resuscitation Guidelines 2010*, Nolan JP, pp. 29-35, Resuscitation Council UK, Retrieved from www.resus.org.uk.

Priori SG, Bossaert LL, Chamberlain DA. et al. (2004). ESC-ERC recommendations for the use of automated external defibrillators (AEDs) in Europe. *European Heart Journal*, Vol. 25, No. 5, (Mar 2004), pp. 437-445.

Valenzuela TD, Roe DJ, Nichol G. et al. (2000). Outcomes of rapid defibrillation by security officers after cardiac arrest in casinos. *New England Journal of Medicine*, Vol. 343, No. 17, (Oct 2000), pp. 1206-1209.

White RD, Asplin BR, Bugliosi TF & Hankins DG. (1996). High discharge survival rate after out-of-hospital ventricular fibrillation with rapid defibrillation by police and paramedics. *Annals of Emergency Medicine*, Vol. 28, No. 5, (Nov 1996), pp. 480-485.

Part 3

Pediatric Defibrillation

11

Implantable-Cardioverter Defibrillator in Pediatric Population

María Algarra, Pablo Santiago, Luis Tercedor, Miguel Álvarez, Rocío Peñas, Francisca Valverde and Abdulreda Abdallah
Arrhythmia Unit. Cardiology Department.
University Hospital Virgen de las Nieves de Granada
Spain

1. Introduction

Implantable cardioverter-defibrillator is largely used as an effective treatment for potentially lethal arrhythmias in adult population. On the contrary, just 1% of devices are implanted in pediatric population worldwide. In our series, 4% of defibrillators implanted between 2000 and 2010 were in children under 18 years of age.

During the last two decades, prevention and treatment decisions in pediatric population have been commonly made on adult data, including device therapy recommendations. Indeed, most pediatric data comes from single-center series and case reports, with no specific clinical trials focused on this population.

The incidence of pediatric sudden cardiac death is estimated at 1.3-8.5:100.000 patients-years (William et al., 1998). Survival of out-hospital cardiac arrest is as low as 8-9% and neurological sequels remain high (Driscoll et al., 1985). Sudden cardiac death in childhood and adolescence is associated with three main cardiovascular conditions: congenital heart diseases, cardiomyopathies, and genetic arrhythmia syndromes. In this setting, implantable defibrillator has become an effective antiarrhythmic therapy in a large variety of structural cardiovascular abnormalities and primary electrical diseases.

Device implantation in children is challenging because of peculiar patient characteristics as age, weight, vascular access and potential somatic growth. Therefore, procedural approach and site of implantation, therapeutic algorithms and early and long-term complications differ from adults. Transvenous approaches could be difficult because of small venous system (Radbill et al., 2010). Abdominal implantation of generator and epicardial leads are frequently needed. Early physical activity and impaired sterile conditions added to individual characteristic are related to more frequent procedural complications (Shah, 2009).

Device dysfunction, i.e. inappropriate therapies may appear frequently, between 11% and 50% of cases, in the settings of sinusal and supraventricular tachycardia or T wave oversensing (Korte et al., 2004). Several algorithms have been used to reduce inappropriate discharges, as QRS discrimination or cardiac rate stability (Barry et al., 2001). Lead complications are related to high physical activity and body surface, significantly higher in patients with body area under 1.2 m2 (OR 4.5) (Shah, 2009).

Psychological impact of defibrillator implantation and discharges during follow up may lead into more frequent depression and anxiety symptoms than in adult patients (Sears et al., 2011). Screening of inherited arrhythmic conditions in relatives of children carrying a defibrillator may be useful to detect potential risk in these relatives. Tomaske et al., 2011, reported 22% appropriate shocks in defibrillators implanted for primary prevention in this population.

2. Sudden cardiac death in children

Sudden cardiac death is defined as an abrupt, unexpected death occurring within 1 hour from the onset of cardiovascular symptoms. In young people, it typically occurs within a few minutes of symptoms onset. Aborted cardiac arrest includes cardiac resuscitation restoring spontaneous circulation. Excluding the Sudden Infant Death Syndrome, that affects children under 1 year, with an incidence around 1-1.5/1.000 infants, sudden death in a young person is a rare event (Gajewski et al., 2010). The estimated incidence of pediatric sudden cardiac death ranges from 1.3 to 8.5 per 100,000 children in the United States (Driscoll et al., 1985) (William et al., 1998). Approximately 20-25% of the deaths occur during sports (Liberthson et al., 1996). In patients with congenital heart disease, this rate increases to 100 deaths per 100,000 patients (O'Connor et al., 1998). Early cardiopulmonary resuscitation and extended availability of automatic external defibrillators could prevent about a quarter of pediatric sudden deaths (Gajewski and Saul, 2010). Since most sudden deaths have a cardiovascular cause, it is theoretically possible to identify patients at risk prior to the event and prevent it (Haskell et al., 2010).

Causes of sudden cardiac death	**Relative incidence (%)**
Hypertrophic cardiomyopathy	36
Increased cardiac mass	10
Coronary arteries anomalies	24
Marfan's Syndrome	6
Congenital heart disease	5
Myocarditis	3
Dilated cardiomyopathy	3
Arrhythmogenic right ventricular dysplasia	3
Ischemic heart disease	2
Commotio cordis	<1

Table 1. Causes of sudden cardiac death in children. Taken from Maron et al. JAMA. 1996.

Most young people with sudden cardiac death have an underlying heart condition, with hypertrophic cardiomyopathy, coronary artery anomalies, arrhythmogenic right ventricular dysplasia and long QT syndrome being commonest in most series (Silka et al., 1991, Maron et al. 1996a).

Hypertrophic cardiomyopathy is the most common cause of sudden unexpected death in childhood, significantly higher in the 8- to 16-year age range than in the 17- to 30-year (Maron et al., 1996a). Disease prevalence is as high as 1 per 500 in young adults (Maron et al., 1996b), (Corrado et al., 1998). Carriers of a genetic mutation may have little or no hypertrophy, especially earlier in life. Sudden death is often exertional and secondary to malignant ventricular arrhythmias. Lipophilic betablocker, disopiramid and implantable cardioverter-defibrillator have demonstrated to increase survival in this population.

Arrhythmia in children with dilated cardiomyopathy is one major clinical manifestation of the disease. The occurrence of arrhythmia is associated with the left ventricular size and heart function and includes ventricular ectopy (Han et al., 2011). An underlying myocarditis is found in 2-15% of patients, rising to 45% in a series of patients under 2 years, with other 25% affected by endomyocardial fibrosis (Meune et al. 2006). Other conditions as infectious, metabolic and neurological diseases have been described as causes of dilated cardiomyopathy. 20-25% of cases are inherited. Dilated cardiomyopathy is progressive, often clinically silent in childhood, and sudden cardiac death may occur prior to development of heart failure symptoms.

Left ventricular hypertrabeculation/noncompaction is a genetic myocardiopathy affecting line-Z skeletal and cardiac contractile proteins. In children, it is found in 0,01% of echocardiographic explorations, meaning 10% of pediatrical cardiomyopathies (Pignatelli et al., 2003). In pediatric population, diagnosis is usually made within first three months of life. Sustained or non-sustained ventricular tachycardia is seen in 40% of patients, and in 14% of patients QT interval is prolonged. Ventricular fibrillation is more frequent in children than in adults (Stöllberger et al., 2010). Almost 20% of patients with ventricular tachycardia or fibrillation have a normal systolic function. Data about long-term follow-up of patients with implanted cardioverter-defibrillator is necessary since indication for prophylactic implantation is still unclear.

The incidence of sudden death in patients with congenital heart disease is about 100/100,000 patient-years (O'Connor et al., 1998). It is higher in cyanotic and left heart obstructive lesions, may be due to arrhythmic, embolic or circulatory phenomena. Certain congenital defects have a higher risk of acquired arrhythmias following repair. The risk of sudden death appears to increase with age and time from surgery. Specifically, tetralogy of Fallot is associated with high incidence of ventricular tachycardia and 0.5% to 6% risk of sudden cardiac death (Gajewski et al., 2010). Patients with both single-ventricle physiology status-post Fontan, and transposition of the great arteries status-post atrial switch also have high acquired arrhythmia rates with increased incidence of sudden cardiac death. These two congenital cardiac conditions may lead to the implantation of a cardioverter-defibrillator as a primary prevention strategy.

Arrhythmogenic right ventricular dysplasia is a rare cause of sudden cardiac death in the United States, but is reported as the most common cause of sudden cardiac death in the young athletes in Italy (Maron et al., 2009), (Corrado et al., 2009). It is a heritable, progressive cardiomyopathy characterized by fatty and fibrous replacement of the myocardium, causing thinning of right ventricular free wall. Although both drug therapy and catheter ablation are occasionally successful, implantation of a defibrillator is usually recommended for patients with significant symptoms.

A variety of conditions can cause primary arrhythmia in young people: Long QT Syndrome, Brugada Syndrome, Catecholaminergic Polymorphic Ventricular Tachycardia, Wolff-Parkinson-White Syndrome, and Congenital Complete Heart Block. Although there are cases in which sudden cardiac death is the first symptom, recurrent syncope often precedes malignant events (Proclemer et al., 2009). Fortunately, the surface 12-lead ECG is abnormal in most cases.

The congenital form of Long QT syndrome is a familial genetic disorder occurring about 1 in 2.500–3.500 individuals (Vincent et al., 1992). It manifests primarily as ventricular repolarization abnormalities caused by cardiac ion-channel mutations. For symptomatic patients, the presenting symptom is usually syncope, due to torsade-de-pointes ventricular tachycardia. The syncope may occur with specific triggers, such as stress, swimming, and loud auditory stimuli, or it may occur when the child is relatively bradycardic, at resting or sleeping (Schwartz et al., 2001). The specific phenotype (LQTS1, LQTS2 and LQTS3) can be predicted from the genetic mutation and may help in the assessment of risk for sudden death or response to therapy (Tester et al., 2005). Main therapy remains beta-blockade, which is less effective for LQTS3. If symptoms recur under beta-blocker therapy, implantation of a cardioverter-defibrillator is generally indicated.

Brugada syndrome is an inherited arrhythmogenic syndrome related to life-threatening ventricular arrhythmia due to a mutation in genes encoding sodium-channels (Miyamoto et al., 2011). Family sudden death history does not predict higher ventricular arrhythmia susceptibility (Delise et al., 2010). Treatment is limited to ICD implantation when symptoms like syncope occur.

Catecholaminergic polymorphic ventricular tachycardia is a genetic arrhythmogenic disease caused by mutations in genes encoding sarcoplasmic calcium ion-channels (Tester et al., 2006). Ventricular ectopy induced by exercise or emotional stress is typically observed. The onset of symptoms typically occurs in childhood and adolescence. Left untreated, Catecholaminergic Polymorphic Ventricular Tachycardia is lethal in 30–50% of patients (Leenhardt et al., 1995). Although beta-blockers are the recommended therapy, many patients present with recurrent arrhythmic symptoms and may need a defibrillator.

3. Cardioverter-defibrillator in pediatric population

3.1 Indications

For the last decade, use of implantable cardioverter-defibrillator in children has increased dramatically. The number of pediatric implants per year has augmented by three-fold. The mean age at implant has decreased significantly (from 13.6 to 12.2 years), and the percentage of patients younger than 5 years of age receiving an implantable defibrillator tended to increase up to 10% (Burns et al., 2011). A large variability in the number of implants per center and year is observed and this situation may have implications for competency and training.

Specific pediatric recommendations have been included in the ACC/AHA/HRS 2008 Guidelines for Device-Based Therapy of Cardiac Rhythm Abnormalities (Ebstein et al., 2008):

Class I	• ICD implantation is indicated in the survivor of cardiac arrest after evaluation to define the cause of the event and to exclude any reversible causes. Level of Evidence : B • ICD implantation is indicated for patients with symptomatic sustained VT in association with congenital heart disease who have undergone hemodynamic and electrophysiological evaluation. Catheter ablation or surgical repair may offer possible alternatives in carefully selected patients. Level of Evidence : C
Class IIa	• ICD implantation is reasonable for patients with congenital heart disease with recurrent syncope of undetermined origin in the presence of either ventricular dysfunction or inducible ventricular arrhythmias at electrophysiological study. Level of Evidence : B
Class IIb	• ICD implantation may be considered for patients with recurrent syncope associated with complex congenital heart disease and advanced systemic ventricular dysfunction when invasive and noninvasive investigations have failed to define a cause. Level of Evidence : C
Class III	• ICD therapy is not indicated for patients who do not have a reasonable expectation of survival with an acceptable functional status for at least 1 year, even if they meet criteria specified in the Class I, IIa, and IIb recommendations above. Level of Evidence : C. • ICD therapy is not indicated for patients with incessant VT or VF. Level of Evidence : C • ICD therapy is not indicated in patients with significant psychiatric illnesses that may be aggravated by device implantation or that may preclude systematic follow-up. Level of Evidence : C • ICD therapy is not indicated for NYHA Class IV patients with drug-refractory congestive heart failure who are not candidates for cardiac transplantation or CRT-D. Level of Evidence : C • ICD therapy is not indicated for syncope of undetermined cause in a patient without inducible ventricular tachyarrhythmias and without structural heart disease. Level of Evidence : C • ICD therapy is not indicated when VF or VT is amenable to surgical or catheter ablation (e.g., atrial arrhythmias associated with the Wolff-Parkinson-White syndrome, RV or LV outflow tract VT, idiopathic VT, or fascicular VT in the absence of structural heart disease). Level of Evidence : C • ICD therapy is not indicated for patients with ventricular tachyarrhythmias due to a completely reversible disorder in the absence of structural heart disease (e.g., electrolyte imbalance, drugs, or trauma). Level of Evidence : B

Table 2.

Indications for implantation of cardioverter-defibrillator in children over last two decades are based on clinical trials designed and performed for adult population. Indications are shifting from secondary to primary prevention. In fact, secondary prevention implants decreased significantly when compared to primary prevention from 77% to 45% (Burns et al., 2011). In the Spanish Registry of Cardioverter-Defibrillator implantation, prophylactic implantation increased from 2006 to 2008 for Arrhythmogenic Right Ventricular Dysplasia and Brugada syndrome, with no increase for Long QT syndrome and hypertrophic cardiomyopathy (Peinado et al., 2008). Primary prevention of sudden cardiac death remains a challenge in which individualized decisions play a mayor role. The low use of cardioverter-defibrillator in pediatric population difficult the assessment of cardioverter-defibrillator survival benefit and long term results.

In 1991, Silka et al. reported a series of 177 patients under 20 years in which a implantable cardioverter-defibrillator was indicated. 75% patients were survivors of sudden cardiac death, 10% had drug-refractory ventricular tachycardia and 10% syncope with positive electrophysiology study for arrythmia-inducibility. Almost 60% had an overt cardiovascular disease, whereas 26% had primary electrical condition and 18% congenital cardiopathy. Hypertrophic and dilated cardiomyopathies, transposition of great arteries and tetralogy of Fallot were commonest structural cardiac diseases. Systolic function was normal in 54% patients, and 48% had some degree of systolic function impairment. Von Berger et al., 2010 reported an updated registry of 210 cardioverter-defibrillators implanted in patients under 30 years-old in seven institutions between October 1992 and January 2007. Heart disease was categorized as electrical (n=90, 42%), cardiomyopathic (n=62, 30%), or congenital heart disease (n=58, 28%).

In the Dutch Registry from 1995 to 2006 (Heersche, 2010), 45 cardioverter-defibrillator were implanted in children and young patients. According to indication, sudden death and ventricular tachycardia patients were similar to the American registry, with a higher rate of electrical conditions (55%) and prophylactic indication (17%). In the electrical disease group, 56% had Long QT syndrome, 25% Idiopathic Ventricular Fibrillation and 19% Brugada Syndrome. Ten Harkell et al., 2006, reported another series of 23 Dutch pediatric defibrillator patients. 22% defibrillators were epicardial and 88% transvenous. The generator was placed in an abdominal position in 35% patients, whereas it was placed in the subpectoral region in 65%. There was no early mortality. Median hospital stay was 5 days.

In our series, 11 cardioverter-defibrillators were implanted between 1995 and 2010 in patients under 18 years, 4% of all implanted defibrillators. 80% defibrillators were implanted for secondary prevention (Ventricular Fibrillation 60%, Ventricular Tachycardia 20%) and 20% were implanted for primary prevention. Cardiac conditions were 40% Long QT Syndrome, 20% congenital cardiopathies, 10% hypertrophic cardiomyopathy, 10% hypertrabeculation/ Noncompactation cardiomyopathy and 20% had no overt structural heart disease. By age, long QT Syndrome was more frequent between younger patients, whereas transposition of Great Arteries was the commonest underlying cardiopathy in 15-18 years-age group. 50% were single chamber devices and 50% dual chambers.

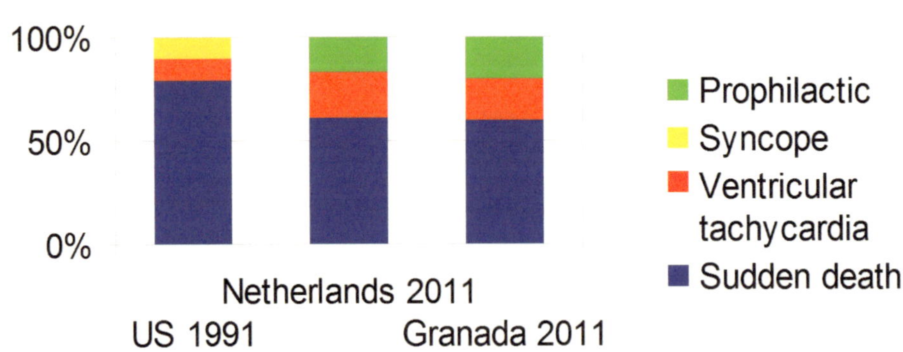

Fig. 1. Comparison of three series of cardioverter-defibrillator implantation according to clinical presentation. Silka et al., 1991. Heersche et al., 2011. Granada, our series.

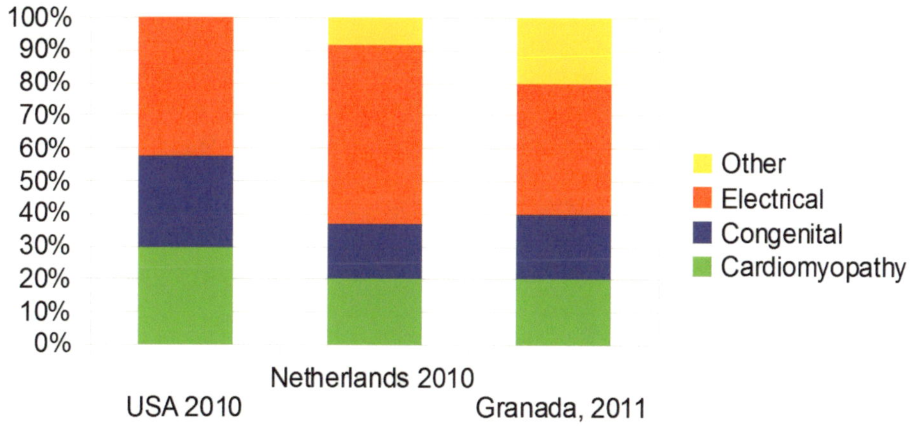

Fig. 2. Comparison of implantable cardioverter-defibrillation cardiac conditions in largest series. USA: Von Berger et al., 2010. Netherlands: Heersche et al., 2010. Granada, our series.

The Italian Registry included pediatric defibrillator use in inherited arrhythmogenic diseases from 2001 to 2006 (Proclemer et el., 2009). For primary prevention, 30% defibrilators were implanted in Hypertrophic Cardiomyopathy, 16% in Arrhythmogenic Right Ventricular Dysplasia, 17% in idiopathic ventricular arrhythmia (they included Brugada Syndrome in this group) and 16% in the Long QT Syndrome. There were 52% single-chamber, 44% dual-chamber, and 5% triple-chamber cardioverter-defibrillators.

In terms of defibrillation energy required in pediatric patients, available data includes only external resuscitation devices. The recommended energy dose had been established in 2 J/kg for the last 30 years, but recent reports may indicate that higher dosages may be more effective and safe. In 2005, the European Resuscitation Council recommended 4 J/kg as initial dose, without escalation for subsequent shocks (Haskell et al., 2010 & Sandroni et al., 2011).

3.2 Implantation techniques

Despite the increasing use of implantable cardioverter-defibrillator in congenital heart patients, specific challenges and implications related to implantation and follow-up are continuously observed. The variability and complexity of congenital pediatric patients make device management a highly individualized art. There are technical issues related to implantation since vascular access and device characteristic may not be suitable for pediatric patient (Chun et al., 2008). Although advances in implantable cardioverter-defibrillator technology are constantly made, the optimal cardioverter-defibrillator implantation technique for pediatric patients has not been established yet. The implantation of cardioverter-defibrillator in pediatric patients has many peculiarities, and there is little information on implant methodology for this population. A statement on training pathways for implantation of cardioverter-defibrillators and cardiac resynchronization therapy devices in pediatric and congenital heart patients was published in 2008 (Saul et al., 2008).

Transvenous implantation in children presents multiple challenges, related to patient body surface and weight, physical activity, increased risk of infections, and long life expectancy. There are no specific electrodes for small vessel diameters, with the consequent risk of venous thrombosis, nor devices adapted to their body surface. The creation of an atrial loop might allow the "elongation" of the lead with the growth. Concerns have been raised about Long-term leads patency, ventricular and valvular dysfunction, venous integrity, cosmetic results and psychological factors. System survival rates are estimated at 91% for the first year from implant, 83% at 24 months and 76% at 36 months (Rabdill et al., 2010).

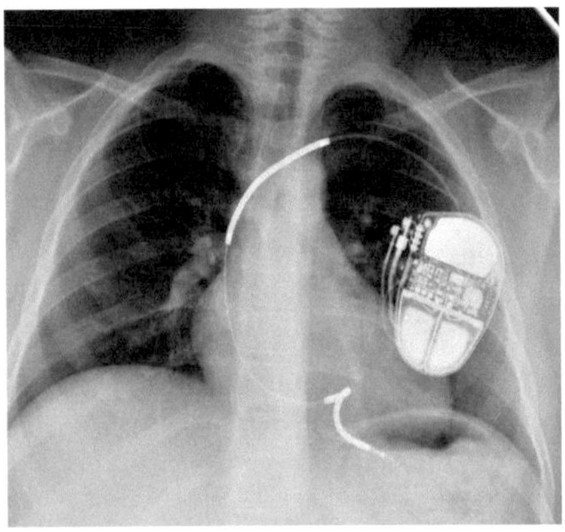

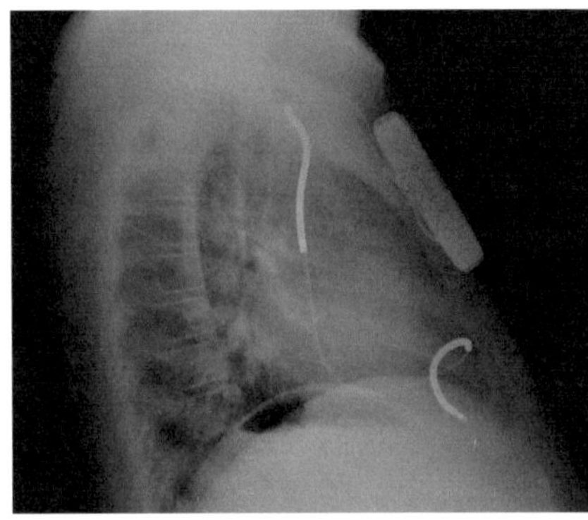

Fig. 1. and 2. Frontal and lateral Rx of a dual-chamber cardioverter-defibrillator in a 10 years-old patient with Brugada Syndrome.

Nontransvenous implantable cardioverter-defibrillator systems include pericardial and subcutaneous coils as alternative approaches in selected pediatric and congenital heart patients who are not candidates for transvenous leads. These nontransvenous systems are more commonly used in younger patients, with smaller body surface area, intracardiac shunts and concurrent thoracotomy surgery or affection of thricuspid valve.

Intrapericardial placement of an ICD coil system can be carried out through a subxiphoid approach and pericardial window without thoracotomy (Tomaske et al., 2008 & Bové et al., 2010). This technique is independent from child size or cardiac status. The defibrillation coil lead is actively fixated in the transverse sinus under fluoroscopic guidance, and the generator placed in a subrectus pocket in the upper abdomen through the same incision. Epicardial system is effective in treating ventricular arrhythmia without inappropriate discharges and no perioperative complications nor early or late deaths have been reported (Hsia et al., 2009). Controversy remains about defibrillation thresholds, since Stephenson et al., described high defibrillation thresholds with epicardial leads (Stephenson et al., 2006) More recently, Silvetti reported, for a 20-months follow-up, impedance stability and acceptable defibrillation thresholds (5-15J) (Silvetti et al., 2007).

Endocardial and epicardial steroid-eluting leads have comparable electrical performances, especially in absence of other congenital heart defects and previous heart surgery, although endocardial pacing shows the best outcomes and should be the first choice in children over 10-15 kg (Chun et al., 2008). System survival is significantly shorter in nontransvenous than in transvenous systems at 12, 24, and 36 months (survival rates at 73%, 55%, and 49%, respectively) (Rabdill et al., 2010). In fact, nontransvenous systems have demonstrated to be an independent predictor of system failure.

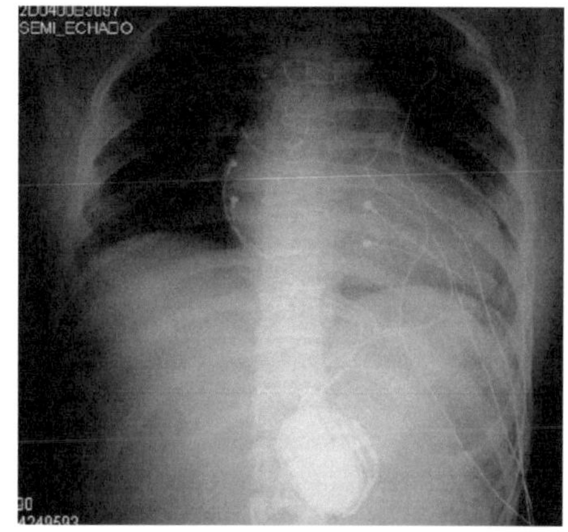

Fig. 3. Dual-chamber epicardial leads cardioverter-defibrillator in a male 6 years-old patient with Tetralogy of Fallot.

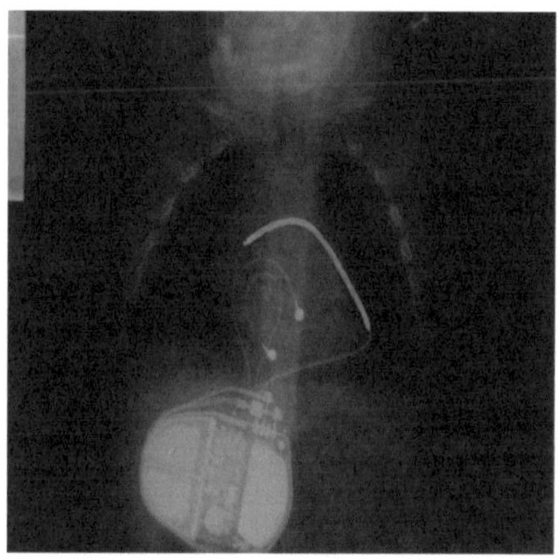

Fig. 4. Single-chamber epicardial cardioverter-defibrillator in a 2 years-old female child with Long QT Syndrome. See abdominal generator implantation, transverse sinus defibrillation coil and epicardial sense and pacing leads.

One increasing option is totally extracardiac implantation. A subcutaneous implantable defibrillator does not require a lead placed on or in the heart (McLeod et al., 2010). It may become an option for children suffering from chronic complications related to transvenous or epicardial leads and inappropriate shocks. High defibrillation thresholds at implant and follow-up are seen (Stephenson et al., 2006). Changing device position from abdominal to a supradiaphragmatic site may solve unsafe elevated discharge impedance and defibrillation threshold during follow-up (Berruezo et al., 2010). The best device configuration reported by Bardy et al., 2010, consisted of a parasternal electrode and a left lateral thoracic pulse generator. This configuration results as effective as a transvenous ICD for terminating induced ventricular fibrillation, albeit with a significantly higher mean energy requirement (35J vs. 11J). 100% ventricular fibrillation detection and 98% cardioversion effectiveness in two consecutive tests confirms its good performance. 100% appropriate shocks have been reported for treating ventricular tachycardia during 10-months follow-up. A low rate of adverse events confirms its safety.

The wearable cardiac defibrillator is an alternative for patients at risk for sudden death who do not fulfill standard criteria for defibrillator implantation or in whom the risk:benefit ratio is equivocal (Everitt et al., 2010). Careful patient selection and education result essential to ensure safety, as noncompliance with wear is common.

3.3 Procedural complications

Implantation procedure complications appear between 14% and 26% (Alexander et al., 2004), (Shah et al., 2009) (Stefanelli et al., 2004). These include pocket infections, pocket hematoma, microdislodgement requiring lead manipulation and electromechanical dissociation. Early electrode dislocation may need reintervention. In young patients, transvenous leads of implantable defibrillator can cause vascular obstruction up to 13%, mainly asymptomatic (Bar-Cohen et al., 2006). Local infection increasing rate may be due to early activity resume and impaired sterile conditions of wound (Link et al., 1999). Most pocket infections are related to local contamination at the time of implantation. Cardiac perforation (Morrison et al., 2009), hemothorax or superior Vena Cava syndrome have been described as implantation early and late complications (Alexander et al., 2010). Postpericardiotomy syndrome is described related to epicardial leads (Stefanelli et al., 2002). No pediatric death has been reported related to implantation procedure.

4. Long-term follow up

4.1 Therapy history

Pediatric defibrillator recipients have significant appropriate shock rates. Antitachycardia pacing therapy is rarely effective and often harmful in young ICD recipients, because this therapy is effective in monomorphic ventricular tachycardia, a rare arrhythmia among

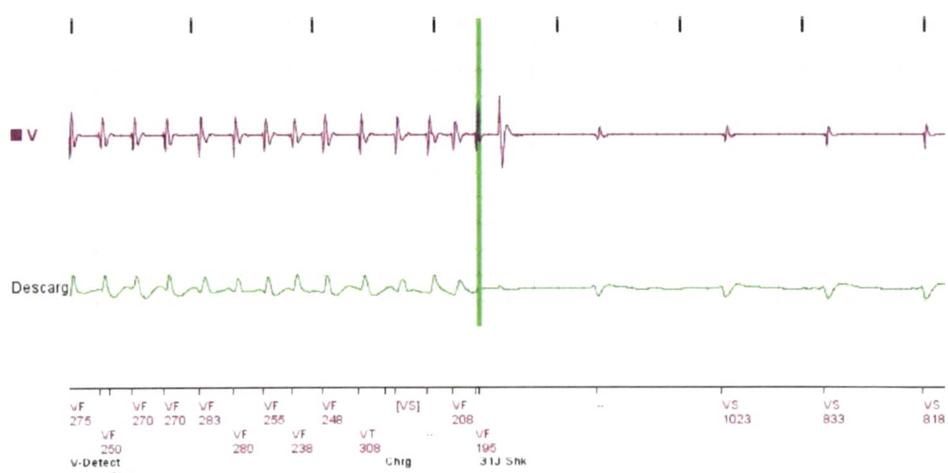

Fig. 5. Appropriate shock delivery for ventricular fibrillation in an 11-years-old female child with hypertrophic cardiomyopathy. See instability in the cycle length of the sensed ventricular electrograms.

children. In most patients, programming ICD for only VF therapy is sufficient. A significant increased rate of appropriate discharges was found in defibrillator devices placed for secondary prevention (52%) versus primary prevention (14%) at 5 years (Von Berger et al., 2011). Therefore, the benefits of an implantable cardioverter-defibrillator remain greater in secondary than in primary prevention patients. In patients with nontransvenous systems, up to 23% receive appropriate shocks (Rabdill et al., 2010). In the Dutch registry, rate of appropriate shocks were reported at 31%, with a significant difference according to patient age (55% for patients under 12 years, 9% for patients between 13 and 18 years old). No difference has been reported in secondary prevention related to age, with rates of approximately 38% appropriate shocks for both groups (Heersche et al., 2010). In a registry of Long QT syndrome from 2002 to 2009, at least 1 appropriate shock was received by 28% of patients during 4 years mean follow-up.

4.2 Device-related complications

Inappropriate discharges, lead-related complications and generator anomalies are the commonest adverse events occurring during follow-up. Lead complications are related to high physical activity and body surface, significantly higher in patients with body area under 1.2 m2 (OR 4.5) (Shah, 2009). Lewandoski et al., 2010 reported 21% complications requiring surgical intervention. In our series, we describe 20% of inappropriate discharges, 20% lead complications and 10% generator anomalies. In the Long-QT-syndrome registry from 2002 to 2009, adverse events occurred in 25% (Schwartz et al., 2009). Serious psychological sequel may reach 43%of patients (Lewandowski et al., 2010).

4.2.1 Inappropriate therapy

Inappropriate discharges are frequent, some of them caused by suboptimal pre-discharge programming of the device (Lewandowski et al., 2010). Reported rates vary sharply in infant series, from 11% to 50% (Botsch et al., 2007), being better defined in adult series (20-30%). Inappropriate shocks occur in the setting of sinusal and supraventricular tachycardia, QRS double-sensing or T-wave oversensing (Korte et al., 2004). Lewandoski et el., 2010 reported inappropriate therapy resulting from T-wave over-sensing in 14%, sinus tachycardia in 5%, fast atrial fibrillation in 8%, and lead insulation disruption in 1%. Several algorithms have been used to reduce inappropriate discharges, as QRS discrimination or cardiac rate stability (Barry et al., 2001). In a multicentric series of 210 young defibrillator recipients from seven institutions, no differences were found in the risk of inappropriate discharges between primary and secondary prevention defibrillators, both rates estimated at approximately 35% within 5 years from implant (Berul et al., 2008). In the Dutch registry, 27% shocks deliveries were inappropriate. In patients with nontransvenous systems, up to 18% receive inappropriate shocks (Rabdill et al., 2010). Congenital patients have higher risk of inappropriate discharges (Williams et al., 1998). A higher rate of inappropriate shocks has been reported in the setting of lead failure than in other conditions causing inappropriate therapies.

4.2.2 Lead and generator specific complications

As a general rule, less leads implanted in children, less complication will occur in the future, and the simplest system (generally, single-chamber), the better outcome (Silvetti et al., 2009).

The second most frequent ICD system-related adverse effect in the pediatric population is ICD lead failure. Lead failures requiring programming or revision interventions have been reported in the range of 7–30% at median follow-up of 2 years in the pediatric literature (Stefanelli et al., 2002 & Berul et al, 2008).

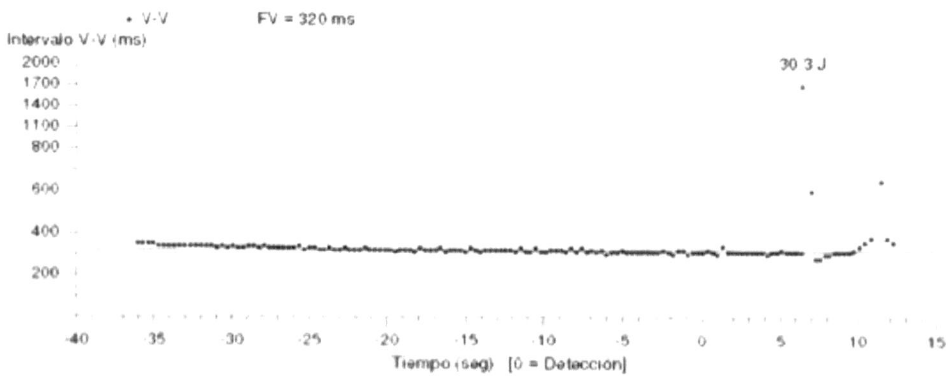

Fig. 6. Inappropriate shock during sinus tachycardia. See the progressive increase of heart rate, stability of cycles length and no further effect of defibrillation discharge.

In the Netherlands Registry, overall complications occurred in 17% patients, 87% related to lead failure (Heersche et al., 2010). Rate of total unanticipated interventions in the nontransvenous group is estimated at 18 per 1.000 person-months versus 6 per 1,000 person-months in the transvenous group (Rabdill et al., 2010). Survival rates for defibrillator leads in children are reported in 89.6% at 5-year, when implantation is made by an expertise operator. Lead failures as lead fraction and insulation failure (Bennett & Tung, 2010) occur mostly within the second year of implantation (Lewandowski et al., 2010). An increase in size was associated with higher risk for lead failure as the proximal shocking electrode ends to become stretched and distorted, leading to lead failure.

Given the finite longevity of current lead designs, lead extraction is an eventuality for a significant subset of pediatric defibrillator patients. Generator elective replacement is the most frequent indication for generator change in the majority of pediatric series.

Longevity is estimated at more than 9 years for a single-chamber defibrillator without permanent pacing, 7 years for a dual-chamber defibrillator pacing 50% of time and 6 years for a resynchronization-defibrillator (Bonney et al., 2010), in clinical practice the predicted generator survival is hardly accomplished.

Apart from lead durability, main indications for removal are vascular obstruction (that requires simultaneous revascularization), increased thresholds, and lead dislocations

(Welisch et al., 2010). Other complications affecting generator are prolonged charge time, early battery depletion, and malfunction during implant testing.

In Dutch series of Harkell et al., 2006, generator replacement was necessary in 18% of patients between 28 and 54 months from implantation. Procedural complications rates are low, according to a review of 203 lead extractions carried out between 2002 and 2008 (Cecchin et al., 2010). No procedure deaths were seen in this series, although removal of non-functional leads bears the risk of vascular disrupture and embolizations. Of this series, 60% of patients had structural heart disease and successful simple extraction was only achievable in 29% of patients (requiring just a nonlocking stylet). Complex extraction techniques include radiofrequency-powered sheath (Zartner et al., 2010). Successful extraction was performed in 80% of all leads and 94% of complex extraction leads (Cecchin et al., 2010). Complications were observed in 5% of patients. Older leads, intraventricular location, and polyurethane insulation were associated with an increased probability of complex extraction. Procedure and x-ray duration correlated to correlated to time from lead implantation.

Cardiac device endocarditis is an infrequent, but potentially lethal complication. Hematogenous seeding of Staphilococcus aureus from a distant focus is the most common etiology in late infections. Cure is achievable in the large majority of patients under an aggressive antimicrobial regime and complete device removal. When the intravascular portion of the lead system cannot be aseptically separated from the pocket, removal of the entire system is essential (Shah, 2009). After device explantation and long-term standard antibiotic treatment to decrease risk for recurrent endocarditis, reimplantation requires additional caution (Mihalcz et al., 2008).

Industry advisories and recalls have an adverse economic, psychosocial and physical impact on pediatric defibrillator patients. Between 2000 and 2005, 25% of implanted defibrillators were affected by industry advisories or recalls (Mahajan et al., 2008), which meant 22% patients undergoing explantation after three years from implant. Just 2 of 89 explanted devices were defective, with loose headers as the unique failure observed.

4.2.3 Progressive increase in defibrillator thresholds

Failure of first cardioverter-defibrillator shock to terminate ventricular tachycardia or fibrillation was reported in 7% of pediatric defibrillator recipients during follow-up, mainly due to chronic rise in defibrillation thresholds (Stefanelli et al., 2002). Rates of significant changes of defibrillation thresholds range 3,2 to 12% (Stephenson et al., 2006 & Brodsky et al., 1999). Epicardial and subcutaneous systems are more likely to present with this complication than transvenous systems.

4.2.4 Electrical storm

Real incidence of electrical storm in pediatric patients is unknown, although Alexander et al., 2004 reported consecutive appropriate shocks in 6% patients. Antiadrenergic medical therapy and amiodarone have been used to treat this complication. Morbidity and hospitalization are direct consequences of this complication.

4.2.5 Death rates

The majority of reported deaths in the pediatric ICD patients appear to be related to intractable arrhythmias. Silka et al., 1991 reported 4% sudden death, 1% due to recurrent ventricular arrhythmias. Alexander et al., 2004 observed 2% sudden deaths in patients with cardioverter-defibrillator, one of them due to intractable ventricular arrhythmia.

Adverse events reported in cardioverter-defibrillator pediatric patients	%
Implantation-related:	14-26
Pocket complications: hematoma, infection	
Lead dislocation	
Cardiac perforation	
Hemothorax	
Venous thrombosis	13
Mid and long term follow-up:	
Inappropriated shocks	11-50
Lead failure	7-30
Generator failure (recalls, advisories)	
Increased defibrillation thresholds	3-12
Electrical storm	
Death	2

Table 3. Early and late complications observed in pediatric defibrillators patients. From Shah, 2009. Blanck-spaces refer to unknown rates.

5. Cost-effectiveness study

Altough more common in adult population, cost-effectiveness studies in pediatric patients are scarce. Because of differences in heart failure etiology, sudden death rates, and defibrillator complication rates, addition of a prophylactic cardioverter-defibrillator to conventional medical management has resulted not cost-effective in children with dilated cardiomyopathy, poor ventricular function, and symptomatic heart failure (Feingold et al., 2010). Total costs were estimated at $433,000 for the defibrillator strategy and $355,000 for the medical management. Although quality adjusted survival was greater in the defibrillator group, the defibrillator strategy was cost-effective only when the annual probability of sudden death exceeded 13%. The low sudden death rates in this population may justify the results. No data is available for other cardiac conditions that may benefit more clearly from the implantation of a cardioverter-defibrillator in pediatric population.

6. Quality of life in children with implantable cardioverter-defibrillator

Psychosocial and quality-of-life outcomes in pediatric patients with implantable cardioverter-defibrillators are poorer than in adult population. Anxiety and depression are highly related to defibrillator therapies. Shock-related anxiety is suspected to be particularly common (Sears et al., 2011). The PedsQL, the Device Severity Index, the ICD and Avoidance Survey provide data about Quality-Of-Life. Pediatric defibrillator patients have similar Quality-Of-Life outcomes to chronic ill children, with exception of lower physical Quality-Of-Life. Parent-observed reports show lower psychosocial and physical QOL than reported by children themselves. Up to 85% of children present with avoidance behaviors from cardioverter-defibrillation implantation, with female children avoiding places more than male. Similar to adult samples, female patients reported lower psychosocial, physical, and cardiac Quality-Of-Life scores. Differently from other series, Sears et al. did not find discharges and medical severity affecting Quality-Of-Life negatively (Sears et al., 2009).

7. References

Alexander ME, Cecchin F, Walsh EP, et al. Implications of implantable cardioverter defibrillator therapy in congenital heart disease and pediatrics. *J Cardiovasc Electrophysiol.* 2004;15:72–76.

Bar-Cohen Y, Berul CI, Alexander ME, Fortescue EB, Walsh EP, Triedman JK, Cecchin F. Age, size, and lead factors alone do not predict venous obstruction in children and young adults with transvenous lead systems. *J Cardiovasc Electrophysiol* 2006;17:754–759.

Bardy GH, Smith WM, Hood MA, Crozier IG, Melton IC, Jordaens L, Theuns D, Park RE, Wright DJ, Connelly DT, Fynn SP, Murgatroyd FD, Sperzel J, Neuzner J, Spitzer SG, Ardashev AV, Oduro A, Boersma L, Maass AH, Van Gelder IC, Wilde AA, van Dessel PF, Knops RE, Barr CS, Lupo P, Cappato R, Grace AA. An entirely subcutaneous implantable cardioverter-defibrillator. *N Engl J Med.* 2010 Jul 1;363(1):36-44.

Barry A., Love M.D., Barret K., Alexander M., Bevilacqua L., Epstein M., Treidman J., Walsh E., Berul C. Supraventricular Arrhythmias in Children and Young Adults with Implantable Cardioverter Defibrillators. *J Cardiovasc Electrophysiol,* 2001; 12: 1097-1101.

Bennett MT, Tung SK. Long-term efficacy of cardiac pacemaker and cardioverter/defibrillators. *J Long Term Eff Med Implants.* 2010;20(3):187-202.

Berruezo A, Zeljko HM, Bartrons J, Mayol J, Prada F, Brugada J. Defibrillation threshold decrease with the supradiaphragmatic extracardiac implantable cardioverter-defibrillator implantation technique. *Europace.* 2010 Nov;12(11):1649-51.

Berul CI, Van Hare GF, Kertesz NJ, Dubin AM, Cecchin F, CollinsKK, Cannon BC, et al. Results of a multicenter retrospective implantable cardioverter-defibrillator registry of pediatric and congenital heart disease patients. J Am Coll Cardiol 2008 Apr 29;51:1685–1691.

Bonney WJ, Spotnitz HM, Liberman L, Silver ES, Ceresnak SR, Hordof AJ, Pass RH. Survival of transvenous ICD leads in young patients. *Pacing Clin Electrophisiol.* 2010 Feb;33(2):186-91.

Botsch MP, Franzbach B, Opgen-Rhein B, Berger F, Will JC. ICD therapy in children and young adults: low incidence of inappropriate shock delivery. Pacing Clin Electrophysiol. 2010 Jun 1;33(6):734-41.

Bové T, François K, De Caluwe W, Suys B, De Wolf D.Effective cardioverter defibrillator implantation in children without thoracotomy: a valid alternative. *Ann Thorac Surg.* 2010 Apr;89(4):1307-9.

Brodsky CM, Chang F, Vlay SC. Multicenter evaluation of implantable cardioverter defibrillator testing after implant: The Postimplant Testing Study (PITS). *Pacing Clin Electrophysiol* 1999;12:1769–1776.

Burns KM, Evans F, Kaltman JR. Pediatric ICD utilization in the United States from 1997 to 2006. *Heart Rhythm.* 2011 Jan;8(1):23-8.

Cecchin F, Atallah J, Walsh EP, Triedman JK, Alexander ME, Berul CI. Lead extraction in pediatric and congenital heart disease patients. *Circ Arrhythm Electrophysiol.* 2010 Oct 1;3(5):437-44.

Cooper JM, Stephenson EA, Berul CI, Walsh EP, Epstein LM. Implantable cardioverter defibrillator lead complications and laser extraction in children and young adults with congenital heart disease: Implications for implantation and management. *J Cardiovasc Electrophysiol* 2003; 14:344–349.

Corrado D, Basso C, Schiavon M, Thiene G. Screening for hypertrophic cardiomyopathy in young athletes. *N Engl J Med.* 1998;339:364–9.

Corrado D, Basso C, Thiene G. Arrhythmogenic right ventricular cardiomyopathy: An update. *Heart.* 2009;95:766–73.

Chun T. Pacemaker and defibrillator therapy in pediatrics and congenital heart disease. *Future Cardiol.* 2008 Sep;4(5):469-79.

Delise P, Allocca G, Marras E, Sitta N, Sciarra L. Brugada syndrome: diagnosis and risk stratification. *G Ital Cardiol* 2010 Oct;11(10 Suppl 1):107S-113S

Driscoll DJ, Edwards WD. Sudden unexpected death in children and adolescents. *J Am Coll Cardiol.* 1985;5:118B–21.

Epstein AE, DiMarco JP, Ellenbogen KA, Estes NA 3rd, Freedman RA, Gettes LS, Gillinov AM, Gregoratos G, Hammill SC, Hayes DL, Hlatky MA, Newby LK, Page RL, Schoenfeld MH, Silka MJ, Stevenson LW, Sweeney MO, Smith SC Jr, Jacobs AK, Adams CD, Anderson JL, Buller CE, Creager MA, Ettinger SM, Faxon DP, Halperin JL, Hiratzka LF, Hunt SA, Krumholz HM, Kushner FG, Lytle BW, Nishimura RA, Ornato JP, Page RL, Riegel B, Tarkington LG, Yancy CW; American College of Cardiology/American Heart Association Task Force on Practice Guidelines (Writing Committee to Revise the ACC/AHA/NASPE 2002 Guideline Update for Implantation of Cardiac Pacemakers and Antiarrhythmia Devices); American Association for Thoracic Surgery; Society of Thoracic Surgeons. ACC/AHA/ HRS 2008 Guidelines for Device-Based Therapy of Cardiac Rhythm Abnormalities : a report on the American College of Cardiology/American Heart Association Task Force on Practice Guidelines (Writing Comitee to Revise the ACC/AHA/NASPE 2002 Guideline Update for Implantation of Cardiac Pacemakers and Antiarrhythmia Devices) developed in collaboration with the American Association for Thoracic Surgery and Society of Thoracic Surgeons. Heart Rhythm. 2008 Jun;5(6):934-55.

Everitt MD, Saarel EV. Use of the wearable external cardiac defibrillation in children, *Pacing Clin Electrophysiol.* 2010 Jun 1; 33(6): 742-6.

Feinglod B, Arora G, Webber SA, Smith KJ.Cost-effectiveness of implantable cardioverter-defibrillators in children with dilated cardiomyopathy. *J Card Fail.* 2010 Sep;16(9):734-41.

Gajewski KK, Saul JP. Sudden cardiac death in children and adolescents (excluding Sudden Infant Death Syndrome). *Ann Pediatr Cardiol.* 2010 Jul;3(2):107-12.

Han YY. Clinical analysis of 68 casos of childhood dilated cardiomyopathy. *Zhongguo Dang Dai Er Ke Za Zhi.* 2011 Feb; 13(2):135-7.

Haskell SE. Defibrillation in children. *J Emerg Trauma Shock.* 2010 Jul;3(3):261-6.

Heersche JH, Blom NA, van de Heuvel F, Blank C, Reimer AG, Clur SA, Witsenburg M, Harkel AD. Implantable Cardioverter Defibrillator therapy for prevention of sudden cardiac death in children in the Netherlands. *Pacing Clin Electrophysiol.* 2010 Feb;33(2):179-85.

Hsia TY, Bradley SM, LaPage MJ, Whelan S, Saul JP, Ringewald JM, Reed JH. Novel minimally invasive, intrapericardial implantable cardioverter defibrillator coil system: a useful approach to arrhythmia therapy in children. *Ann Thorac Surg.* 2009 Apr;87(4):1234-8.

Korte T, Koditz H, Niehaus M, Paul T, Tebbenjohanns J. High incidence of appropriate and inappropriate ICD therapies in children and adolescents with implantable cardioverter defibrillator. *Pacing Clin Electrophysiol* 2004;27:924–932.

Leenhardt A, Lucet V, Denjoy I, Grau F, Ngoc DD, Coumel P. Catecholaminergic polymorphic ventricular tachycardia in children. A 7-year follow-up of 21 patients. *Circulation.* 1995; 91:1512–9.

Lewandowski M, Sterlinski M, Maciag A, Syska P, Kowalik I, Szwed H, Chojnowska L, Przybylski A. Long-term follow-up of children and young adults treated with implantable cardioverter-defibrillator: the authors' own experience with optimal implantable cardioverter-defibrillator programming. *Europace.* 2010 Sep;12(9):1245-50.

Liberthson RR. Sudden death from cardiac causes in children and young adults. *N Engl J Med.* 1996;334:1039–44

Link MS, Hill SL, Cliff DK, Swygman CA, Foote CB, Homoud MK, Wang PJ, et al. Comparison of frequency of complications of implantable cardioverter defibrillators in children versus adults. *Am J Cardiol* 1999;83:263–266.

Mahajan T, Dubin AM, Atkins DL, Bradley DJ, Shannon KM, Erickson CC, Franklin WH, Cecchin F, Berul CI; Members of Pediatric and Congenital Electrophysiology Society. Impact of manufacturer advisories and FDA recalls of implantable cardioverter defibrillator generators in pediatric and congenital heart disease patients. *J Cardiovasc Electrophysiol.* 2008 Dec;19(12):1270-4.

Maron BJ, Thompson PD, Puffer JC, McGrew CA, Strong WB, Douglas PS, et al. Cardiovascular preparticipation screening of competitive athletes. A statement for health professionals from the Sudden Death Committee (clinical cardiology) and Congenital Cardiac Defects Committee (cardiovascular disease in the young), American Heart Association. *Circulation.* 1996;94:850–6.

Maron BJ, Shirani J, Poliac LC, Mathenge R, Roberts WC, Mueller FO. Sudden death in young competitive athletes. Clinical, demographic, and pathological profiles. *JAMA* 1996; 276:199-204.

Maron BJ, Haas TS, Doerer JJ, Thompson PD, Hodges JS. Comparison of U.S. And Italian experiences with sudden cardiac deaths in young competitive athletes and implications for preparticipation screening strategies. *Am J Cardiol.* 2009 Jul 15;104(2):276-80

McLeod KA, McLean. Implantation of a fully subcutaneous ICD in children. *Pacing Clin Electrophysiol.* 2010 Aug 17.

Meune C, Van Berlo JH, Anselme F, Bonne G, Pinto YM, Duboc D. Primary prevention of sudden death in patients with lamin A/C gene mutations. *N Engl J Med.* 2006;354:209–10.

Mihálcz A, Földesi C, Szili-Török T. Implantation of subcutaneous defibrillator in a patient treated for recidive endocarditis, previously operated for tetralogy of Fallot. *Orv Hetil.* 2008 Jun 8;149(23):1067-9.

Miyamoto A, Hayashi H, Makiyama T, Yoshino T, Mizusawa Y, Sugimoto Y, Ito M, Xue JQ, Murakami Y, Horie M. Risk determinants in individual with a spontaneous Type 1 Brugada syndrome ECG . *Circ J.* 2011 Mar 25;75(4):844-51.

Morrison TB, Ackerman MJ, Rea RF. Subacute perforation of the St. Jude Riata implantable cardioverter-defibrillator lead: a report of two pediatric cases. *Pediatr Cardiol.* 2009 Aug;30(6):834-6.

O'Connor FG, Kugler JP, Oriscello RG. Sudden death in young athletes: Screening for the needle in a haystack. *Am Fam Physician.* 1998;57:2763–70.

Peinado R, Torrecilla EG, Ormaetxe J, Alvarez M, Cózar R, Alzueta J; Working Group on Implantable Cardioverter-Defibrillators. Spanish Implantable Cardioverter-Defibrillator Registry. Fourth Official Report of the Spanish Society of Cardiology Working Group on Implantable Cardioverter-Defibrillators (2007). *Rev Española Cardiol.* 2008 Nov;61(11):1191-203.

Pignatelli RH, McMahon CJ, Dreyer WJ, et al. Clinical characterization of left ventricular noncompaction in children: a relatively common form of cardiomyopathy. *Circulation* 2003; 108:2672-78.

Proclemer A, Ghidina M, Facchin D, Rebellato L, Corrado D, Gasparini M, Gregori D. Use of implantable cardioverter-defibrillator in inherited arrhythmogenic diseases: data from Italian ICD Registry for the years 2001-6. *Pacing Clin Electrophysiol.* 2009 Apr;32(4):434-45.

Radbill AE, Triedman JK, Berul CI, Fynn-Thompson F, Atallah J, Alexander ME, Walsh EP, Cecchin F. System survival of nontransvenous implantable cardioverter-defibrillators compared to transvenous implantable cardioverter-defibrillators in pediatric and congenital heart disease patients. *Heart Rhythm* 2010;7(2):193-8.

Sandroni C, Nolan J. ERC 2010 Guidelines for adult and pediatric resucitation: summary of mayor changes. *Minerva Anestesiol.* 2011 Feb;77(2):220-6.

Saul JP, Epstein AE, Berul CI, Dick M 2nd, Dimarco JP, Friedman RA, Rosenthal E, Stephenson Ea, Vetter VL, American College of Cardiology; American Heart Association; Heart Rhythm Society; Pediatric and Congenital Electrophysiology Society. Heart Rhythm Society/Pediatric and Congenital Electrophysiology Society Clinical Competency Statement: training pathways for implantation of cardioverter-defibrillators and cardiac resynchronization therapy devices in pediatric and congenital heart patients. *Heart Rhythm.* 2008 Jun;5(6):926-33.

Schwartz PJ, Stramba-Badiale M, Crotti L, Pedrazzini M, Besana A, Bosi G, et al. Prevalence of the congenital long-QT syndrome. *Circulation.* 2009;120:1761–7.

Schwartz PJ, Priori SG, Spazzolini C, Moss AJ, Vincent GM, Napolitano C, et al. Genotype-phenotype correlation in the long-QT syndrome: Gene-specific triggers for life-threatening arrhythmias. *Circulation.* 2001;103:89–95

Schwartz PJ, Spazzolini C, Priori SG, Crotti L, Vicentini A, Landolina M, et al. Who are the long-QT syndrome patients who receive an implantable cardioverter-defibrillator and what happens to them?: Data from the European Long-QT Syndrome Implantable Cardioverter-Defibrillator (LQTS ICD) Registry. *Circulation* 2010;122:1272-82.

Sears SF, St Amant JB, Zeigler V. Psychosocial Considerations for Children and Young Adolescents with Implantable Cardioverter Defibrillators: An Update. *Pacing Clin Electrophysiol.* 2009 Jul; 32 Suppl 2:S80-2.

Sears SF, Hazelton AG, St Amant J, Matchett M, Kovacs A, Vazquez LD, Fairbrother D, Redfearn S, Hanisch D, Dubin A, Cannon BC, Fishbach P, Kanter R, Bryant RM. Quality of Life in Pediatric Patients With Implantable Cardioverter Defibrillators. *Am J Cardiol.* 2011 Apr 1;107(7):1023-7.

Shah MJ. Implantable cardioverter defibrillator-related complications in the pediatric population. *Pacing Clin Electrophysiol.* 2009 Jul;32 Suppl 2:S71-4.

Silvetti MS. Pacemaker and implantable cardioverter defibrillator implantation in pediatric patients. *Minerva Cardioangiol.* 2007 Dec;55(6):803-13.

Silka MJ. Sudden death due to cardiovascular disease during childhood. *Pediatr Ann.* 1991;20:360–7.

Stefanelli CB, Bradley DJ, Leroy S, Dick M 2nd, Serwer GA, Fischbach PS. Implantable cardioverter defibrillator therapy for life threatening arrhythmias in young patients. *J Intervent Cardiac Electrophysiol* 2002; 6:235–244.

Stephenson EA, Batra AJ, Knilans TK, Gow RM, Gradaus R, Balaji S, Dubin AM, et al. A Multicenter experience with novel implantable cardioverter defibrillator configurations in the pediatric and congenital heart disease populations. *J Cardiovasc Electrophysiol* 2006; 17:41–46.

Stöllberger C, Finsterer J. Arrhythmia and left ventricular hypertrabeculation/ noncompactation. *Cur Pharm Des.* 2010; 16(26): 2880-94.

Harkel AD, Blom NA, Reimer AG, et al. Implantable cardioverter defibrillator implantation in children in The Netherlands. *Eur J Pediatr* 2005; 164:436-441.

Tester DJ, Will ML, Haglund CM, Ackerman MJ. Compendium of cardiac channel mutations in 541 consecutive unrelated patients referred for long QT syndrome genetic testing. *Heart Rhythm.* 2005;2:507–17.

Tester DJ, Arya P, Will M, Haglund CM, Farley AL, Makielski JC, et al. Genotypic heterogeneity and phenotypic mimicry among unrelated patients referred for catecholaminergic polymorphic ventricular tachycardia genetic testing. *Heart Rhythm.* 2006;3:800–5.

Tomaske M, Gerritse B, Kretzers L, Pretre R, Dodge-Khatami A, Rahn M, Bauersfeld U. A 12-year experience of bipolar steroid-eluting epicardial pacing leads in children. *Ann Thorac Surg.* 2008 May; 85(5): 1704-11.

Tomaske M, Keller DI, Bauersfeld U. Sudden cardiac death: clinical evaluation of paediatric family members. *Europace.* 2011 Mar;13(3):421-6. 2010 Jul;3(3):261-6.

Vincent GM, Timothy KW, Leppert M, Keating M. The spectrum of symptoms and QT intervals in carriers of the gene for the long-QT syndrome. *New Engl J Med.* 1992;327:846–52.

Von Bergen NH, Atkins DL, Dick M 2nd, Bradley DJ, Etheridge SP, Saarel EV, Fischbach PS, Balaji S, Sreeram N, Evans WN, Law IH. Multicenter Study of the Effectiveness of Implantable Cardioverter Defibrillators in Children and Young Adults With Heart Disease. *Pediatr Cardiol.* 2011 Jan 6.

Welisch E, Cherlet E, Crespo-Martinez E, Hansky B.A single institution experience with pacemaker implantation in a pediatric population over 25 years. *Pacing Clin Electrophysiol.* 2010 Sep;33(9):1112-8.

William R. Wilson, MD, Georgia E. Greer, MSN, and Blair P. Grubb, MD. Implantable Cardioverter-Defibrillators in Children: A Single-Institutional Experience. *Ann Thorac Surg* 1998;65:775– 8.

Zartner PA, Wiebe W, Toussaint-Goetz N, Schneider MB. Lead removal in young patients in view of lifelong pacing. *Europace*. 2010 May;12(5):714-8.

12

ICD Implantations in the Pediatric and Young Adult Population

Ten Harkel Arend DJ and Blom Nico A
Leiden University Medical Center, Department of Pediatric Cardiology, Leiden, The Netherlands

1. Introduction

Large clinical trials in adult patients at risk for sudden cardiac death (SCD) have proven the efficacy of implantable cardioverter defibrillator (ICD) therapy for both secondary and primary prevention of SCD (Moss et al., 1996). In 1989, the first use of ICDs in young patients was reported (Kral et al., 1989). Since this initial report, ICD therapy has become increasingly important as a treatment approach in the pediatric population, despite the lack of randomized pediatric ICD studies. Nevertheless, children still present only 1% of all ICD recipients. The first large study of ICD implantations in patients below the age of 20 years was reported by Silka et al in 1993 (Silka et al., 1993). Since then many retrospective cohorts describing the clinical outcome of pediatric ICD therapy have been published. (Eicken et al., 2006; Ten Harkel et al., 2005; Heersche et al., 2010). More recently, two large multicenter studies evaluating the clinical outcome of ICD therapy in pediatrics and adults with congenital heart disease, including more than 200 children were published (Berul et al., 2008; Von Bergen et al., 2011). These studies have similar results, showing that ICD therapy in children appears to be effective, but with a higher rate of inappropriate shock therapy and complications as compared with adult series. The growing number of ICD implantations in children has now been followed by a decrease in the number of complications (Burns et al., 2011). Despite the lack of large randomized trials, efforts have been made to develop guidelines for ICD therapy in children. Recommendations for ICD therapy in primary and secondary prevention of SCD in adults have been formalized in the 2006 ACC/AHA guidelines (Zipes et al., 2006). Class I indications in pediatric and congenital heart disease (CHD) patients include aborted SCD without reversible cause. Sustained ventricular tachycardia (VT) associated with structural heart disease may be an ICD indication if not amenable to ablation or surgical resection (Blom 2008; Berul 2009; Zipes et al., 2006). In the following we will discuss the role of ICD treatment in children and young adults within different disease entities with an increased risk of SCD: 1) primary electrical heart disease; 2) cardiomyopathy, either hypertrophic or dilated; 3) operated or unoperated congenital heart disease. Finally, we will discuss the effect of ICD therapy on the quality of life and the different modalities of programming and implantation.

2. Primary electrical heart disease

Among the various disorders, presently known as primary electrical heart disease, the long-QT syndrome is by far the most prevalent among young patients. The congenital long-QT syndrome (LQTS) is a genetic channelopathy with variable penetrance and characterized by prolongation of the QT interval on the electrocardiogram. It is associated with increased propensity for polymorphic ventricular tachy-arrhythmias and SCD in young individuals with normal cardiac morphology (Goldenberg et al., 2010). To date, more than 500 mutations have been identified in 12 LQTS genotypes, with the LQTS type 1 (LQT1) and LQTS type 2 (LQT2) genotypes accounting for nearly 90% of identified cases. Although there is a continuous growth in the number of ICDs used to prevent fatal outcome associated with life-threatening arrhythmic episodes in LQTS patients the identification of patients that will profit most of ICD implantation remains a challenge. Long QT syndrome without symptoms is increasingly recognized as family members are screened. It has, however, been studied that the risk of death does not increase by the death of a sibling (Kaufman et al., 2008) It is, therefore, important that the decision to implant a defibrillator is based on the own risk factors of an LQTS patient (Kaufman et al., 2008). Previous studies of highly symptomatic patients were more worrisome. In the era of genetic testing and device implantation, overall mortality is low with treatment. Device therapy, although effective, is not without complications and should be reserved for high-risk patients (Etheridge et al., 2007).

The first-line treatment of patients with LQTS remains the use of beta-blockers. These have been shown to be very effective especially in LQT1 and LQT2 patients in the prevention of cardiovascular events. However, in large studies a substantial number of LQTS patients were not treated by beta-blockers before ICD implantation. (Goldenberg et al., 2010). In high-risk patients beta-blockers reduce the risk of adverse events by about 70% (Goldenberg et al., 2010). These findings underscore the fact that beta-blocker therapy should be routinely administered in all high risk LQT1 and LQT2 patients without contraindications as a first line measure (Goldenberg et al., 2010). Patients with syncope during beta-blocker therapy are at high risk of life-threatening events, and ICD therapy should be considered in these patients. The risk of beta-blocker failure is highest in young children and in women (Jons et al., 2010).

There is a continuous growth in the number of ICDs in this patient group (Schwartz & Crotti 2008). Potentially, life-saving therapies were rendered at a 5% to 6% per year rate among those selected for ICD therapy. Similar inappropriate shock frequencies were also noted. Secondary prevention, genotype, and QTc predicted those most likely to receive appropriate therapy. In a recent study about ICD implantations in LQTS patients Schwartz et al showed that especially among the LQT3 subtype many patients were asymptomatic before ICD implantation, and probably did not need one (Schwartz et al., 2010). They showed that some patients in whom an ICD was implanted the supposed high risk was questionable. Although the ICD implant frequency is greatest among LQT3 patients, the greatest save rate has occurred among LQT2 women who were assessed to be at high risk (Horner et al., 2010).

However, when used in a high-risk LQTS population, ICD therapy seems to be a safe option (Monnig et al., 2005). Risk factors for appropriate ICD shocks are longer QTc intervals and being survivors of a cardiac arrest. However, betablockers should always be added to ICD therapy, while some patients might benefit from additional antibradycardia pacing, prolonged detection time, and a rate-smoothing algorithm to prevent recurrent episodes (Monnig et al., 2005).

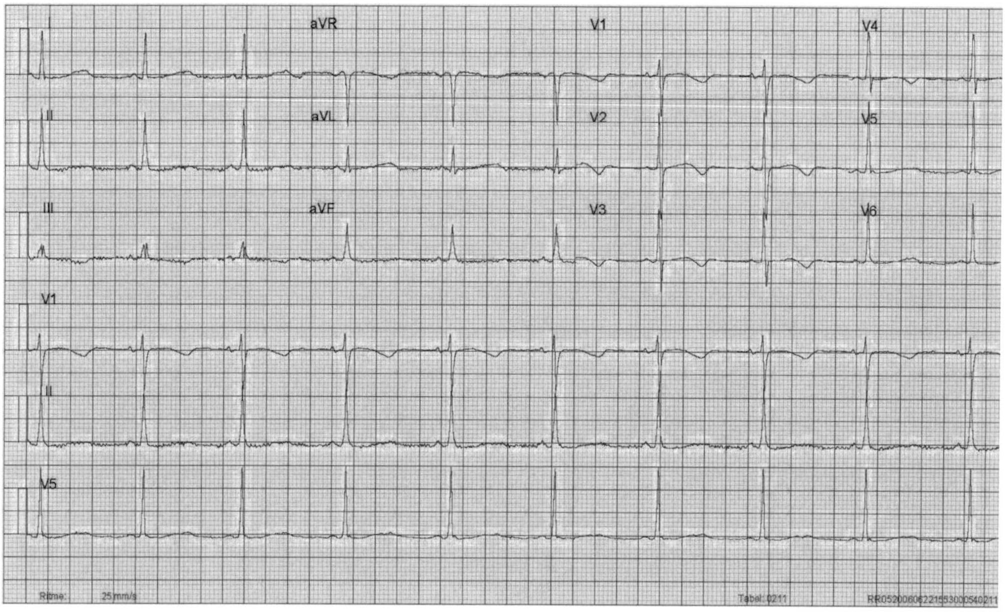

Fig. 1. Electrocardiogram of a 20-year old woman with the long-QT syndrome. A prolongation of the QT-interval of 520 msec is shown (normally less than 440 msec).

3. Hypertrophic cardiomyopathy

ICDs have proven effective in preventing SCD in young hypertrophic cardiomyopathy (HCM) patients with appropriate intervention rates of 11% for secondary and 4% for primary prevention, despite massive left ventricular (LV) hypertrophy, LV outflow obstruction, diastolic dysfunction or microvascular ischemia. Targeting candidates for prophylactic ICD therapy can be complex, compounded by the unpredictability of the arrhythmogenic substrate, the absence of a dominant risk factor, and difficulty in assembling randomized trials. However, a single major risk factor is often sufficient to justify an ICD, although additional markers and other disease features can resolve ambiguous decision-making. Nevertheless, the absence of all risk factors does not convey absolute immunity to SCD. However, when presenting with a normal electrocardiogram the patients seem at lower risk for cardiac events (McLeod et al., 2009).

Until now, there is, however, no consensus as to the indication for primary prevention with ICD implantation in children (Ostman-Smith 2010). Especially a high rate of inappropriate shocks up to 27% and a complication rate up to 17% necessitate careful considerations when an ICD implantation is to be planned in the pediatric age group (Ostman-Smith 2010).

The primary prevention risk factors in HCM are 1) family history of HCM related SCDs. When a high risk population that received primary prevention with ICD implantation was studied the number of appropriate shocks during follow-up did not differ between those with a family history of HCM related SCD, whether as an isolated risk factor or combined with other risk factors (Bos et al., 2010); 2) episodes of unexplained, recent syncope; 3) massive LV hypertrophy >30 mm; 4) nonsustained VT on ambulatory 24-hour Holter ECGs;

5) hypotensive or attenuated blood pressure response to exercise (Maron 2010). In addition, Gimeno et al recently showed that ventricular arrhythmias during exercise increased the risk of SCD as well (Gimeno et al., 2009). However, patients who survive cardiac arrest may remain asymptomatic for prolonged periods after the first cardiac event, underscoring the unpredictability of the arrhythmogenic substrate in these patients.

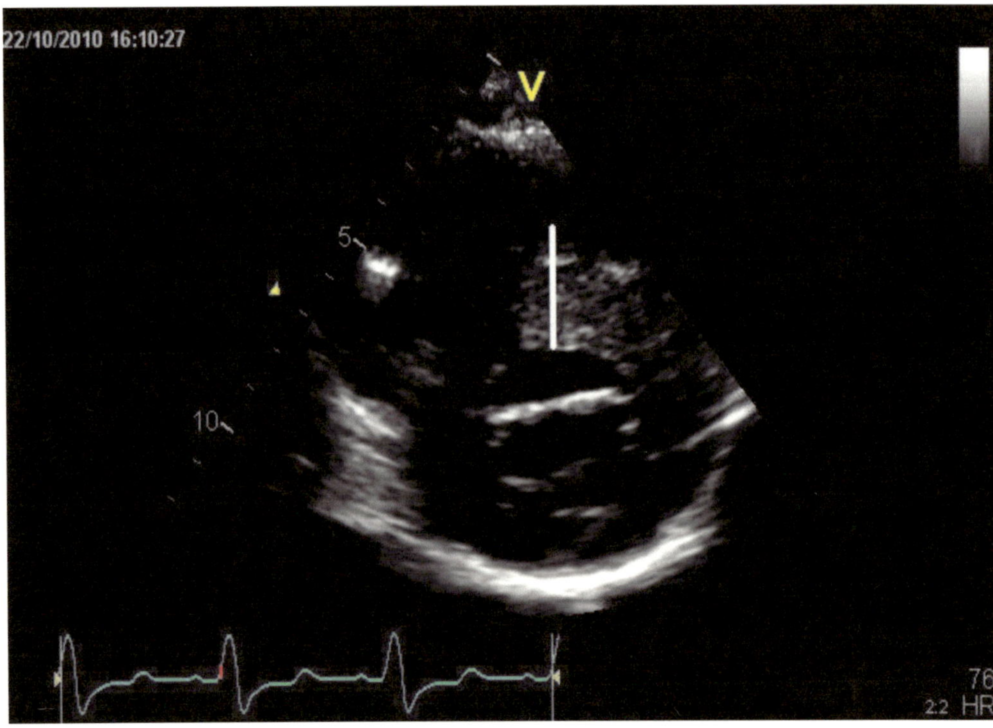

Fig. 2. Short axis of the left ventricle by echocardiography of a 14-year old boy with hypertrophic cardiomyopathy. There is a thickness of 30 mm (normally less than 11 mm).

In children, the risk of non-sudden cardiac death is as high as sudden cardiac death. Extreme left ventricular hypertrophy and a blunted blood pressure response to exercise are risk factors (Decker et al., 2009). Risk factors for SCD are extreme left ventricular hypertrophy on the electrocardiogram and a septal thickness over 190% of normal, with a sensitivity of 91% and a specificity of 78% (Ostman-Smith et al., 2005). Children may be at risk for SCD already at young age, and should therefore be screened early in hypertrophic cardiomyopathy families (Ostman-Smith et al., 2008).

When evaluating HCM patients who underwent ICD placement the number of complications is considerable (Lin et al., 2009). In the study of Lin et al 181 patients with a mean age of 44 years were investigated. During a follow-up period of 5 years, 65 patients (36%) had a total of 88 device related complications including 42 (23%) patients with inappropriate shocks. Younger age and atrial fibrillation were associated with an increased risk of inappropriate ICD discharges. It is concluded that the high incidence of complications should be taken into account when considering ICD implantation in a high-risk HCM patient (Lin et al., 2009).

4. Congenital heart disease

Although most patients who are being operated for their congenital heart disease presently survive their surgery and lead a relatively normal life, a substantial portion of patients develop symptoms of heart failure or rhythm abnormalities in due time. In adult patients with ischemic or non-ischemic cardiomyopathy an LV ejection fraction below 30% is considered a clear indication for primary prevention with ICD implantation (Moss et al., 2002; Bardy et al., 2005). Risk stratification for primary prevention remains highly complex and is usually individualized, based on a variety of surgical, hemodynamic, electrocardiographic, and electrophysiologic factors (McLeod et al., 2010). However, some authors advocate that also for patients with congenital heart disease an LV ejection fraction below 30% as single risk factor is sufficient reason to implant an ICD (Silka & Bar-Cohen 2008), which is argued by others (Triedman 2008). Since the overall rate of SCD is 5 to 10 times lower than that observed in high-risk cardiomyopathy patients, the life expectancy in CHD patients is much larger. Furthermore, in CHD patients vascular access is often difficult, and the rate of device associated cardiac events and lead-failure is much higher, and they have variable cardiac anatomy. Therefore, the results of the large ICD trials cannot simply be extrapolated to the population of CHD patients. Other risk factors have to be taken into account before deciding to implant an ICD (Triedman 2008). With the increasing knowledge of rhythm abnormalities in congenital heart disease and the emergence of interventional electrophysiologic techniques some ventricular arrhythmias can be treated by catheter ablation (Walsh 2007). ICD implantation remains to be limited to otherwise untreatable rhythm abnormalities.

In a study of Yap et al more than 60% of the patients with an ICD and a congenital heart disease had a tetralogy of Fallot (Yap et al.,. 2007). However, the overall complication rate in the Fallot patients was higher as compared to other congenital heart defects, the number of inappropriate shocks was high (40%), while the number of appropriate shocks was low as compared to other patients (18% versus 33%). When compared with an older ICD population with dilated cardiomyopathy (DCM), the Tetralogy of Fallot patients were more likely to have experienced oversensing (45 vs. 13%; $P < 0.02$), inappropriate anti-tachycardia pacing delivery (20 vs. 2%; $P < 0.05$), and inappropriate cardioversion (25 vs. 4%; $P = 0.06$) and less likely to receive appropriate therapies (Witte et al., 2008). On the other hand, Khairy et al studied 121 Fallot patients who received an ICD for primary (N=68) or secondary (N=53) prevention. During follow-up the number of appropriate shocks was considerable (30% of patients). This was, however, at the cost of a 5.8% yearly incidence of inappropriate shocks, and the occurrence of complications in 36 patients, mostly (70%) lead-related (Khairy et al., 2008). In Fallot patients with unstable ventricular tachycardia, their rhythm abnormalities may in some patients be treated by catheter ablation (Kriebel et al., 2007).

5. ICD programming

In children with ICDs, the risk of inappropriate shock therapy is significantly higher as compared to adult studies. Pediatric ICD series with mean intervals of follow-up between 29 and 51 months have reported 20% to 50% inappropriate shock therapy. These shocks may have a negative impact on the quality of life, and can induce secondary arrhythmias.

	Tomaske 2008	Stephenson 2006	Kriebel 2006	Cannon 2006
Number	15	22	8	8
Age (yr)	12.5	8.9	0.3-8	1-29
Weight (kg)	36.5	25.5	4-29	
Follow-up (mo)	22	29	14.5	22
Appr Shocks	4	7	2	2
Inappr Shocks	3	4	0	3
Revision	4	7	2	3

Table 1. Outcomes of extracardiac ICD implantations in young patients and patients with congenital heart disease. Results are comparable to transvenous approaches.

Inappropriate shocks in children are mostly caused by sinus tachycardia or supraventricular tachycardia. High sinus rates up to 200 per minute are not uncommon in children and patients with congenital heart disease have a high incidence of atrial arrhythmias, mostly intraatrial reentrant tachycardia. Implantation of a dual chamber ICD system can potentially reduce the incidence of inappropriate discharges attributable to the misclassification of sinus tachycardia or supraventricular tachycardia as a ventricular event. In a recent multicenter study the difference of appropriate and inappropriate shocks in a single chamber or dual chamber device in patients <30 years old was investigated (Lawrence et al., 2009). The authors found no differences between single chamber or dual chamber systems regarding the occurrence of appropriate or inappropriate shocks, irrespective of underlying cardiovascular disorder or type of ICD system. (Lawrence et al., 2009). T-wave sensing is another important cause of inappropriate shock therapy especially in the group of patients with long QT syndrome. Exercise tests are required to obtain maximal heart rate and to evaluate T wave sensing during high heart rates. QRS discrimination or atrial discrimination algorithms can be helpful tools to prevent some of these problems. β-blockade can also be a practical therapy to avoid inappropriate ICD shock for supraventricular tachycardias or sinus tachycardia. However, the most important measure to reduce inappropriate shocks is careful ICD programming of the individual child with regard to detection rate and time immediately after ICD implantation. In a recent article several programming tips have been given (Khairy & Mansour 2011). Since sinus tachycardia and supraventricular tachycardia may have frequencies as high as 200 bpm, most young patients have a ventricular fibrillation zone programmed up to 220 bpm. Concerning detection times there is a compromise between overtreating otherwise self-terminating events and delaying therapy for potentially unstable arrhythmias. Detection times as long as 18 of 24 intervals or even 30 of 40 intervals have been advocated with no increase in adverse events. Antitachycardia pacing (ATP) has been shown to be effective in the majority of congenital heart disease patients, thereby lowering the number of shocks.

Although routine testing of the defibrillation threshold (DFT) is not necessary during follow-up of pediatric ICD patients, any clinical change or problem should be evaluated immediately and DFT testing should also be considered in this situation. (Theuns & Gold, 2010). In young children with subcutaneous ICD systems regular DFT testing should be considered during growth.

6. Complications

There seem to be differences in the frequency of ICD-related complications between children and adults. However, due to the small number of patients in pediatric series it is difficult to estimate the true incidence of ICD related complications in children. (Shah et al., 2009). Implantation procedure-related complications include pocket infection, pocket hematoma, microdislodgement requiring lead manipulation , hemothorax, superior vena cava syndrome, pneumonia, electromechanical dissociation requiring cardiopulmonary resuscitation and second degree burns from repeated external rescue shocks (Shah et al., 2009). Especially the number of infections seem to be higher in children as compared to adults (Link et al., 1999). The most common ICD system related adverse effect is the high incidence of inappropriate shocks and a high incidence of lead failures in children. Inappropriate shocks are usually related to the occurrence of sinus tachycardia, supraventricular tachycardia, T wave oversensing or QRS complex double sensing. Lead failures are strongly related to the size of the patient. The youngest and smallest patients have the highest risk of lead complications. Furthermore, higher levels of exercise and activity in the pediatric population may increase the amount of lead problems.

7. Mode of ICD implantation

In children or young patients with congenital heart defects it is often not possible to make use of routine transvenous ICD systems. Underlying causes are the size of the patient or structural heart diseases with residual intracardiac shunts and abnormal systemic venous pathways. Various modifications have been used to implant ICDs in patients with limited venous access (Cannon et al., 2006; Bove et al., 2010; Greene et al., 2004; Kriebel et al., 2006; Stephenson et al., 2006; Tomaske et al., 2008). These include subcutaneous patches, epicardial and pleural lead positioning, use of the subxiphoid incision, or direct transatrial approach. It is important that the technique used is individualized in the diverse population of children and young patients with congenital heart disease in need for ICD placement (Stephenson et al., 2006). Recently, Radbill et al compared the use of transvenous ICDs with nontransvenous systems in a group of pediatric and congenital heart disease patients (Radbill et al., 2010). Although no differences were reported considering appropriate or inappropriate shocks there was a significantly higher amount of ICD system failure in the nontransvenous group. System survival at 12, 24, and 36 months was 73%, 55% and 49% in the nontransvenous group compared to 91%, 83% and 76% in the transvenous group. Causes of system failure in the nontransvenous group included pace-sense lead failure, shock coil failure, generator migration, and loosened set-screw connection.

Recently, the search for avoidance of transvenous lead placement has resulted in the development of an entirely subcutaneous ICD system (Bardy et al., 2010). The system consists of a parasternal electrode and a left lateral thoracic pulse generator. In a trial of 55 adult patients it was shown as effective in terminating ventricular tachyarrhythmias with little complications during a 10-month follow-up period. This subcutaneous ICD system can also be used in older children and has been reported in two children of 10 and 12 years old (34 and 35 kg body weight) (McLeod and McLean 2010). In both children this device was implanted without complications, and no adverse events occurred during an 8- and 5-month follow-up period (McLeod & McLean 2010).

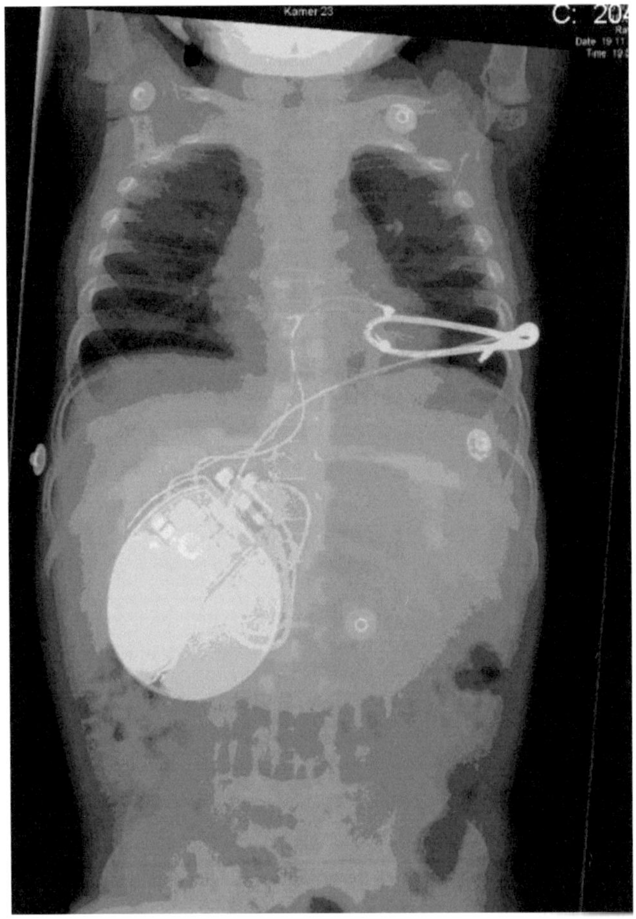

Fig. 3. Chest X-ray of a 6-month old child with an ICD. The active can is placed abdominally, and the pacing wires are placed epicardially. A subcutaneous patch is in use for eventual shocks.

Another approach is the placement of the ICD in the axilla. The usual infraclavicular placement of a transvenous ICD can cause a quite visible scar with a suboptimal cosmetic result. Furthermore, straps can rub and cause irritation at this site (Collins et al., 2009; Rausch et al., 2010). In a large retrospective review it was shown that there were no differences between the axillary and infraclavicular technique in implant characteristics, lead longevity, implant complications, lead fractures or dislodgements, inappropriate ICD discharges, or device infections (Rausch et al., 2010).

8. Home monitoring

Since 2000 a remote control system was introduced for the follow-up of ICD patients. Through this system data from the implanted device are transmitted to a website once a day as well as immediately following an arrhythmia. By this method changes in ICD function, lead problems, and asymptomatic arrhythmias can be detected earlier without the patient actually visiting the hospital. It has been shown that the events as send by the home monitoring system show excellent comparability to the data as obtained by standard clinical evaluation (Perings et al., 2011). The home monitoring system can detect several, otherwise asymptomatic episodes enhancing prompt detection of for instance lead problems and facilitates management decisions (Varma et al., 2010). Most patients show a high level of acceptance and satisfaction of this new system after a mean follow-up period of 1 year, with only some refusing the home monitoring (Ricci et al., 2010). Until now, however, this system has mostly been used in the adult population, and data about the appropriateness in pediatrics are as yet lacking.

9. Quality of life

With the increasing number of ICDs in young patients the psychological effects has been studied as early as 1996 (Dubin et al., 1996). Nearly 75% of the patients felt their health was good to excellent with 40% reporting improvement since ICD implantation. All felt capable of performing daily activities (Dubin et al., 1996).

The implantation of an ICD has a great impact on the quality of life of these patients. These psychological effects have sofar been investigated by many authors (Herrmann et al., 1997). The poor psychosocial outcome in these patients may be related to the underlying cardiovascular condition (Burke et al., 2003), or it may be the effect of surviving an out of hospital cardiac arrest, not related to the treatment received (Kamphuis et al., 2002). It has been found that the lasting psychological distress will not dissipate spontaneously or naturally and that psychosocial intervention may be warranted (Kamphuis et al., 2003). The most common psychological problems are depression and anxiety. Depressive symptoms persist over time, and are associated with a higher incidence of shock therapy (Suzuki et al., 2010). However, concerns about the ICD has been found a predictor of psychological morbidity independently of the number of shocks (Pedersen et al., 2005). On the other hand, Luyster et al found no relation between number of shocks and anxiety (Luyster et al., 2006). They found especially a higher level of perceived resource loss to be associated with higher levels of both anxiety and depression (Luyster et al., 2006).

The growing pediatric ICD population stresses the need to evaluate the quality of life in this group of ICD recipients. Adult patients with ICDs show significantly worse psychological and physical functioning. Behavioral changes have been reported such as reduced activity, avoidance, depression, and anxiety, especially in those who had received ICD shocks. These finding in adults could not be confirmed in a recent study in a group of pediatric ICD recipients. In this study, cardiac illness severity and ICD shock therapy were not significantly associated with anxiety, depression, quality of life, or family functioning.

Recently, we have also evaluated health-related quality of life study in 30 Dutch pediatric ICD recipients using different quality of life questionnaires. This study showed that pediatric ICD recipients showed more problems in the domains of motor functioning, sleep, work/school, negative emotions, and anxiety. Furthermore, worry and anxiety were significantly associated with the number of ICD shocks (unpublished data). These findings indicate that avoidance or reduction of inappropriate shocks is one of the most important steps to improve quality of life. Furthermore, it emphasizes the need of proper guidance and, if necessary, implementation of psychological interventions. Screening for cardiovascular diseases may have its own impact, Children who were genetically tested carriers showed to have a reduced psychological well-being (Smets et al., 2008).

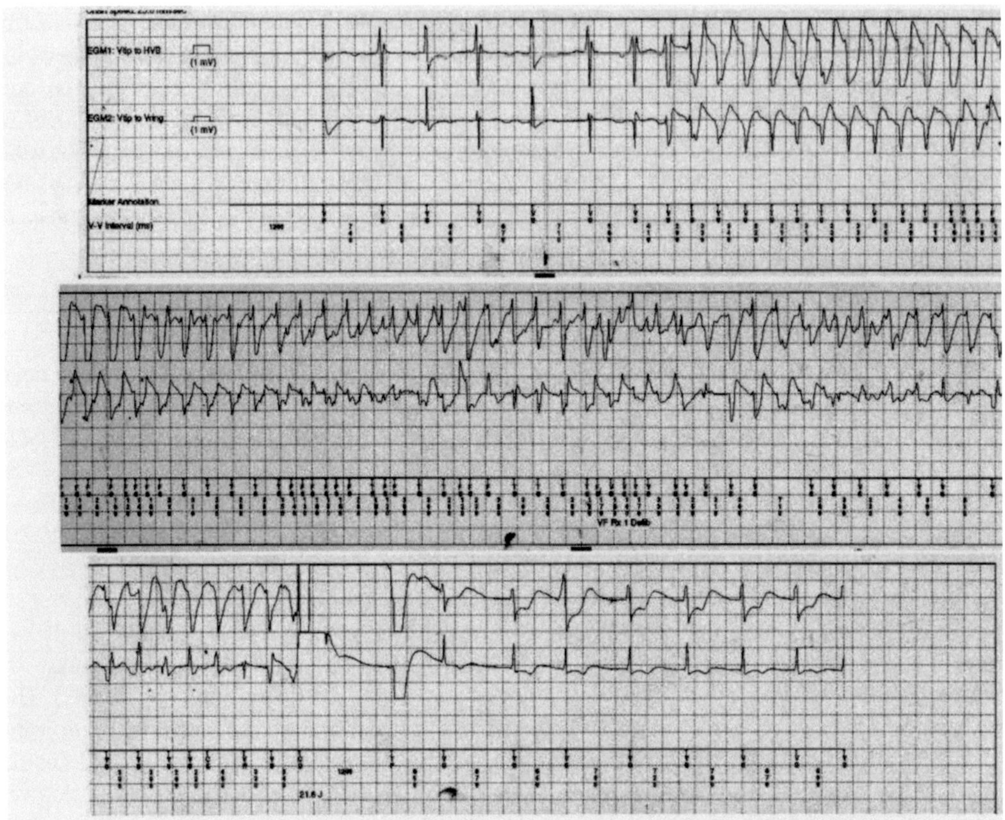

Fig. 4. An ICD strip of an appropriate shock is shown. Fast ventricular tachycardia is followed by a 21-J shock which terminated the tachycardia. This is followed by an escape rhythm with broad QRS complexes.

10. Conclusions

ICD implantations are increasingly performed in children and young adults with a variety of underlying cardiac disorders. Although the effectiveness of ICD therapy in this specific population is good, there are concerns about the high number of inappropriate shocks and lead problems. New developments include the complete subcutaneous device and home monitoring systems. Although the overall quality of life usually is good, several patients need psychological support, and this support has to be included in regular follow-up programs.

11. References

Bardy GH, Lee KL, Mark DB, Poole JE, Packer DL, Boineau R, Domanski M, Troutman C, Anderson J, Johnson G, McNulty SE, Clapp-Channing N, Davidson-Ray LD, Fraulo ES, Fishbein DP, Luceri RM, Ip JH. (2005) Sudden Cardiac Death in Heart Failure Trial (SCD-HeFT) Investigators. Amiodarone or an implantable cardioverter-defibrillator for congestive heart failure. *N Engl J Med* 352: 225–237.

Bardy GH, Smith WM, Hood MA, Grozier IG, Melton IC, Jordaens L, Theuns D, Park RE, Wright DJ, Connelly DT, Fynn SP, Murgatroyd FD, Sperzel J, Neuzner J, Spitzer SG, Ardashev AV, Oduro A, Boersma L, Maass AH, Van Gelder IC, Wilde AA, Van Dessel PF, Knops RE, Barr CS, Lupo P, Cappato R, Grace AA. (2010) An entirely subcutaneous implantable cardioverter-defibrillator *New Engl J Med* 363:36-44.

Berul CL. (2009) Implantable cardioverter defibrillator criteria for primary and secondary prevention of pediatric sudden cardiac death. *PACE* 32:S67-S70.

Berul CL, Van Hare GF, Kertesz NJ, Dubin AM, Cecchin F, Collins KK, Cannon BC, Alexander ME, Triedman JK, Walsh EP, Friedman RA. (2008) Results of a multicenter retrospective implantable cardioverter-defibrillator registry of pediatric and congenital heart disease patients. *J Am Coll Cardiol* 51:1685-1691.

Blom NA. (2008) Implantable cardioverter-defibrillators in children. *PACE* 31:S32-S34.

Bos JM, Maron BJ, Ackerman MJ, Haas TS, Sorajji P, Nishimura RA, Gersh BJ, Ommen SR. (2010) Role of family history of sudden death in risk stratification and prevention of sudden death with implantable defibrillators in hypertrophic cardiomyopathy. *Am J Cardiol* 106:1481-1486.

Botsch MP, Franzbach B, Opgen-Rhein B, Berger F, Will JC. (2010) ICD therapy in children and young adults: low incidence of inappropriate shick delivery. *PACE* 33:734-741.

Bove T, Francois K, De Caluwe W, Suys B, De Wolf D. (2010) Effective cardioverter defibrillator implantation in children without thoracotomy: a valid alternative. *Ann Thorac Surg* 89:1307-1309.

Burke JL, Hallas CN, Clark-Carter D, White D, Connelly D. (2003) The psychosocial impact of the implantable cardioverter defibrillator: A meta-analytic review. *British Journal of Health Psychology* 8:165-178.

Burns KM, Evans F, Kaltman JR. (2011) Pediatric ICD utilization in the United States from 1997 to 2006. *Heart Rhythm* 8:23-28.

Cannon BC, Friedman RA, Fenrich AL, Fraser CD, McKenzie ED, Kertesz NJ. (2006) Innovative techniques for placement of implantable cardioverter defibrillator leads in patients with limited venous access to the heart. *PACE* 29:181-187.

Collins KK, Runciman M, Rausch CM, Schaffer MS. (2009) Toward improved cosmetic results: a novel technique for the placement of a pacemaker or internal cardioverter/ defibrillator generators in the axilla of young patients. *Pediatr Cardiol* 30:1157-1160.

Daubert JP, Zareba W, Rosero SZ, Budzikowski A, Robinson JL, Moss AJ. (2007) Role of implantable cardioverter defibrillator therapy in patients with long QT syndrome. *Am Heart J* 153:553-558.

Decker JA, Rossano JW, Smith O, Cannon B, Clunie SK, Gates C, Jefferies JL, Kim JJ, Price JF, Dreyer WJ, Towbin JA, Denfield SW. (2009) Risk factors and mode of death in isolated hypertrophic cardiomyopathy in children. *J Am Coll Cardiol* 54:250-254.

DeMaso DR, Lauretti A, Spieth L, Van Der Feen JR, Jay KS, Gauvreau K, Walsh EP, Berul CI. (2004) Psychosocial factors and quality of life in children and adolescents with implantable cardioverter-defibrillators. *Am J Cardiol* 93:582-587.

Dubin AM, Batsford WP, Lewis RJ, Rosenfeld LE. (1996) Quality-of-life in patients receiving implantable cardioverter defibrillators at or before age 40. *PACE* 19:1555-1559.

Eicken A, Kolb C, Lange S, Brodherr-Heberlein S, Zrenner B, Schreiber C, Hess J. (2006) Implantable cardioverter defibrillator (ICD) in children. *Int J Cardiol* 107:30-35.

Etheridge SP, Sanatani S, Cohen MI, Albaro CA, Saarel EV, Bradley DJ. (2007) Long QT syndrome in children in the era of implantable defibrillators. *J Am Coll Cardiol* 50:1335-1340.

Gimeno JR, Tome-Esteban M, Lofiego C, Hurtado J, Pantazis A, Mist B, Lamblase P, McKenna WJ, Elliott PM. (2009) Exercise-induced ventricular arrhythmias and risk of sudden cardiac death in patients with hypertrophic cardiomyopathy. *Eur Heart J* 30:2599-2605.

Goldenberg I, Bradley J, Moss A, McNitt S, Polonsky S, Robinson JL, Andrews M, Zareba W. (2010) Beta-blocker efficacy in high-risk patients with the congenital long-QT syndrome types 1 and 2: implications for patient management. *J Cardiovasc Electrophysiol* 21:893-901.

Greene AE, Moak JP, Di Russo G, Berger JT, Heshmat Y, Kuehl KS. (2004) Transcutaneous implantation of an internal cardioverter defibrillator in a small infant with recurrent myocardial ischemia and cardiac arrest simulating sudden infant death syndrome. *PACE* 27:112-116.

Heersche JHM, Blom NA, Van de Heuvel F, Blank C, Reimer AG, Clur SA, Witsenburg M, Ten Harkel ADJ. (2010) Implantable cardioverter defibrillator therapy for prevention of sudden cardiac death in children in The Netherlands. *PACE* 33:179-185.

Herrmann C, von zur Mühen F, Buss U, Kemper S, Wantzen C, Gonska BD. (1997) Standardized assessment of psychological well-being and quality-of-life in patients with implanted defibrillators. *PACE* 20:95-103.

Horner JM, Kinoshita M, Webster TL, Haglund CM, Friedman PA, Ackerman MJ. (2010) Implantable cardioverter defibrillator therapy for congenital long QT syndrome: a single-center experience. *Heart Rhythm* 7:1616-1622.

Jons C, Moss AJ, Goldenberg I, Liu J, McNitt S, Zareba W, Qi M, Robinson JL. (2010) Risk of fatal arrhythmic events in long QT syndrome patients after syncope. *J Am Coll Cardiol* 55:783-788.

Kamphuis HCM, de Leeuw JRJ, Derksen R, Hauer R, Winnubst JAM. (2002) A 12-month quality of life assessment of cardiac arrest survivors treated with or without an implantable cardioverter defibrillator. *Europace* 4:417-425.

Kamphuis HCM, de Leeuw JRJ, Derksen R, Hauer RNW, Winnubst JAM. (2003) Implantable cardioverter defibrillator recipients: quality of life in recipients with and without ICD shock delivery: A prospective study. *Europace* 5:381-389.

Kaufman ES, McNitt S, Moss AJ, Zareba W, Robinson JL, Hall WJ, Ackerman MJ, Benhorin J, Locati ET, Napolitano C, Priori SG, Schwartz PJ, Towbin JA, Vincent GM, Zhang L. (2008) Risk of death in the long QT syndrome when a sibling has died. *Heart Rhythm* 5:831-836.

Khairy P & Mansour F. (2011) Implantable cardioverter-defibrillators in congenital heart disease: 10 programming tips. *Heart Rhythm.*

Khairy P, Harris L, Landzberg MJ, Viswanathan S, Barlow A, Gatzoulis MA, Fernandes SM, Beauchesne L, Therrien J, Chetaille P, Gordon E, Muhll IV, Cecchin F. (2008) Implantable cardioverter-defibrillatos in tetralogy of Fallot. *Circulation* 117:363-370.

Kral MA, Spotnitz HM, Hordof A, Bigger JT Jr, Steinberg JS, Livelli FD Jr. (1989) Automatic implantable cardioverter defibrillator implantation for malignant ventricular arrhythmias associated with congenital heart disease. *Am J Cardiol.* 63:118-9.

Kriebel T, Ruschewski W, Gonzalez M, Walter K, Kroll J, Kampmann C, Heinemann M, Schneider H, Paul T. (2006) ICD implantation in infants and small children. The extracardiac technique. *PACE* 29:1319-1325.

Kriebel T, Saul JP, Schneider H, Sigler M, Paul T. (2007) Radiocontact mapping and radiofrequency catheter ablation of fast and hemodynamically unstable ventricular tachycardia after surgical repair of tetralogy of Fallot. *J Am Coll Cardiol* 50:2162-2168.

Lawrence D, Von Bergen N, Law IH, Bradley DJ, Dick II M, Frias PA, Streiper MJ, Fischbach PS. (2009) Inappropriate ICD discharges in single-chamber versus dual-chamber devices in the pediatric and young adult population. *J Cardiovasc Electrophysiol* 20:287-290.

Lin G, Nishimura RA, Gersh BJ, Phil D, Ommen SR, Ackerman MJ, Brady PA. (2009) Device complications and inappropriate implantable cardioverter defibrillator shocks in patients with hypertrophic cardiomyopathy. *Heart* 95:709-714.

Link MS, Hill SL, Cliff DL, Swygman CA, Foote CB, Homoud MK, Wang PJ, Estelli M, Berul CI. (1999) Comparison of frequency of complications of implantable cardioverter-defibrillators in children versus adults. *Am J Cardiol* 83:263-266.

Luyster FS, Hughes JW, Waechter D, Josephson R. (2006) Resource Loss Predicts Depression and Anxiety Among Patients Treated With an Implantable Cardioverter Defibrillator. *Psychosom Med* 68:794-800.

Maron BJ. (2010) Risk stratification and role of implantable defibrillators for prevention of sudden death in patients with hypertrophic cardiomyopathy. *Circ J* 74:2271-2282.

Maron BJ, Haas TS, Shannon KM, Almquist AK, Hodges JS. (2009) Long-term survival after cardiac arrest in hypertrophic cardiomyopathy. *Heart Rhythm* 6:993-997.

McLeod KA & McLean A. (2010) Implantation of a fully subcutaneous ICD in children. *PACE* 1-4.

McLeod CJ, Ackerman MJ, Nishimura RA, Tajik AJ, Gersh BJ, Ommen SR. (2009) Outcome of patients with hypertrophic cardiomyopathy and a normal electrocardiogram. *J Am Coll Cardiol* 54:229-233.

McLeod CJ, Kapa S, Asirvatham SJ. (2010) Implantable cardioverter-defibrillator therapy in congenital heart disease. *Expert Rev Med Devices* 7:1-3.

Monnig G, Kobe J, Loher A, Eckardt L, Wedekind H, Scheld HH, Haverkamp W, Milberg P. Breithardt G, Schulze-Bahr E, Bocker D. (2005) Implantable cardioverter-defibrillator therapy in patients with congenital long-QT syndrome: a long-term follow-up. *Heart Rhythm* 2:497-504.

Moss AJ, Zareba W, Hall WJ, Klein H, Wilber DJ, Cannon DS, Daubert JP, Higgins SL, Brown MW, Andrews ML; Multicenter Automatic Defibrillator Implantation Trial II Investigators. (2002) Prophylactic implantation of a defibrillator in patients with myocardial infarction and reduced ejection fraction. *N Engl J Med.* 346: 877–883.

Moss AJ, Hall WJ, Cannon DS, Daubert JP, Higgins SL, Klein H, Levine JH, Saksena S, Waldo AL, Wilber D, Brown MW, Heo M. (1996) Improved survival with an implanted defibrillator in patients with coronary disease at high risk for ventricular arrhythmia. Multicenter Automatic Defibrillator Implantation Trial Investigators. *N Engl J Med.* 335:1933-40.

Ostman-Smith I, Wettrell G, Keeton B, Riesenfeld T, Holmgren D, Ergander U. (2005) Echocardiographic and electrocardiographic identification of those children with hypertrophic cardiomyopathy who should be considered at high-risk of dying suddenly. *Cardiol Young* 15:632-642.

Ostman-Smith I, Wettrell G, Keeton B, Holmgren D, Ergander U, Gould S, Bowker C, Verdicchio M. (2008) Age- and gender-specific mortality rates in childhood hypertrophic cardiomyopathy. *Eur Heart J* 29:1160-1167.

Ostman-Smith I. (2010) Hypertrophic cardiomyopathy in childhood and adolescence – strategies to prevent sudden death. *Fundam Clin Pharmacol* 24:637-652.

Pedersen SS, van Domburg RT, Theuns DAMJ, Jordaens L, Erdman RAM. (2005) Concerns about the implantable cardioverter defibrillator: A determinant of anxiety and depressive symptoms independent of experienced shocks. *Am Heart J* 149:664-669.

Perings C, Bauer WR, Bondke HJ, Mewis C, James M, Bocker D, Broadhurst P, Korte T, Toft E, Hintringer F, Clementy J, Schwab JO. (2011) Remote monitoring of implantable-cardioverter defibrillator: results from the reliability of IEGM online interpretation (RIONI) study. *Europace* 13:221-229.

Radbill AE, Triedman JK, Berul CI, Fynn-Thompson F, Atallah J, Alexander ME, Walsh EP, Cecchin F. (2010) System survival of nontransvenous implantable cardioverter-defibrillators compared to transvenous implantable cardioverter-defibrillators in pediatric and congenital heart disease patients. *Heart Rhythm* 7:193-198.

Rausch CM, Hughes BH, Runciman M, Law IH, Bradley DJ, Sujeev M, Duke A, Schaffer M, Collins KK. (2010) Axillary versus infraclavicular placement for endocardial heart rhythm devices in patients with pediatric and congenital heart disease. *Am J Cardiol* 106:1646-1651.

Ricci RP, Morichelli L, Quarta L, Sassi A, Porfill A, Laudadio MT, Gargaro A, Santini M. (2010) Long-term patient acceptance of and satisfaction with implanted device remote monitoring. *Europace* 12:674-679.

Schwartz PJ & Crotti L. (2008) Ion channel diseases in children: manifestations and management. *Curr Opin Cardiol* 23:184-191.

Schwartz PJ, Spazzolini C, Priori SG, Crotti L, Vicentini A, Landolina M, Gasparini M, Wilde AAM, Knops RE, Denjoy I, Toivonen L, Monnig G, Al-Fayyadh M, Jordaens L, Borggrefe M, Holmgren C, Brugada P, De Roy L, Hohnloser SH, Brink PA. (2010) Who are the Long-QT syndrome patients who receive an implantable cardioverter-defibrillator and what happens to them? Data from the European Long-QT syndrome implantable cardioverter-defibrillator (LQTS ICD) registry. *Circulation* 122:1272-1282.

Sears SF, Burns JL, Handberg E, Sotile WM, Conti JB. (2001) Young at heart: understanding the unique psychosocial adjustment of young implantable cardioverter defibrillator recipients. *PACE* 24:1113-1117.

Sears SF, St.Amant JB, Zeigler V. (2009) Psychosocial considerations for children and young adolescents with implantable cardioverter defibrillators: an update. *PACE* 32:S80-82.

Shah MJ. (2009) Implantable cardioverter defibrillator-related complications in the pediatric population. *PACE* 32:S71-S74.

Silka MJ, Kron J, Dunnigan A, Dick M 2nd. (1993) Sudden cardiac death and the use of implantable cardioverter-defibrillators in pediatric patients. The Pediatric Electrophysiology Society. *Circulation.* 87:800-7.

Silka MJ & Bar-Cohen Y. (2008) Should patients with congenital heart disease and a systemic ventricular ejection fraction less than 30% undergo prophylactic implantation of an ICD? Patients with congenital heart disease and a systemic ventricular ejection fraction less than 30% should undergo prophylactic implantation of an implantable cardioverter defibrillator. *Circ Arrhythmia Electrophysiol* 298-306.

Smets EMA, Stam MMH, Meulenkamp TM, Van Langen IM, Wilde AAM, Wiegman A, De Wert GM, Tibben A. (2008) Health-related quality of life of children with a positive carrier status for inherited cardiovascular diseases. *Am J Med Genet Part A* 146A:700-707.

Stephenson EA, Batra AS, Knilans TK, Gow RM, Gradaus R, Balaji S. (2006) A multicenter experience with novel implantable cardioverter defibrillator configuration in the pediatric and congenital heart disease population. *J Cardiovasc Electrophysiol* 17:41-46.

Suzuki T, Shiga T, Kuwahara K, Kobayashi S, Suzuki S, Nishimura K, Suzuki A, Ejima K, Manaka T, Shoda M, Ishigooka J, Kasanuki H, Hagiwara N. (2010) Prevalence and persistence of depression in patients with implantable cardioverter defibrillators: a 2-year longitudinal study. *PACE* 33:1455-1461.

Ten Harkel ADJ, Blom NA, Reimer AG, Tukkie R, Sreeram N, Bink-Boelkens MTE. (2005) Implantable cardioverter defibrillator implantation in children in The Netherlands. *Eur J Pediatr* 164:436-441.

Theuns DAMJ & Gold MR. (2010) Defibrillator threshold testing at implantation: can we predict the patient with a high defibrillation threshold? *Europace* 12:309-310.

Tomaske M, Pretre R, Rahn M, Bauersfeld U. (2008) Epicardial and pleural lead ICD systems in children and adolescents maintain functionally over 5 years. *Europace* 10:1152-1156.

Triedman JK. (2008) Should patients with congenital heart disease and a systemic ventricular ejection fraction less than 30% undergo prophylactic implantation of an ICD? Implantable cardioverter defibrillator implantation guidelines based solely on left ventricular ejection fraction do not apply to adults with congenital heart disease. *Circ Arrhythmia Electrophysiol* 1:307-316.

Varma N, Michalski J, Epstein AE, Schweikert R. (2010) Automatic remote monitoring of implantable cardioverter-defibrillator lead and generator performance . The lumos-T safely reduces routine office device follow-up (TRUST) trial. *Circ Arrhythm Electrophysiol* 3:428-436.

Von Bergen NH, Atkins DL, Dick II M, Bradley DJ, Etheridge SP, Saarel EV, Fischbach PS, Balaji S, Sreeram N, Evans WN, Law IH. (2011) Multicenter study of the effectiveness of implantable cardioverter defibrillators in children and young adults with heart disease. *Pediatr Cardiol* 32:399-405.

Walsh EP. (2007) Interventional electrophysiology in patients with congenital heart disease. *Circulation* 115:3224-3234.

Witte KK, Pepper CB, Cowan JC, Thomson JD, English KM, Blackburn ME. (2008) Implantable cardioverter-defibrillator therapy in adult patients with tetralogy of Fallot. *Europace* 10:926-930.

Yap SC, Roos-Hesselink JW, Hoendermis ES, Budts W, Vliegen HW, Mulder BJM, Van Dijk APJ, Schalij MJ, Drenthen W. (2007) Outcome of implantable cardioverter defibrillators in adults with congenital heart disease: a multicenter study. *Eur Heart J* 28:1854-1861.

Zipes DP, Camm AJ, Borggrefe M, Buxton AE, Chaitman B, Fromer M, Gregoratos G, Klein G, Moss AJ, Myerburg RJ, Priori SG, Quinones MA, Roden DM, Silka MJ, Tracy C, Smith SC Jr, Jacobs AK, Adams CD, Antman EM, Anderson JL, Hunt SA, Halperin JL, Nishimura R, Ornato JP, Page RL, Riegel B, Blanc JJ, Budaj A, Dean V, Deckers JW, Despres C, Dickstein K, Lekakis J, McGregor K, Metra M, Morais J, Osterspey A, Tamargo JL, Zamorano JL (2006). American College of Cardiology/American Heart Association Task Force; European Society of Cardiology Committee for Practice Guidelines; European Heart Rhythm Association; Heart Rhythm Society.ACC/AHA/ESC 2006 Guidelines for Management of Patients With Ventricular Arrhythmias and the Prevention of Sudden Cardiac Death: a report of the American College of Cardiology/American Heart Association Task Force and the European Society of Cardiology Committee for Practice Guidelines (writing committee to develop Guidelines for Management of Patients With Ventricular Arrhythmias and the Prevention of Sudden Cardiac Death): developed in collaboration with the European Heart Rhythm Association and the Heart Rhythm Society. *Circulation* 114:e385-484.

13

AED for Paediatric Use, Implications in the Design of Shock Advice Algorithms

Sofia Ruiz de Gauna, Jesus Ruiz, Unai Irusta and Elisabete Aramendi
University of the Basque Country
Spain

1. Introduction

Sudden cardiac death (SCD) is the single most important cause of death in the adult population of the industrialised world (Jacobs et al., 2004). It is estimated that SCD accounts for an average of 100 to 200 deaths per 100 000 adults over 35 years and represents 50 % of all heart-related death (Myerburg, 2001). Most sudden cardiac arrests occur out of hospital, and the annual incidence of out of hospital cardiac arrest (OHCA) treated by emergency medical services in the US is 55 per 100 000 population (Myerburg, 2001).
Ventricular fibrillation (VF) is the initial rhythm in 40 % of cardiac arrest cases (Rea et al., 2004). Survival rates in untreated VF cardiac arrest decrease by 7 to 10 % per minute (Larsen et al., 1993; Valenzuela et al., 1997), as the heart function deteriorates. Although many victims present VF or ventricular tachycardia (VT) at the time of collapse, by the time the first ECG is recorded the rhythm has deteriorated to asystole (Waalewijn et al., 2002). The estimated survival rate in all cases of OHCA is a poor 8.4 %, but rises to 17.7 % when the victim presents VF as initial rhythm (Rea et al., 2004). Consequently, early intervention is critical for the survival of OHCA victims.
In the early 1990s, the American Heart Association (AHA) established the *chain of survival* metaphor to describe the sequence of actions to treat OHCA. The chain of survival consists of four links: *early access, early cardiopulmonary resuscitation, early defibrillation and early advanced cardiac life support*. Defibrillation is normally administered using an automated external defibrillator (AED). The AED analyses the rhythm acquired through two electrode pads and delivers an electrical shock if a lethal ventricular arrhythmia – VF or rapid VT – is detected. The shock advice algorithm (SAA) of an AED analyses the ECG to discriminate shockable from non-shockable rhythms. Given a database of classified ECG records, the performance of the SAA is evaluated in terms of the proportion of correctly identified shockable – *sensitivity* – and non-shockable – *specificity* – rhythms, which must exceed the minimum values set by the AHA (Kerber et al., 1997).
SCD is 10 times less frequent in children than in adults. However, only in the US, an estimated 16 000 children die each year from sudden cardiac arrest (Sirbaugh et al., 1999). Moreover, the social and emotional impact of the death of a child is enormous because of the greater life expectancy. Paediatric cardiac arrest constitutes less than 10 % of all OHCA, and cardiac arrest due to arrhythmias is also less frequent in children than in adults. VF is the initially recorded

rhythm in 3.8 - 19 % of paediatric OHCA cases, and more importantly, VF is the arrhythmia associated with the highest survival rate (Biarent et al., 2005).

As late as 2000, no conclusive study existed on the use of AED in children under 8 years of age. By 2003 the International Liaison Committee on Resuscitation (ILCOR) recommended the use of AED in children 1–8 years of age (Samson et al., 2003), based on the evidence provided in two independent studies (Atkinson et al., 2003; Cecchin et al., 2001). Since 2005 the Resuscitation guidelines[1] reflect the need of adapting AED for paediatric use. This involves adjusting the defibrillation pads and the defibrillation energy dose, but also, demonstrating that the SAA are accurate in the detection of paediatric arrhythmias. In fact, the first studies on the use of AED in children showed that two adult SAA from commercial AED accurately identified many paediatric rhythms (Atkinson et al., 2003; Cecchin et al., 2001). The specificity for non-shockable rhythms and the sensitivity for VF were above the values recommended by the AHA. However, those studies failed to meet AHA criteria for shockable paediatric VT. In 2008, a third study showed that a SAA designed for adult patients did not meet AHA criteria for non-shockable paediatric supraventricular tachycardia (SVT) (Atkins et al., 2008).

SAA are based on the combination of several discrimination parameters computed from the surface ECG. There are differences in rate, amplitude and ECG wave morphology between paediatric and adult rhythms (Aramendi et al., 2010; Cecchin et al., 2001; Rustwick et al., 2007). The faster heart rates and shorter QRS durations of paediatric rhythms produce differences in the values of the discrimination parameters which may affect the performance of SAA designed for adult use. Some of these differences have been previously assessed (Aramendi et al., 2010; Irusta et al., 2008; Ruiz de Gauna et al., 2008). However, based on the thorough analysis presented in this chapter, adequate strategies can be defined to either adapt (Atkins et al., 2008; Irusta & Ruiz, 2009) or redesign adult SAA algorithms to be valid also for paediatric use.

The discrimination parameters analysed in this study quantify features of the ECG signal in three domains: slope, frequency and time. The parameters are computed for a database of more than 1900 ECG records from adult and paediatric patients. Section 2 describes the database in terms of numbers of rhythms and patients, as well as the ECG record sources and the rhythm classification process. Then, in section 3 paediatric and adult heart rates are compared for the different age groups. The differences in the values of the discrimination parameters between adult and paediatric rhythms are assessed in section 4. The differences are quantified in terms of the statistical distributions of the values of the parameters, both for shockable and non-shockable rhythms. Emphasis is made on the influence of the age group on the values of the parameters. Then, the discriminative power of each parameter is assessed through the Receiver Operating Characteristic (ROC) curve and the sensitivity/specificity values. The analysis reveals important aspects that must be addressed when a SAA is adapted or designed for paediatric use. Finally, section 5 discusses strategies to design reliable SAA for adults and children and puts forward the main conclusions extracted from the study.

2. Collecting ECG recordings from adult and paediatric patients

The framework for the assessment of AED SAA was established by an AHA statement in 1997 (Kerber et al., 1997). The statement describes the composition of the databases used to

[1] The latest version of the guidelines was released in 2010 (Biarent et al., 2010).

develop and test SAA, including the types of rhythms and the minimum number of records per rhythm type. It also defines the minimum sensitivities and specificities of SAA for those rhythm types, these values are compiled in table 1. Furthermore, the statement mentions that although a database can contain several records from the same patient there can only be one record of each rhythm type per patient.

Currently there exist no public database of ECG records compliant with the AHA statement. Each AED manufacturer compiles its own data, which must include paediatric rhythms if the AED will treat children. However, the studies describing paediatric databases (Atkins et al., 2008; Atkinson et al., 2003; Cecchin et al., 2001) report less shockable rhythms than those specified by the AHA because paediatric ventricular arrhythmias are scarce.

In this study we use a database composed of adult and paediatric ECG records collected from in- and out-of-hospital sources. Three cardiologists assigned a rhythm type and a shock/no-shock recommendation to each record. For potentially shockable rhythms, the criteria to determine the shock/no-shock recommendation were: the patient is unresponsive, has no palpable pulse, and an unknown age (Cecchin et al., 2001). Diagnostic discrepancies among the reviewers were further discussed, and a consensus decision for the shock/no-shock diagnosis was agreed after the assessment of the risks of each potential recommendation.

The database contains shockable rhythms (VF and rapid VT) and the most representative non-shockable rhythms: Normal Sinus Rhythm (NSR) and SVT. SVT were treated separately because adult SAA have been shown to misdiagnose high rate paediatric SVT (Atkins et al., 2008). Furthermore, VT should only be shocked when its rate exceeds a threshold. In fact, the AHA statement allows the manufacturer to specify this threshold because tolerance to VT varies widely among patients. We considered VT shockable for rates above 150 bpm in adults and 20 bpm above age-matched normal rate in children (Atkinson et al., 2003). Table 1 is a summary of the database, where the paediatric data is divided in three age groups: under 1

		Paediatric			AHA goal	
Rhythms	**Adult**	<1y	1y–8y	>8y	Records	Sens/Esp
Shockable						
Coarse VF [a]	374 (374)	3 (1)	18 (11)	37 (10)	200	90 %
Rapid VT	200 (200)	8 (4)	39 (19)	19 (13)	50	75 %
Non-shockable						
NSR	292 (292)	14 (13)	312 (280)	214 (161)	100	99 %
SVT	89 (89)	38 (29)	147 (103)	137 (104)	30	95 %
Total	**955 (820)**	**63 (39)**	**516 (357)**	**407 (216)**	–	–

[a] Peak-to-peak amplitude above 200μV.

Table 1. Number of records per rhythm class in the adult and paediatric databases, the number of patients is indicated in parenthesis. The AHA statement sets the minimum figures per rhythm class, both in terms of number of records to test SAA and sensitivity/specificity scores of the SAA.

year (infants), 1–8 years of age (ILCOR recommendation) and above 8 years. All records were stored with a common format, and a sampling frequency of $f_s = 250\,\text{Hz}$.
The following sections describe the origin and the characteristics of the adult and paediatric records.

2.1 ECG records from adult patients

The adult database contains 955 records from 820 patients, 574 non-shockable records from 541 patients and 381 shockable records from 351 patients. The database is fully compliant with the AHA statement for the rhythm categories used in this study. The mean duration of the records was 13.0 ± 5.3 s, 15.4 ± 4.2 s for the non-shockable and 11.4 ± 5.4 s for the shockable records.
The adult records were obtained from three sources. 251 non-shockable and 63 shockable records were extracted from Public ECG databases[2]. The adult data also includes 127 shockable and 325 non-shockable records from in-hospital electrophysiology (EP) studies and intensive care units obtained at two Spanish hospitals (Basurto and Donostia hospitals). Finally, the database contains 3 non-shockable and 186 shockable out-of-hospital records from the Spanish emergency services in Madrid and the Basque Country.
Public databases are available in digital format with different sampling rates and storage formats. In-hospital data was gathered in digital format (Prucka Cardiolab and EP-Tracer systems) or as printed ECG paper strips. All the out-of-hospital data came in paper format from AED printouts.

2.2 ECG records from paediatric patients

The paediatric database contains 986 records from 612 paediatric and adolescent patients aged between 1 day and 20 years (mean age 7.1 ± 4.5 years). There are 862 non-shockable records from 579 patients and 124 shockable records from 49 patients. The mean duration of the records was 13.7 ± 9.0 s, 14.1 ± 9.3 s for the non-shockable and 10.9 ± 4.9 s for the shockable records.
Although the non-shockable portion of the database is compliant with the AHA statement, the shockable portion is not. There are only 58 VF from 22 patients and 66 VT from 36 patients, well below the 250 fatal ventricular arrhythmias (200 VF and 50 VT) specified in the AHA statement. Furthermore in the paediatric database rhythm repetition – one patient contributing more than one record within a rhythm type – was allowed when the morphology of the rhythms was sufficiently different. A low number of ventricular arrhythmias and rhythm repetition ease the terms imposed by the AHA statement, however all studies on the use of AED in children have followed this path due to the scarceness of paediatric ventricular arrhythmias (Atkins et al., 2008; Atkinson et al., 2003; Cecchin et al., 2001).
All the paediatric records were collected in-hospital, from archived paper and digital EP studies (Prucka Cardiolab and EP-Tracer systems). The records were retrospectively obtained in five Spanish hospitals: Cruces, Donostia, La Paz , Gregorio Marañón and San Joan de Deu. The accurate discrimination of SVT and VT based on a single lead ECG is hard in the paediatric case (Irusta & Ruiz, 2009). In fact, there were a number of paediatric SVT and VT cases were the consensus decision between the cardiologists was not possible, Fig. 1 shows four

[2] The MIT-BIH arrhythmia, the AHA and the Creighton University Ventricular Tachyarrhythmia databases.

examples. Discrepancies were resolved by adopting the original interpretation from the physician aware of the clinical history of the patient. This interpretation is more reliable but it is only available when records are obtained from documented EP studies. For out-of-hospital records a consensus decision is the only alternative.

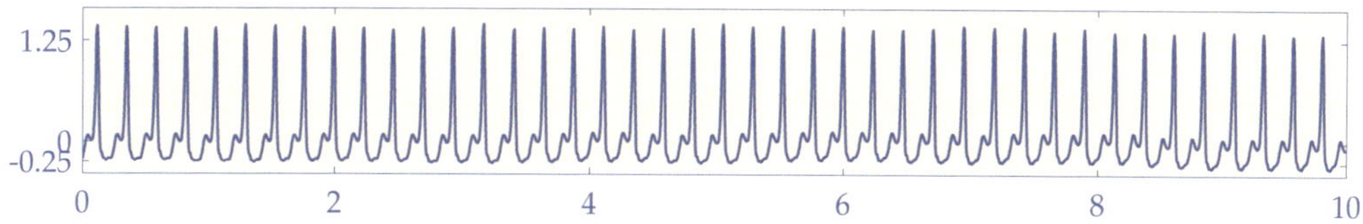

(a) Paediatric SVT with disagreements in diagnosis (Rate 255 bpm).

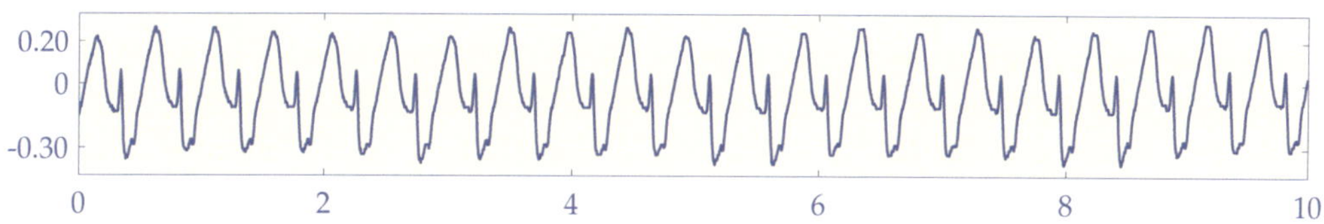

(b) Paediatric SVT with disagreements in diagnosis (Rate 125 bpm).

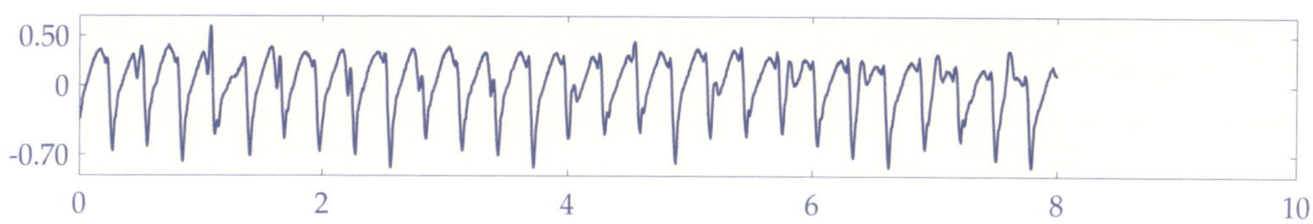

(c) Paediatric VT with disagreements in diagnosis (Rate 210 bpm).

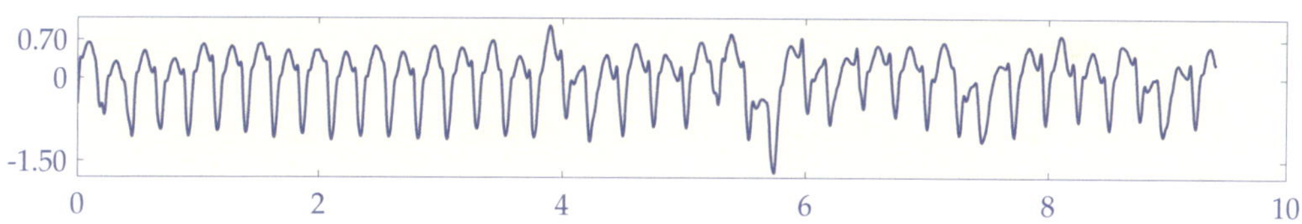

(d) Paediatric VT with disagreements in diagnosis (Rate 255 bpm).

Fig. 1. Examples of paediatric VT and SVT with disagreements in the cardiologists' classification. In these cases, the diagnosis from the rhythm source was adopted.

3. Analysis of the heart rate

A well-known ECG difference between children and adults is the heart rate. Normal heart rate changes with age, from the neonatal period, through infancy, childhood and adolescence. To maintain the cardiac output in neonates and infants, higher heart rates compensate smaller stroke volumes. As a result of the maturation of the cardiovascular system, the stroke volume increases so the heart rate lowers maintaining the overall cardiac output (Chan et al., 2008). In this section we report the heart rates of the NSR, SVT and VT records from our database. VF records were excluded from the analysis because VF is an irregular ventricular rhythm characterized by the absence of QRS complexes and a well defined heart rate. First, QRS complexes were automatically detected[3] and the results were visually inspected and corrected when necessary. We computed the heart rate (HR) for each record as the inverse of the mean time-interval between consecutive beats (QRS complexes). The result was expressed in beats per minute (bpm).

Fig. 2 shows the HR distributions for the non-shockable (NSR and SVT) and the VT rhythms for all patients (a), the paediatric group (b) and the adult group (c). There is a remarkable overlap between the HR of the non-shockable and the VT records caused by the high rate of the non-shockable paediatric rhythms. In the adult case, the HR values of non-shockable rhythms and VT are well separated. This demonstrates that a shock/no-shock discrimination approach depending on the HR is not efficient when paediatric rhythms are included, although it can be useful for the adult group.

Table 2 presents the mean HR per rhythm category for the different age groups. As expected, HR decreases with age. Our results are in line with the literature, although the age categories do not match strictly (Chan et al., 2008; Finley & Nugent, 1995). SVT records have a mean HR of 187 bpm, higher than the 131 bpm obtained for the adult group. The mean HR of SVT in infants (under 1 year) is lower than the figures reported in the literature: > 220 bpm (Chan et al., 2008) or between 260-300 bpm (Schwartz et al., 2002). For the 1–8 years of age group, the mean HR of SVT is comparable to the >180 bpm reported by Chan et al. The mean HR is similar for adult and paediatric VT, and is above 200 bpm for all age groups. The overlap in HR between non-shockable and VT rhythms observed in Fig. 2 is therefore caused by the high rates of paediatric SVT. This overlap is best seen in Fig. 3 which shows the HR distributions of the paediatric VT and SVT.

		Paediatric			
Rhythms	**Adult**	Total	<1y	1y–8y	>8y
Non-shockable					
NSR	74 (15)	98 (21)	122 (19)	102 (19)	90 (20)
SVT	131 (32)	187 (40)	186 (45)	194 (39)	180 (39)
Shockable					
VT	241 (58)	232 (54)	226 (31)	247 (57)	206 (46)
VF	–	–	–	–	–

Table 2. Mean HR (standard deviation in parenthesis) expressed in bpm for the adult and the paediatric records. There are no HR values for VF because it is not possible to associate a heart rate to a VF rhythm.

In conclusion, the higher heart rates of paediatric rhythms have important implications in the design of SAA. Paediatric SVT with rates close to or above those of rapid VT may be wrongly classified as shockable, therefore decreasing the specificity of the SAA.

In the next section we analyse how well several parameters discriminate shockable from non-shockable rhythms. Our purpose is not to define a SAA by optimizing the sensitivity and specificity for the records in our database. On the contrary, we study the possibility of defining

[3] All the signal processing and measurements for this study were made with Matlab (MathWorks, Natick, MA)

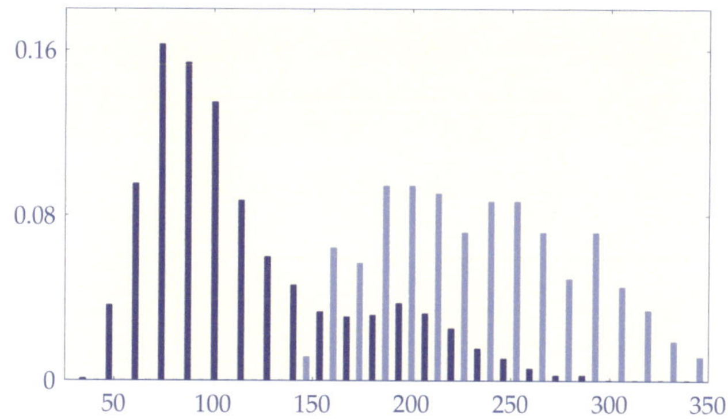

(a) HR distribution of the non-shockable (■) and shockable VT (■) records in the complete database.

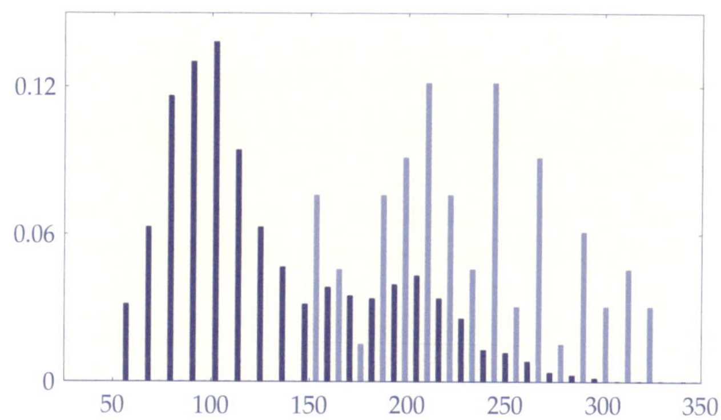

(b) HR distribution of the non-shockable (■) and shockable VT (■) records in the paediatric database.

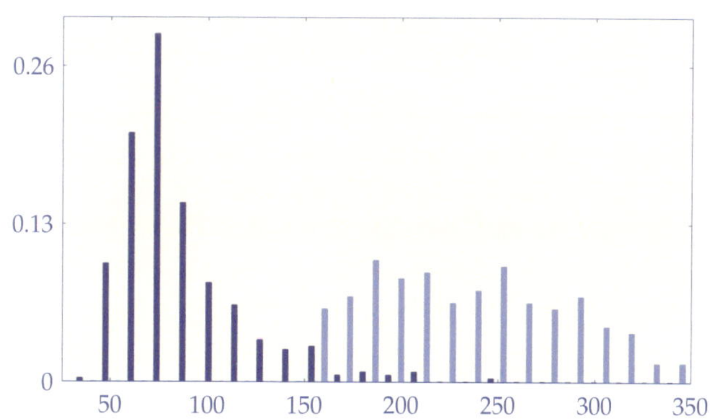

(c) HR distribution of the non-shockable (■) and shockable VT (■) records in the adult database.

Fig. 2. HR distributions for all the records, the adult records and the paediatric records.

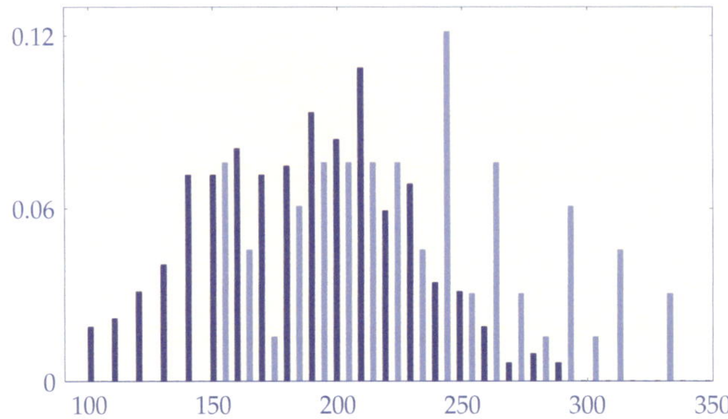

Fig. 3. HR distribution for the paediatric SVT (■) and VT records (■).

different features that will serve to discriminate fatal ventricular arrhythmias regardless of the patient age, i.e., paediatric or adult. Those parameters must therefore be as independent as possible from the HR.

4. Parameters for the shock/no-shock discrimination

The basic principle of any SAA is the definition of a set of features that will serve to discriminate fatal ventricular arrhythmias, i.e. shockable rhythms. These features quantify distinctive characteristics of the rhythms, generally better observed by transforming the time domain representation of the ECG into a new analysis domain. For example, non-shockable rhythms have larger bandwidths and more harmonic content because of the fast-changing QRS complexes. This information is easily observed in the frequency domain representation of the ECG. Other characteristics, such as the rapid variation of the ECG waveform during QRS complexes are better observed in the slope domain.

In this section, we describe a set of four parameters and analyse their ability to accurately identify shockable arrhythmias regardless the age of the patient. One feature is computed in the slope domain; two in the frequency domain and the last one in the time domain. The parameters were computed using ECG segments of 3.2 s duration, and a maximum of 3 segments per record were used.

Each parameter is first analytically defined and then the idea behind the parameter is illustrated through an example from our database. Then, we compute the ROC curve for the parameter to quantify its potential ability to discriminate shockable from non-shockable rhythms. Emphasis is made on how well the parameter discriminates SVT from VT in the paediatric case. Finally, we show different graphical examples corresponding to border-line cases, for which the discrimination efficiency decreases.

4.1 Slope domain: slope bandwidth

In a normal sinus rhythm the ECG varies slowly most of the time, during QRS complexes however the ECG changes very rapidly. These differences in the rate of variation of the ECG permit the identification of QRS complexes in the normal ECG. In our context, we want to quantify the differences between non-shockable rhythms, with narrow QRS complexes, and shockable rhythms, with either wide QRS complexes (VT) or no QRS complexes at all (VF).

We have defined a parameter named *slope bandwidth* (sBW) to identify the presence of QRS complexes in the slope domain.
First, each 3.2 s ECG segment is preprocessed with an order 10 Butterworth band-pass filter (0.5 - 30 Hz). Then, the slope of the ECG is estimated as the first difference of the preprocessed ECG, $x_{ecg}[n]$. Since we are only interested in the relative magnitude of the slope, the first difference is squared and normalized to amplitude one.

$$x_d[n] = (x_{ecg}[n+1] - x_{ecg}[n])^2 \quad (1)$$

$$\overline{x_d}[n] = \frac{x_d[n]}{max\{x_d[n]\}} \quad (2)$$

ECG segments with QRS complexes will show large differences in the values of $\overline{x_d}[n]$, with peaks around the QRS complexes and valleys for the intervals when the ECG changes slowly. On the contrary, the values of $\overline{x_d}[n]$ are more evenly distributed for shockable rhythms because there are no narrow fast changing QRS complexes.
To quantify these differences we define the sBW parameter as the 25th percentile (P_{25}) of the values of $\overline{x_d}[n]$ scaled by a factor of 1000:

$$sBW = 1000 \cdot P_{25} \quad (3)$$

The value of sBW will be small when narrow QRS complexes are present and large when wide QRS complexes or no QRS complexes are present. Fig. 4 shows the $\overline{x_d}[n]$ waveforms for a non-shockable (a) and a shockable segment (b); the figure illustrates how representing the ECG in the slope domain enhances the presence of QRS complexes.
Table 3 presents the mean sBW per rhythm category for the adult and paediatric records, including the 1–8 years of age group. The average sBW results show a clear separation between the shockable and the non-shockable segments for each age category. As expected, sBW is much larger for VT and VF segments, because shockable rhythms have more evenly distributed amplitudes in the slope domain. However, the mean sBW value for paediatric VT is significantly lower than for adult VT (8.85 versus 17.99). Furthermore, SVT rhythms have larger sBW values, particularly in the paediatric case. Consequently, the least accurate discrimination based on the slope domain occurs between paediatric VT and SVT.
The shock/no-shock discrimination power of sBW is assessed in terms of its ROC curve, shown in Fig. 5. The ROC curve depicts the proportion of correctly classified shockable segments (sensitivity) against the proportion of wrongly classified non-shockable segments (1-specificity) as the classification threshold (the value of sBW) varies. The optimal operating point (OOP) was selected to maximize the detection accuracy (number of correct decisions), which produced a 95.5 % sensitivity and 97.2 % specificity.
Although the global discrimination results are good a detailed analysis reveals that the SVT/VT discrimination is poorer. The SVT/VT discrimination results for the OOP obtained for the complete database were: 96.5 % VT sensitivity and 94.8 % SVT specificity in adults and 84.6 % VT sensitivity and 92.2 % SVT specificity in children.
Fig. 6 shows two examples of misclassified VT paediatric segments (the group with lowest performance). The VT segment in panel (a) presents spiky noise that can be interpreted as QRS

complexes. The VT segment in panel (b) shows abrupt descents with large slopes, therefore is classified as non shockable.

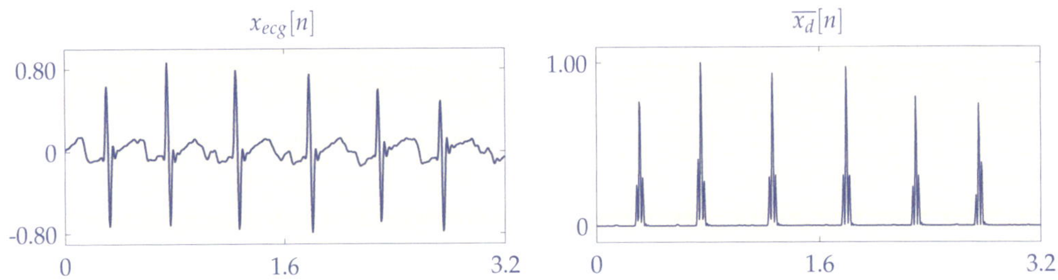

(a) SVT segment. Large differences in the slope produce low sBW values (0.06).

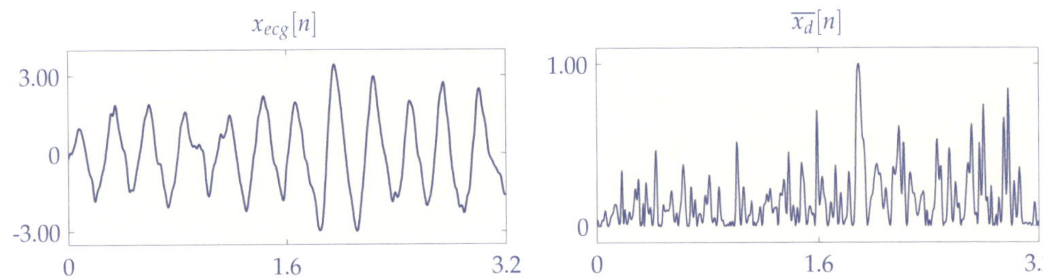

(b) VF segment. Fast ventricular activity with an evenly distributed slope produce high sBW values (34.21).

Fig. 4. Differences in the distribution of the slope, $\overline{x_d}[n]$, between shockable and non-shockable segments.

			Paediatric	
Rhythms	**All patients**	**Adult**	Total	1y–8y
Non-shockable				
NSR	0.18 (0.35)	0.22 (0.50)	0.16 (0.22)	0.16 (0.21)
SVT	0.76 (1.27)	0.65 (1.28)	0.80 (1.26)	0.79 (0.99)
Shockable				
VT	15.80 (17.24)	17.99 (18.58)	8.85 (9.01)	8.52 (8.77)
VF	10.66 (7.05)	10.74 (7.20)	10.15 (6.00)	9.40 (4.57)

Table 3. Mean sBW (standard deviation in parenthesis) for the adult and the paediatric records.

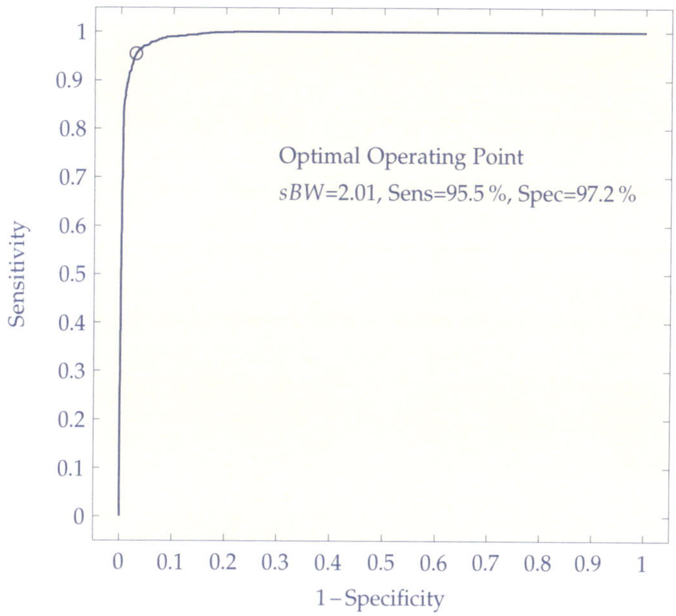

Fig. 5. ROC curve for the shock/no-shock discrimination based on the sBW parameter.

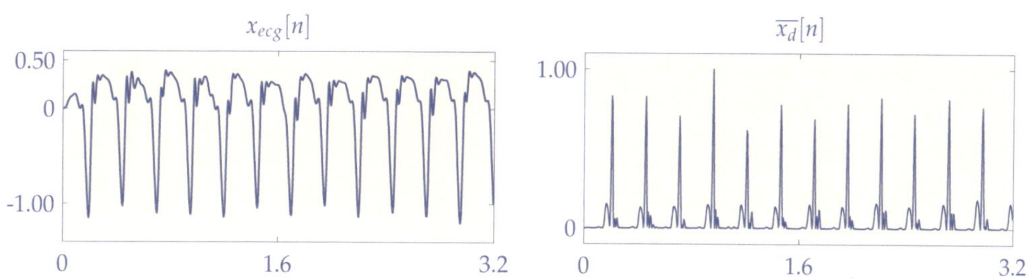

(a) VT segment with QRS like activity ($sBW = 0.55$).

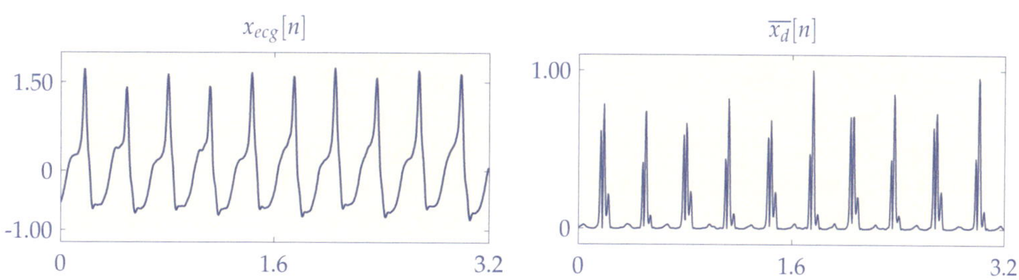

(b) VT segment with abrupt descents provoking large slopes ($sBW = 0.98$).

Fig. 6. Examples of paediatric VT segments misclassified in terms of the sBW parameter.

4.2 Frequency domain: dominant power and high power content

There are important differences in the power spectral density (PSD) between shockable and non-shockable rhythms. VT presents regular ventricular beats that frequently appear as a sinus-like waveform; its power spectral distribution is therefore concentrated around the frequency of the ventricular rate, the dominant frequency. VF is a more irregular rhythm so it has a wider band power distribution. Non-shockable rhythms, SVT or NSR, are very repetitive in time, and present complex waveforms consisting of a P wave, a QRS complex and T wave. Their power is distributed among the harmonics of the heart rate, and occupies a much larger bandwidth than for shockable rhythms. We have defined two frequency domain features to quantify these differences.

First, each 3.2 s ECG segment is preprocessed with an order 10 Butterworth band-pass filter (0.5 - 30 Hz). Then, we apply a Hanning window with no overlap to the segment and compute the FFT of the windowed ECG segment, $X_{ecg}(f)$. The PSD is estimated as the square of the amplitude of the FFT normalised to a unit area under the curve:

$$PSD(f) = \frac{|X_{ecg}(f)|^2}{\sum_{f=0}^{f=30} |X_{ecg}(f)|^2} \tag{4}$$

The first parameter, named P_D, measures how concentrated the spectrum is around the frequency for which the PSD is maximum, the dominant frequency f_D. P_D is the relative power content in a B_f=1.2 Hz bandwidth symmetrically distributed around f_D:

$$P_D(\%) = 100 \cdot \sum_{f_D - B_f/2}^{f_D - B_f/2} PSD(f) \tag{5}$$

The second parameter measures the power content of the high frequencies. For a cutoff frequency $f_H = 12.5$ Hz, the relative power content above f_H is:

$$P_H(\%) = 100 \cdot \sum_{f=12.5}^{f=30} PSD(f) \tag{6}$$

Fig. 7 shows examples of the PSD for the four type of rhythms, and the graphical description of the two parameters used to quantify these differences. VT rhythms concentrate most of the power around f_D, consequently P_D is large and P_H is small. For VF rhythms the power concentrates in a wider band around f_D and the power content in the high frequencies is higher than for VT. On the contrary, rhythms with narrow QRS complexes distribute their power around several harmonics of the heart rate, P_D is therefore smaller and P_H larger than for shockable rhythms. The differences in the spectral separation of the harmonics between NSR and SVT rhythms are explained by the larger heart rates of SVT.

Tables 4 and 5 list the mean P_D and P_H for the adult and paediatric records, including the 1–8 years of age group. There is a significant difference in the values of P_H between adult and paediatric NSR segments. This difference is due to the influence of heart rate in the power content above a fixed f_H. Children have faster normal rates, the harmonics of the heart rate are therefore at higher frequencies and the value of P_H is larger. In any case, these values are well-above those obtained for the shockable segments.

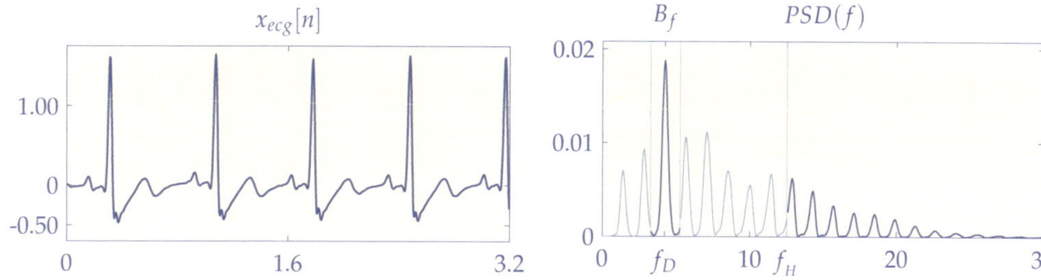

(a) NSR segment. Narrow QRS complexes produce a large harmonic content, and the power content of the high frequencies is large: $P_D = 17.8\%$ and $P_H = 23.1\%$.

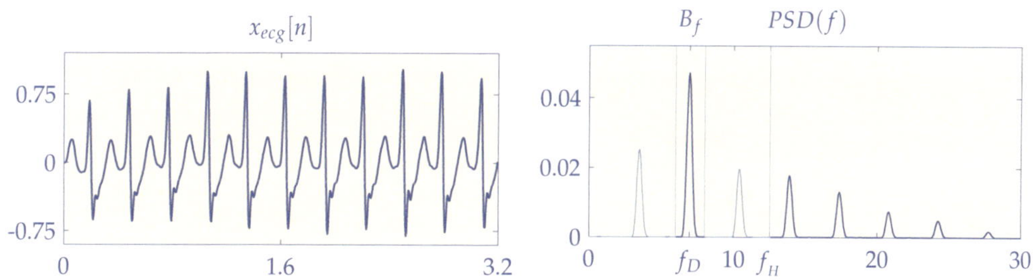

(b) SVT segment. Narrow QRS complexes produce a large harmonic content but at higher frequencies due to the larger heart rates: $P_D = 33.5\%$ and $P_H = 33.8\%$.

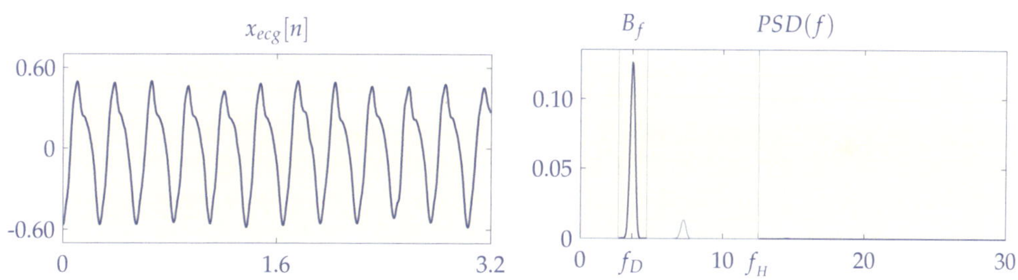

(c) VT segment. Most of the power is concentrated around f_D and there is very little power in the high frequencies: $P_D = 89.1\%$ and $P_H = 0.49\%$.

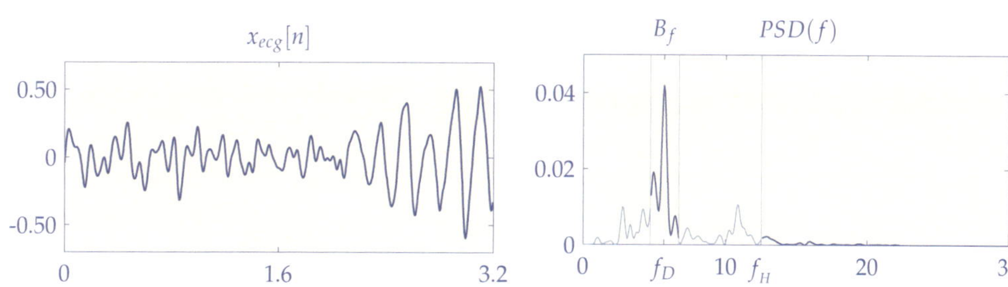

(d) VF segment. The power concentrates around f_D but with a wider band power distribution, the power content of the high frequencies is low: $P_D = 31.6\%$ and $P_H = 7.2\%$.

Fig. 7. Examples of the PSD for the four types of rhythms. The differences in the PSD are reflected in the values of the P_D and P_H parameters.

Rhythms	All patients	Adult	Paediatric	
			Total	1y–8y
Non-shockable				
NSR	19.4 (8.8)	20.2 (9.6)	19.0 (8.2)	18.7 (8.2)
SVT	32.6 (14.4)	28.9 (14.6)	33.7 (14.2)	35.1 (13.8)
Shockable				
VT	82.4 (10.2)	83.5 (10.1)	79.0 (9.8)	79.5 (9.1)
VF	58.2 (18.6)	58.3 (18.4)	57.0 (20.0)	46.2 (19.8)

Table 4. Mean P_D (standard deviation in parenthesis) for the adult and the paediatric records.

Rhythms	All patients	Adult	Paediatric	
			Total	1y–8y
Non-shockable				
NSR	27.2 (14.4)	21.6 (13.4)	30.5 (13.4)	33.0 (12.1)
SVT	28.4 (15.0)	25.3 (16.9)	29.3 (14.3)	28.8 (14.0)
Shockable				
VT	2.0 (2.1)	1.6 (1.9)	3.1 (2.3)	3.3 (2.4)
VF	2.5 (3.0)	2.2 (2.4)	4.3 (5.2)	4.1 (3.5)

Table 5. Mean P_H (standard deviation in parenthesis) for the adult and the paediatric records.

The shock/no-shock discrimination power of P_D and P_H is assessed in terms of their ROC curves, shown in Figs. 8 and 9. The sensitivity and specificity for the OOP were 83.4 % and 92.4 % for the P_D parameter, and 93.4 % and 89.6 % for the P_H parameter, respectively. Table 6 shows the sensitivity and the specificity in the SVT/VT discrimination for the OOP threshold, both for the adult and the paediatric groups. The P_D parameter has a very high VT sensitivity for the paediatric (100 %) and adult (99.0 %) cases[4], at the expense of a very poor SVT specificity (79.0 % and 85.8 %, respectively). However, in the same conditions, the P_H parameter presents a contrary behaviour for the paediatric (79.6 % sensitivity vs 95.6 % specificity) and adult cases (94.9 % sensitivity vs 82.4 % specificity).

SVT/VT discrimination	P_D		P_H	
	Paediatric	**Adult**	**Paediatric**	**Adult**
VT sensitivity	100 %	99.0 %	79.6 %	95.0 %
SVT specificity	79.0 %	85.8 %	95.6 %	82.4 %

Table 6. SVT/VT discrimination based on the spectral parameters for the adult and the paediatric cases.

[4] VF rhythms are therefore responsible for the total sensitivity decrease, as their values are close to the SVT values, see Table 4.

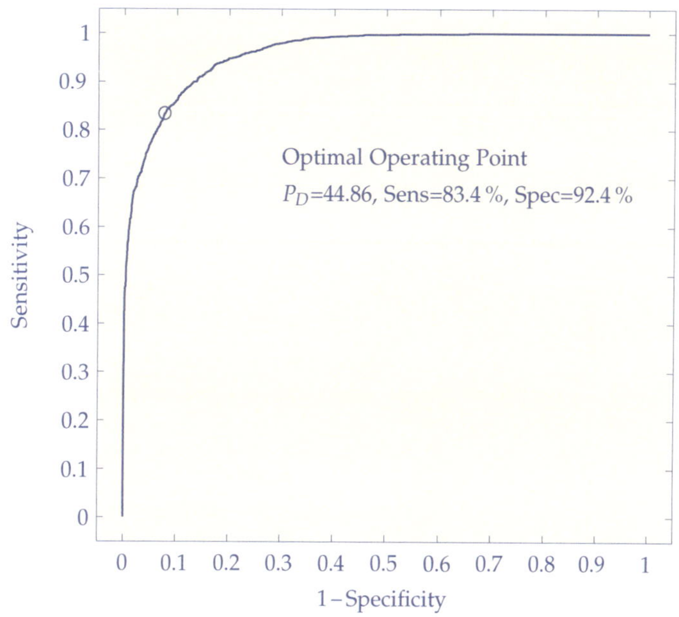

Fig. 8. ROC curve for the shock/no-shock discrimination based on the P_D parameter.

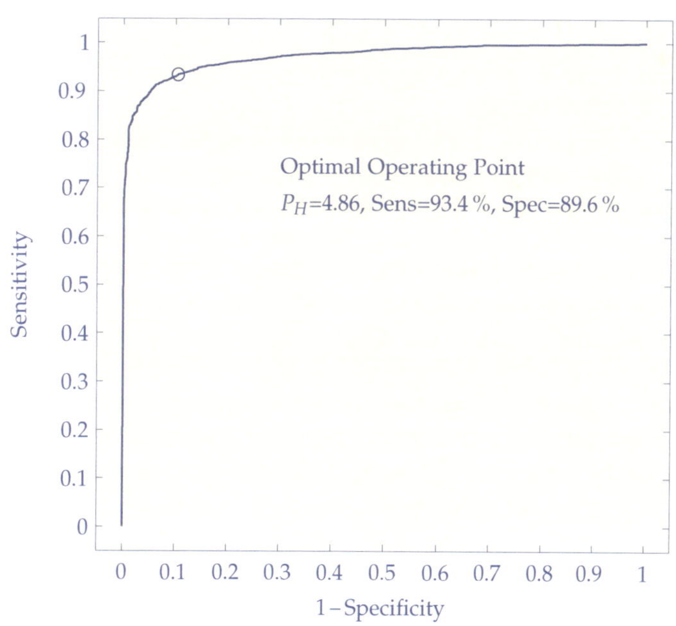

Fig. 9. ROC curve for the shock/no-shock discrimination based on the P_H parameter.

Fig. 10 shows one example of misclassification for each parameter in the frequency domain. The SVT segment shown in panel (a) has a large harmonic content; however, its power content around f_D is still high (P_D=67.7 %). The VT segment in panel (b) has a very high heart rate (395 bpm, 6.6 Hz), its second harmonic falls above f_H and P_H is therefore large.

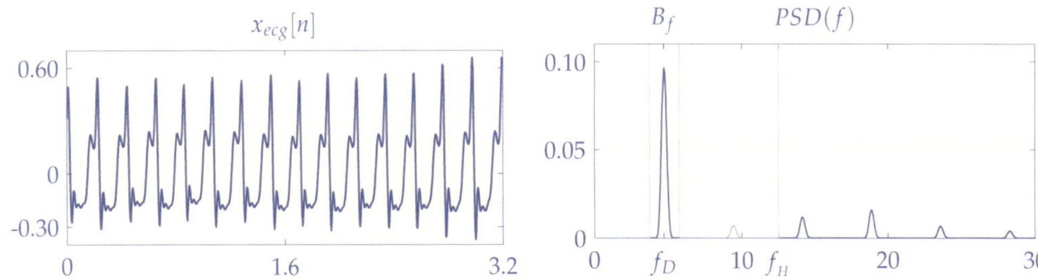

(a) SVT segment with a large power content around the fundamental frequency, $P_D = 67.7\%$.

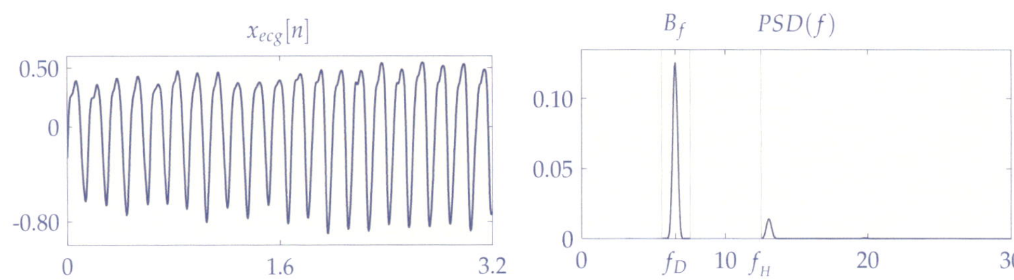

(b) VT segment. Fast rate, a significant second harmonic power content above f_H, $P_H = 11.1\%$.

Fig. 10. Examples of misclassification in the frequency domain parameters.

4.3 Time domain: baseline content

A normal ECG with well defined QRS complexes has long ECG intervals around the baseline or isoelectric line. These intervals shorten as the heart rate increases. For shockable rhythms, on the contrary, the proportion of time spent by the ECG around the baseline is low because of the fast ventricular activity. This difference between non-shockable and shockable rhythms is related to the presence or absence of QRS complexes. We have defined a parameter named *baseline content* (bC). The purpose is not to accurately estimate the isoelectric content but rather to define a parameter that enhances the differences between rhythms with large and small isoelectric contents.

First, each 3.2 s ECG segment is preprocessed with an order 10 Butterworth band-pass filter (5 - 30 Hz). The unusually large low cutoff frequency was selected to eliminate P and T waves, highlighting the presence of QRS complexes and maximizing the baseline effect. The preprocessed ECG is then normalised so that the maximum absolute value of the amplitude of $x_{ecg}[n]$ is one,

$$\overline{x_{ecg}}[n] = \frac{x_{ecg}[n]}{max\{|x_{ecg}[n]|\}} \tag{7}$$

The bC parameter is computed in the time domain as the proportion of the samples of $\overline{x_{ecg}}[n]$ in the ± 0.1 range. Fig. 11 shows an example of the calculation of this parameter. Segments

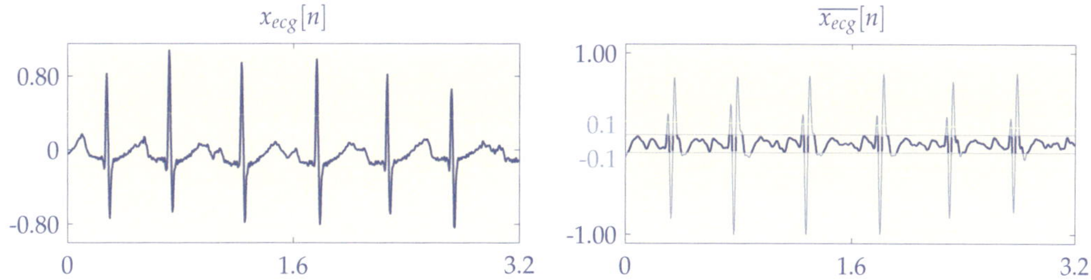

(a) SVT segment. Long isoelectric intervals between QRS complexes; $bC = 0.75$

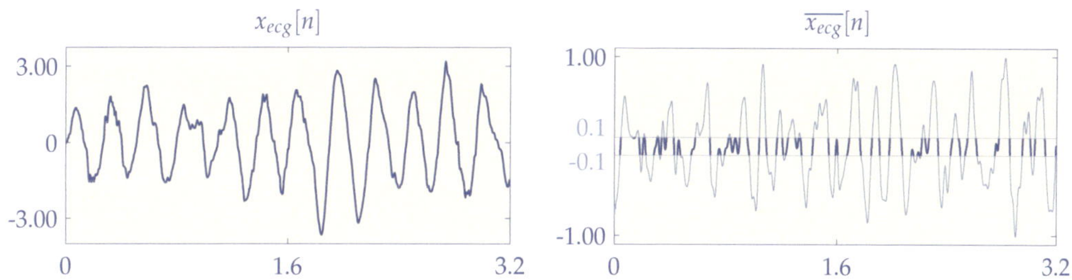

(b) VF segment. Fast ventricular activity with low isoelectric content; $bC = 0.20$

Fig. 11. Differences in the value of bC for shockable and non-shockable segments. The waveform of the normalised preprocessed ECG, $\overline{x_{ecg}}(n)$, is very distorted because of the large low cutoff frequency of the preprocessing filter.

with QRS complexes contain a large proportion of samples in the ± 0.1 range, bC is therefore large. On the other hand, fast ventricular arrhythmias present evenly distributed amplitudes and bC is small.

Table 7 presents the mean bC per rhythm category for the adult and paediatric records, including the 1–8 years of age group. For each rhythm type, the differences in the value of bC between the age groups are small. The largest difference occurs between adult and paediatric SVT, and is caused by the large difference in HR reported in table 2. As in the other two domains paediatric SVT is the most difficult to discriminate rhythm.

The shock/no-shock discrimination power of bC is assessed in terms of the ROC curves, shown in Fig. 12. The total sensitivity and specificity for the OOP were 91.1 % and 92.0 %. Again the SVT/VT discrimination, particularly for paediatric patients, remains a problem. Paediatric VT sensitivity is good, 93.2 %, the SVT specificity however is a poor 72.2 %. The figures are better in the adult case, 95.5 % VT sensitivity and 85.8 % SVT specificity, although far from reliable for a SAA.

Fig. 13 shows two examples of misclassified SVT paediatric segments. The SVT segment in panel (a) presents large T waves, the baseline content is therefore low. The SVT segment in panel (b) shows a similar effect for a faster rate.

Rhythms	All patients	Adult	Paediatric	
			Total	1y–8y
Non-shockable				
NSR	0.65 (0.13)	0.67 (0.14)	0.64 (0.13)	0.65 (0.12)
SVT	0.40 (0.14)	0.49 (0.16)	0.37 (0.13)	0.35 (0.11)
Shockable				
VT	0.17 (0.07)	0.16 (0.07)	0.19 (0.06)	0.17 (0.05)
VF	0.21 (0.07)	0.21 (0.07)	0.22 (0.06)	0.23 (0.07)

Table 7. Mean *bC* (standard deviation in parenthesis) for the total, the adult and the paediatric records, including the 1–8 years old subgroup.

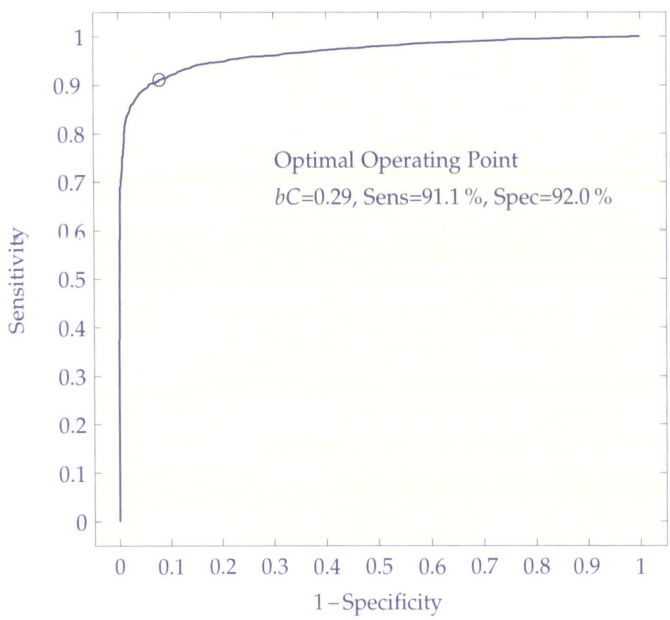

Fig. 12. ROC curve for the shock/no-shock discrimination based on the *bC* parameter.

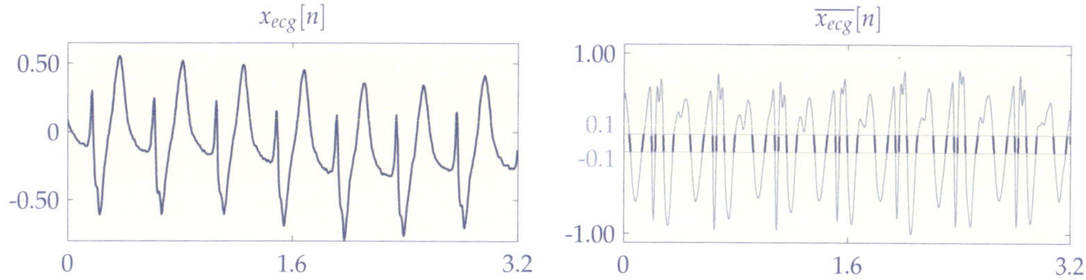

(a) SVT segment with large T waves ($bC = 0.08$) .

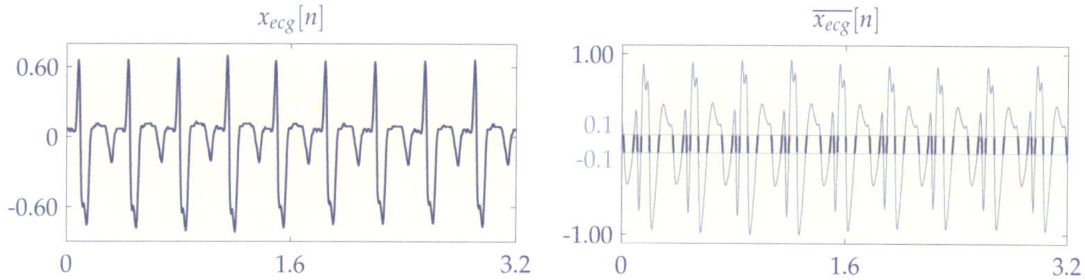

(b) SVT segment with low baseline content ($bC = 0.09$) .

Fig. 13. Examples of paediatric SVT segments misclassified in terms of the bC parameter.

5. Discussion and conclusions

The ILCOR recommended the use of AED in children 1–8 years of age in 2003. Two independent studies provided the scientific evidence for this recommendation (Atkinson et al., 2003; Cecchin et al., 2001). These contributions demonstrated that two adult algorithms from commercial AED accurately identified paediatric non-shockable rhythms and paediatric VF. In both studies, the overall specificity was above 99 % and the VF sensitivity above 95 %. However, both studies failed in the accurate classification of rapid VT; Cecchin et al. reported a 71 % VT sensitivity, and the results from Atkinson et al. were not significant because their database only contained three instances of shockable VT. These two studies represent the first alternative for the design of SAA adapted for paediatric use, which consists on proving that a SAA designed for adult patients is suitable for paediatric patients

The differences between paediatric and adult arrhythmias might explain the poor VT sensitivity results; in particular, the higher rates of paediatric SVT. A related problem is that, as indicated in the ILCOR statement, heart rate oriented SAA designed for adult patients might identify high rate paediatric SVT as shockable. Atkins et al. (Atkins et al., 2008) addressed this difficulty when they showed how an SAA designed for adult patients failed to accurately identify non-shockable paediatric SVT, the SVT specificity was 87 %. They increased the SVT specificity to 99.6 % by applying specific detection criteria to paediatric rhythms. This study proposes a second alternative for the design of paediatric SAA, namely changing the detection criteria fixed for adult patients to accurately detect paediatric arrhythmias.

The current literature only covers ventricular arrhythmia detection algorithms developed and tested using arrhythmias from adult patients, and the validation of complete AED SAA in children. In this work, we have analysed the feasibility of a third alternative, oriented to the design of a SAA but including adult and paediatric rhythms in the design of the algorithm. Consequently, a significant database of adult and paediatric arrhythmias is needed from the early stages of the process. Obtaining shockable paediatric arrhythmias is particularly challenging because fatal ventricular arrhythmias are scarce in children. We describe the process of gathering and classifying a database of adult and paediatric rhythms compliant with the AHA statement. This laborious and complex task involved emergency services, hospitals and, in particular, expert cardiologists to classify the records and biomedical engineers to manage and store the data.

We have dedicated a section to analyse the heart rate of the records in our database, and to asses the differences in heart rate between children and adults. Our analysis shows that the discrimination of shockable rhythms based on the heart rate may be accurate with adult patients but not valid for children, due to the higher rates of paediatric SVT. Consequently, rate-oriented SAA designed for adults will present a low specificity for paediatric SVT, which confirms the findings of Atkins et al (Atkins et al., 2008).

The core of the chapter is dedicated to the analysis of the ECG in the slope, time and frequency domains. We define four easily computable parameters to quantify the differences between shockable and non-shockable rhythms. These parameters were designed to be independent of the heart rate and therefore less influenced by the age of the patient.

After the analysis, we conclude that the parameters are to a great degree independent of the heart rate. There are, however, small differences between paediatric and adult patients for some rhythm types. For example, the average value of the sBW parameter for VT is different in adults and children. We have quantified the discrimination capacity of the four parameters in terms of their ROC curves. As anticipated, there are some borderline cases between paediatric SVT and VT. In fact, the accurate discrimination of paediatric SVT is a key aspect when adapting adult AED algorithms for paediatric use. Following this line, Irusta and Ruiz proposed a SVT/VT discrimination algorithm that could be incorporated to adult and paediatric AED (Irusta & Ruiz, 2009).

Although the performance of each parameter is not sufficient for a reliable shock/no-shock discrimination, the parameters can be efficiently combined to accurately identify non-shockable rhythms with narrow QRS complexes. However, a SAA valid for adult and paediatric patients based on this strategy must incorporate several additional algorithms which fall beyond the scope of this work. Those algorithms include: an algorithm for the detection of non-shockable rhythms with low electrical activity such as asystole or idioventricular rhythms, an algorithm to discriminate VF (always shockable) from VT (shockable above a rate threshold) and the protective addition of a SVT/VT discrimination algorithm to avoid shock diagnoses for fast paediatric SVT.

6. References

Aramendi, E., Irusta, U., Pastor, E. et al. (2010). ECG spectral and morphological parameters reviewed and updated to detect adult and paediatric life-threatening arrhythmia., *Physiological Measurement* 31(6): 749–761.

Atkins, D. L., Scott, W. A., Blaufox, A. D. et al. (2008). Sensitivity and specificity of an automated external defibrillator algorithm designed for pediatric patients., *Resuscitation* 76(2): 168–174.

Atkinson, E., Mikysa, B., Conway, J. A. et al. (2003). Specificity and sensitivity of automated external defibrillator rhythm analysis in infants and children., *Ann Emerg Med* 42(2): 185–196.

Biarent, D., Bingham, R., Eich, C. et al. (2010). European Resuscitation Council Guidelines for Resuscitation 2010 Section 6. Paediatric life support., *Resuscitation* 81(10): 1364–1388.

Biarent, D., Bingham, R., Richmond, S. et al. (2005). European Resuscitation Council guidelines for resuscitation 2005. Section 6. Paediatric life support., *Resuscitation* 67 Suppl 1: S97–133.

Cecchin, F., Jorgenson, D. B., Berul, C. I. et al. (2001). Is arrhythmia detection by automatic external defibrillator accurate for children?: Sensitivity and specificity of an automatic external defibrillator algorithm in 696 pediatric arrhythmias., *Circulation* 103(20): 2483–2488.

Chan, T. C., Sharieff, G. Q. & Brady, W. J. (2008). Electrocardiographic manifestations: pediatric ECG., *J Emerg Med* 35(4): 421–430.

Finley, J. P. & Nugent, S. T. (1995). Heart rate variability in infants, children and young adults., *J Auton Nerv Syst* 51(2): 103–108.

Irusta, U. & Ruiz, J. (2009). An algorithm to discriminate supraventricular from ventricular tachycardia in automated external defibrillators valid for adult and paediatric patients., *Resuscitation* 80(11): 1229–1233.

Irusta, U., Ruiz, J., Aramendi, E. & de Gauna, S. R. (2008). Amplitude, frequency and complexity features in paediatric and adult ventricular fibrillation., *Resuscitation* 77: S53–S53.

Jacobs, I., Nadkarni, V., Bahr, J. et al. (2004). Cardiac arrest and cardiopulmonary resuscitation outcome reports: update and simplification of the Utstein templates for resuscitation registries., *Circulation* 110(21): 3385–3397.

Kerber, R. E., Becker, L. B., Bourland, J. D. et al. (1997). Automatic external defibrillators for public access defibrillation: recommendations for specifying and reporting arrhythmia analysis algorithm performance, incorporating new waveforms, and enhancing safety. A statement for health professionals from the American Heart Association Task Force on Automatic External Defibrillation, Subcommittee on AED Safety and Efficacy., *Circulation* 95(6): 1677–1682.

Larsen, M. P., Eisenberg, M. S., Cummins, R. O. & Hallstrom, A. P. (1993). Predicting survival from out-of-hospital cardiac arrest: a graphic model., *Ann Emerg Med* 22(11): 1652–1658.

Myerburg, R. J. (2001). Sudden cardiac death: exploring the limits of our knowledge., *J Cardiovasc Electrophysiol* 12(3): 369–381.

Rea, T. D., Eisenberg, M. S., Sinibaldi, G. & White, R. D. (2004). Incidence of EMS-treated out-of-hospital cardiac arrest in the United States., *Resuscitation* 63(1): 17–24.

Ruiz de Gauna, S., Ruiz, J., Irusta, U. & Aramendi, E. (2008). Parameters affecting shock decision in pediatric automated defibrillation., *Proc. Computers in Cardiology*, pp. 929–932.

Rustwick, B., Geheb, F., Brewer, J. & Atkins, D. (2007). Electrocardiographic characteristics for automated external defibrillator algorithms are different between children and adults., *Circulation* 116.

Samson, R. A., Berg, R. A., Bingham, R. et al. (2003). Use of automated external defibrillators for children: an update: an advisory statement from the pediatric advanced life support task force, International Liaison Committee on Resuscitation., *Circulation* 107(25): 3250–3255.

Schwartz, P. J., Garson, A., Paul, T. et al. (2002). Guidelines for the interpretation of the neonatal electrocardiogram. A task force of the European Society of Cardiology., *Eur Heart J* 23(17): 1329–1344.

Sirbaugh, P. E., Pepe, P. E., Shook, J. E. et al. (1999). A prospective, population-based study of the demographics, epidemiology, management, and outcome of out-of-hospital pediatric cardiopulmonary arrest., *Ann Emerg Med* 33(2): 174–184.

Valenzuela, T. D., Roe, D. J., Cretin, S. et al. (1997). Estimating effectiveness of cardiac arrest interventions: a logistic regression survival model., *Circulation* 96(10): 3308–3313.

Waalewijn, R. A., Nijpels, M. A., Tijssen, J. G. & Koster, R. W. (2002). Prevention of deterioration of ventricular fibrillation by basic life support during out-of-hospital cardiac arrest., *Resuscitation* 54(1): 31–36.

Part 4

ICD Implications

14

Role of Implantable Cardioverter Defibrillators for Dialysis Patients

Marlies Ostermann
King's College London, Guy's & St Thomas' Hospital
United Kingdom

1. Introduction

The number of patients suffering from chronic kidney disease (CKD) and end-stage renal disease (ESRD) is increasing worldwide (Ansell et al., 2007; National Institutes of Health, 2009). Mortality is high with cardiac disease being the primary cause of death, especially in long-term dialysis patients (84.5 per 1000 patient years) (National Institutes of Health, 2009). Yearly mortality is ~4% in dialysis patients younger than 20 years but rises gradually to 35% in patients older than 65 years. Ventricular arrhythmias account for >60% of all sudden cardiac deaths (SCD) (Bleyer et al., 2006; Eknoyan et al., 2002; Wanner et al., 2005). A retrospective analysis of the Multicenter Automatic Defibrillator Implantation Trial showed a correlation between renal function and risk of SCD (Goldenberg et al., 2006). For each 10 unit reduction in estimated glomerular filtration rate (eGFR), the risk of all-cause mortality and SCD increased by 16% and 17%, respectively.

Outcome after a cardiac arrest is poor. Most dialysis patients die immediately or within 30 days after a cardiac arrest (Herzog et al., 2005). Measures aimed at modifying risk factors and preventing this catastrophic outcome are urgently needed (De Bie et al., 2009; Passman et al., 2011; Young, 2011).

2. Risk factors for sudden cardiac death

In the general population, ischaemic heart disease and moderate to severe left ventricular systolic dysfunction are the major risk factors for SCD (National Institutes of Health, 2009). CKD patients often suffer from significant cardiovascular morbidity (hypertension, diabetes, vascular disease). However, the exact pathophysiology of SCD in dialysis patients is not fully understood and includes risk factors specifically related to end-stage renal disease. Left ventricular hypertrophy (LVH) is one potential factor. It is very common in dialysis patients and often accompanied by microvascular disease and marked interstitial fibrosis which is more pronounced than in non-renal patients with similar degrees of LVH (Amann et al., 1998). Other cardiac abnormalities associated with CKD are functional and structural changes of intramyocardial arteries, reduced capillary density and abnormalities of myocardial metabolism leading to reduced myocardial perfusion reserve (Amann & Ritz, 1997). Increased sympathetic activity has also been identified as a cause for the increased risk of SCD (Nishimura et al., 2010). Recent hospitalization, malnutrition, inflammatatory processes and use of catheter for dialysis access are also markers of increased risk (Pun et al., 2011).

Several studies have reported a temporal relationship between SCD and the haemodialysis procedure (Bleyer et al., 2006; Karnik et al., 2001; Pun et al., 2011). Reports suggest that 20-30% of dialysis treatments are complicated by intradialytic hypotension. Electrocardiographic, isotopic and echocardiographic investigations have confirmed that periods of subclinical myocardial ischaemia and myocardial stunning occur during haemodialysis (Selby & McIntyre, 2007). Large fluid and electrolyte shifts, low dialysis dose and low pre-dialysis potassium levels are contributing factors (Bleyer et al., 2006; Karnik et al., 2001; Port et al., 2002 Pun et al., 2011). Rates of SCD per dialysis session range from 3.4 in 100.000 to 7.0 in 100.000 dialysis sessions in the outpatient setting and to 12.5 in 100.000 dialysis sessions in hospital-based haemodialysis units (Bleyer et al., 2006; Lafrance et al., 2006). Cardiac arrests are more common on the first dialysis day after a 2-day hiatus (Davis et al., 2008). The risk is particularly high during and immediately after haemodialysis rather than pre-dialysis. Concomitant beta-blocker therapy is beneficial. The risk also declines after renal transplantation.

Data on the incidence of SCD in patients treated with peritoneal dialysis is sparse. Wang et al reported a 25% incidence of SCD in 230 peritoneal dialysis patients which is similar to that in haemodialysis patients (Wang et al., 2010). As fewer abrupt electrolyte shifts occur with peritoneal dialysis than with haemodialysis, it supports the hypothesis that SCD in dialysis patients is predominantly caused by abnormalities of the myocardium common in ESRD rather than the type of dialysis.

3. Interventions to reduce the risk of sudden cardiac death

3.1 Medical interventions

There is evidence from observational and interventional studies that beta-blocker therapy improves outcome in dialysis patients, especially after a cardiac arrest (Cice et al., 2003; Foley et al., 2002; Pun et al., 2007). However, despite this benefit, less than 30% of haemodialysis patients are prescribed beta-blocker therapy (Abbott et al., 2004).

The role of statins in preventing SCD in dialysis patients remains uncertain. The 4D study evaluated the effectiveness of atorvastatin in 1255 haemodialysis patients with diabetes mellitus and found no beneficial effect on cardiovascular mortality, non-fatal myocardial infarction and stroke despite a reduction in LDL cholesterol (Wanner et al., 2005). In contrast, a meta-analysis by Strippoli et al demonstrated that statin therapy in CKD patients significantly reduced lipid concentrations and led to a 20% reduction in non-fatal cardiovascular events (Strippoli et al., 2008). There was no benefit on all-cause mortality.

3.2 Role of implantable cardioverter defibrillator for primary prophylaxis

In patients suffering from reduced left ventricular ejection fraction (LVEF), implantable cardioverter defibrillators (ICD) have emerged as the most effective treatment to reduce the risk of SCD. ICD implantation is recommended for the primary prevention of sudden cardiac death in patients with Class II and III congestive heart failure and decreased LVEF. In patients with refractory heart failure, cardiac resynchronization therapy has been shown to improve symptoms, reduce hospitalizations, and reduce mortality. However, patients with advanced CKD were excluded from most ICD trials despite the fact that the prevalence of left ventricular dysfunction in dialysis patients is reported to be in the vicinity of 14% (Mark et al., 2006).

Data from retrospective analyses showed that CKD patients treated with an ICD for primary prophylaxis against SCD had better outcomes compared to CKD patients treated with conventional therapy alone (Hager et al., 2010). However, there is evidence that ICD efficacy is dependent on renal function. 958 patients with left ventricular dysfunction who had undergone ICD placement for primary prevention of SCD were stratified into 5 groups according to their CKD stage. The median survival time for patients with stage I to V was 78, 90, 80, 42 and 21 months, respectively ($p<0.0001$), and the likelihood of death at 1 year was significantly greater for patients with CKD stage IV or V than for those with stage I. Goldenberg et al came to similar conclusions in their retrospective analysis of patients enrolled into the Multicenter Automatic Defibrillator Implantation Trial (Goldenberg et al., 2006). ICD therapy was only associated with a survival benefit in patients with eGFR ≥ 35 ml/min/1.73m^2 but not in patients with eGFR <35ml/min/1.73m^2. Using a decision analysis model of primary prevention ICD implantation, Amin et al showed that ICD implantation in patients with CKD stage V was only favoured in those aged <65 years (Amin et al., 2008).
The benefit of ICD therapy in dialysis patients is questionable. To date, no randomized clinical trials have been performed in this area. Khan et al reported the impact of ICDs on survival in 78 patients with advanced CKD of whom 45 patients were on dialysis (Khan et al., 2010). In the dialysis cohort, ICD therapy did not impact survival whereas in CKD patients not on dialysis, survival was significantly better in patients with an ICD (2-year survival 80% versus 54%; $p=0.027$). This benefit persisted after adjusting for gender, race, eGFR, digoxin use and presence of coronary heart disease, heart failure, or hypertension.
A meta-analysis on the outcome of patients with an ICD included data of 7 studies with a total of 2516 patients and 89 patients receiving dialysis (Sakhuja et al., 2009). Despite an ICD, dialysis patients had a 2.7 fold higher mortality compared to those not on dialysis. The authors came to the conclusion that ICD therapy did not appear to close the mortality gap between dialysis patients and those not receiving dialysis. This lack of benefit from ICDs in patients with advanced CKD may be explained by more advanced coronary artery disease, concomitant left ventricular hypertrophy, higher propensity for electrolyte imbalances and higher infection risk, all leading to increased susceptibility to arrhythmias and refractoriness to treatment (Dasgupta et al., 2007; Wase et al., 2004). Another proposed mechanism for the reduced benefit may be resistance to ICD therapy with declining renal function. Wase et al found that >35% of dialysis patients had elevated defibrillation thresholds compared to <10% among patients without CKD (Wase et al., 2004).

3.3 Role of implantable cardioverter defibrillator for secondary prophylaxis

Despite the lack of benefit of ICDs in primary prevention of SCDs in dialysis patients, there may be a role for ICDs for secondary prevention in survivors of a cardiac arrest. Retrospective data showed that in patients who survived for 30 days after a cardiac arrest, the median survival in the ICD group was 26 months compared to 11 months in the non-ICD group (Herzog et al., 2005). However, only 8% of the dialysis patients who survived a cardiac arrest episode in fact underwent implantation of an ICD. Patients with an unfavorable clinical status post arrest were excluded.
Considering the high incidence of cardiac deaths in dialysis patients and the cost-effectiveness of ICDs seen in patients with normal or mildly impaired renal function, there is a need for further clinical trials in patients with advanced CKD. Three critical issues

remain: whether there is a role for ICDs in dialysis patients, how to identify those patients who would benefit most from such therapies, and how to achieve even greater prevention, especially primary prevention. Results from "The Implantable Cardioverter Defibrillator in Dialysis patients (ICD2) study" are awaited (De Bie et al., 2008). This prospective randomised controlled study is the first trial which evaluates the possible benefit of prophylactic ICD therapy for the primary prevention of sudden cardiac death in dialysis patients aged 55-80 years with 4-year follow up data.

4. Conclusions

Advanced CKD is associated with a high risk of SCD. Prophylactic ICD implantation has a beneficial role in patients with eGFR > 35ml/min/m^2 but there is less evidence for its use in dialysis patients. Until the results of future trials are available, clinical management needs to focus on preventive strategies, including regular review of the dialysis prescription, avoidance of rapid electrolyte shifts and frequent evaluation of concomitant medication, especially cardioprotective drugs.

5. References

Abbott, KC.; Trespalacios, F.C.; Agodoa, L.Y.; Taylor, A.J. & Bakris, G.L. (2004). Beta-blocker use in long-term dialysis patients: association with hospitalised heart failure and mortality. *Arch Intern Med*, Vol.164, pp. 2465-2471

Amann, K. & Ritz, E. (1997). Cardiac disease in chronic uremia: pathophysiology. *Adv Ren Replace Ther*, Vol.4, pp. 212-224

Amann, K.; Rychlik, I.; Miltenberger-Milteny, G. & Ritz, E. (1998). Left ventricular hypertrophy in renal failure. *Kidney Int Suppl*, Vol.68, pp.S78-S85

Amin, M.S.; Fox, A.D.; Kalahasty, G.; Shepard, R.K.; Wood, M.A. & Ellenbogen, K.A. (2008). Benefit of primary prevention implantable cardioverter-defibrillators in the setting of chronic kidney disease: a decision model analysis. *J Cardiovasc Electrophysiol*, Vol.12, pp.1-6

Ansell, D.; Feehally, J.; Feest, T.G.; Tomson, C.; Williams, A.J. & Warwick, G. (2007). UK Renal Registry Report 2007, Bristol, UK: *UK Renal Registry*

Bleyer, A.J.; Hartman, J.; Brannon, P.C.; Reeves-Daniel, A.; Satko, S.G. & Russell, G. (2006). Characteristics of sudden death in hemodialysis patients. *Kidney Int*, Vol.69, pp.2268-2273

Cice, G.; Ferrara, L.; D'Andrea, A.; D'Isa, S.; Di Benedetto, A., Cittadini, A.; Russo, P.E.; Golino, P. & Calabro, R. (2003). Carvedilol increases two-year survival in dialysis patients with dilated cardiomyopathy: a prospective placebo-controlled trial. *J Am Coll Cardiol*, Vol.41, pp.1438-1444

Dasgupta, A.; Montalvo, J.; Medendorp, S.; Lloyd-Jones, D.M.; Ghossein, C.; Goldberger, J. & Passman, R. (2007). Increased complication rates of cardiac rhythm management devices in ESRD patients. *Am J Kidney Dis*, Vol.49, pp.656-663

Davis, T.R.; Young, B.A.; Eisenberg, M.S.; Rea, T.D.; Copass, M.K. & Cobb, L.A. (2008). Outcome of cardiac arrests attended by emergency medical services staff at community outpatient dialysis centers. *Kidney Int*, Vol.73, pp.933-939

De Bie, M.K.; Lekkerkerker, J.C.; van Dam, B.; Gaasbeek, A.; van Buren, M.; Putter, H.; van Erven, L.; Bax, J.J.; Schalij, M.J.; Rabelink, T.J. & Jukema, J.W. (2008). Prevention of sudden cardiac death: rationale and design of the Implantable Cardioverter Defibrillators in Dialysis patients (ICD2) Trial - a prospective pilot study. *Curr Med Res Opin*, Vol.24, pp.51-2157

De Bie, M.K.; Van Dam, B.; Gaasbeek, A.; van Buren, M.; van Erven, L.; Bax, J.J.; Schalij, M.J.; Rabelink, T.J. & Jukema, J.W. (2009). The current status of interventions aiming at reducing sudden cardiac death in dialysis patients. *Eur Heart J*, Vol.30, pp.1559-1564

Eknoyan, G.; Beck, G.J.; Cheung, A.K.; Daugirdas, J.T.; Greene, T.; Kusek, J.W.; Allon, M.; Bailey, J.; Delmez, J.A.; Depner, T.A.; Dwyer, J.T.; Levey, A.S.; Levin, N.W.; Milford, E.; Ornt, D.B.; Rocco, M.V.; Schulman, G.; Schwab, S.J.; Teehan, B.P.; Toto, R. & Hemodialysis (HEMO) Study Group. (2002). Effect of dialysis dose and membrane flux in maintenance hemodialysis. *N Engl J Med*, Vol.347, pp.2010-2019

Foley, R.N.; Herzog, C.A. & Collins, A.J. (2002). Blood pressure and long-term mortality in United States hemodialysis patients: ESRDS Waves 3 and 4 Study. *Kidney Int*, Vol.62, pp.1784-1790

Goldenberg, I.; Moss, A.J.; McNitt, S.; Barsheshet, A.; Gray, D.; Andrews, M.L.; Brown, M.W.; Zareba, W.; Sze, E.; Solomon, S.D.; Pfeffer, M.A. & Multicenter Automatic Defibrillator Implantation Trial--Cardiac Resynchronization Therapy Investigators. (2006). Relations among renal function, risk of sudden cardiac death, and benefit of the implanted cardiac defibrillator in patients with ischemic left ventricular dysfunction. *Am J Cardiol*, Vol.98, pp.485-490

Hager, C.S.; Jain, S.; Blackwell, J.; Culp, B.; Song, J. & Chiles, C.D. (2010). Effect of renal function on survival after implantable cardioverter defibrillator placement. *Am J Cardiol*. Vol.106, pp.1297-1300

Herzog, C.A.; Li, S.; Weinhandl, E.D.; Strief, J.W.; Collins, A.J. & Gilbertson, D.T. (2005). Survival of dialysis patients after cardiac arrest and the impact of implantable cardioverter defibrillators. *Kidney Int*, Vol.68, pp.818-825

Karnik, J.A.; Young, B.S.; Lew, N.L.; Herget, M.; Dubinsky, C.; Lazarus, J.M. & Chertow, G.M. (2001). Cardiac arrest and sudden death in dialysis units. *Kidney Int*, Vol.60, pp.350-357

Khan, F.; Adelstein, E. & Saba, S. (2010). Implantable cardioverter defibrillator confer survival benefit in patients with renal insufficiency but not in dialysis-dependent patients. *J Interv Card Electrophysiol*, Vol.28, pp.117-123

Lafrance, J.P.; Nolin, L.; Senecal, L. & Leblanc, M. (2006). Predictors and outcome of cardiopulmonary resuscitation (CPR) calls in a large haemodialysis unit over a seven-year period. *Nephrol Dial Transplant*, Vol.21, pp.1006-1012

Mark, P.B.; Johnston, N.; Groenning, B.A.; Foster, J.E.; Blyth, K.G.; Martin, T.N.; Steedman, T.; Dargie, H.J. & Jardine, A.G. (2006). Redefinition of uremic cardiomyopathy by contrast-enhanced cardiac magnetic resonance imaging. *Kidney Int*, Vol.69, pp.1839-1845

Nishimura, M.; Tokoro, T.; Nishida, M.; Hashimoto, T.; Kobayashi, H.; Yamazaki, S.; Imai, R.; Okino, K.; Iwamoto, N.; Takahashi, H. & Ono, T. (2010). Sympathetic overactivity and sudden cardiac death among hemodialysis patients with left ventricular hypertrophy. *Int J Cardiol*, Vol. 142, pp.80-86

Passman, R. & Herzog, C.A. (2011). Sudden cardiac death: stratifying risk in dialysis patients. *Nat Rev Nephrol*, Vol.7, pp.133-135

Port, F.K.; Ashby, V.B.; Dhingra, R.K.; Roys, E.C. & Wolfe, R.A. (2002). Dialysis dose and body mass index are strongly associated with survival in hemodialysis patients. *J Am Soc Nephrol*, Vol.13, pp.1061-1066

Pun, P.H.; Lehrich, R.W.; Smith, S.R. & Middleton, J.P. (2007). Predictors of survival after cardiac arrest in outpatient hemodialysis clinics. *Clin J Am Soc Nephrol*, Vol.2, pp.491-500

Pun, P.H.; Lehrich, R.W.; Honeycutt, E.F.; Herzog, C.A. & Middleton, J.P. (2011). Modifiable risk factors associated with sudden cardiac arrest within hemodialysis clinics. *Kidney Int*, Vol.79, pp.218-27

Sakhuja, R.; Keebler, M.; Lai, T.S.; McLaughlin, G. C.; Thakur, R. & Bhatt, D.L. (2009). Meta-analysis of mortality in dialysis patients with an implantable cardioverter defibrillator. *Am J Cardiol*, Vol.103, pp.735-741

Selby, N.M. & McIntyre, C.W. (2007). The acute cardiac effects of dialysis. *Semin Dial*, Vol.20, pp.220-228

Strippoli, G.F.; Navaneethan, S.D.; Johnson, D.W.; Perkovic, V.; Pellegrini, F.; Nicolucci, A. & Craig, J.C. (2008). Effects of statins in patients with chronic kidney disease: meta-analysis and meta-regression of randomised controlled trials. *BMJ*, Vol.336, pp.645-651

National Institutes of Health. (2009). U.S. Renal Data System. Annual Data Report: *Atlas of Chronic Kidney Disease and End-Stage Renal Disease in the United States*. Bethesda, MD: National Institute of Diabetes and Digestive and Kidney Diseases; Bethesda, Maryland, USA, 2009

Wang, A.Y.; Lam, C.W.; Chan, I.H.; Wang, M.; Lui, S.F. & Sanderson, J.E. (2010). Sudden cardiac death in end-stage renal disease patients: a 5-year prospective analysis. *Hypertension*, Vol.56, pp.210-216

Wanner, C.; Krane, V.; März, W.; Olschewski, M.; Mann, J.F.; Ruf, G.; Ritz, E. & German Diabetes and Dialysis Study Investigators. (2005). Atrovastatin in patients with type 2 diabetes mellitus undergoing hemodialysis. *N Engl J Med*, Vol.353, pp.238-248

Wase, A.; Basit, A.; Nazir, R.; Jamal, A.; Shah, S.; Khan, T.; Mohiuddin, I.; White, C.; Saklayen, M. & McCullough, P.A. (2004). Impact of chronic kidney disease upon survival among implantable cardioverter-defibrillator recipients. *J Interv Card Electrophysiol*, Vol.11, pp.199-204

Young, B.A. (2011). Prevention of sudden cardiac arrest in dialysis patients: can we do more to improve outcomes? *Kidney Int*, Vol.79, pp.147-149

15

Cardiac Rehabilitation for Patients with an Implantable Cardioverter Defibrillator

Alan Robert Denniss and Robert Zecchin
Westmead Hospital and University of Western Sydney, Sydney, Australia

1. Introduction

Patients with an implantable cardioverter defibrillator (ICD) are not routinely referred to Cardiac Rehabilitation (CR) due to fears that exercise may induce ventricular tachyarrhythmias. Meta analyses and systematic reviews have shown that a CR program with an exercise component can improve survival, as well as non-fatal disease manifestations, functional capacity and quality of life (QOL) in patients with previous myocardial infarction or cardiac surgery (Ades 2001; Lewin et al., 2001; Wenger 2008).
Whether the same is true for patients with an ICD is not clear, especially as these patients may have ischaemic or non-ischaemic causes for their propensity for ventricular tachyarrhythmias, and are more likely to need treatment for heart failure. There is evidence that exercise programs can improve functional status and counter deconditioning in cardiac patients with heart failure (Smart and Marwick 2004).
Most previous studies which have examined the safety of exercising ICD patients have been small, with less than 100 patients in their studies (Belardinelli et al., 2006; Chinnaiyan et al., 2007; Dougherty et al., 2008; Fan et al., 2009; Fitchet et al., 2003; Vanhees et al., 2004) . A notable exception was the HF-ACTION cohort, in which 1285 patients had an ICD implanted before or during the trial and had at least one exercise test performed after ICD implantation (Keteylan et al., 2009). This large study clearly demonstrated the safety of exercise testing in ICD patients, but did not show the changes in workloads achievable during the course of a CR program, or examine QOL issues.
Exercise capacity at treadmill testing, expressed as peak metabolic equivalents (METS), has been shown to be of prognostic significance (Kokkinos et al., 2007), with each 1 MET increase in exercise capacity being associated with a 13% decrease in mortality (mean follow-up 7.5 years). This data suggests that exercise programs should aim to improve functional capacity in cardiac patients, and endeavour to help sustain this level of functional improvement over time.

2. Study aims

The current study was designed to document the safety and benefits of CR, which included exercise training and testing, in patients with an ICD. In addition to documenting morbidity and mortality associated with the CR program, the study examined the increase in functional capacity achievable over the course of the CR program, as well as the potential improvements possible in QOL measures during the program.

3. Methodology

Consecutive patients with an ICD who entered a single comprehensive tertiary CR program in Sydney, Australia, from 1997 to 2010 were included. Prospective data was analyzed including demographics, past medical history, cardiac risk factors, medications, exercise days, dropout status, left ventricular ejection fraction by gated heart pool scan (LVEF,%), functional capacity, QOL and outcome indicators, program morbidity, and 1 year mortality post CR.

Exercise capacity was assessed in all patients by functional testing at the beginning of the CR program, and an exercise program, including both aerobic and resistive exercise regimes, was prescribed. All ICD patients were exercised with a wireless monitor linked to a central computer. Exercise capacity after the 6 week CR program was also assessed in patients completing the program.

All patients had education, assessment and counselling sessions as well as exercise training as previously described (Briffa et al., 2009; Zecchin et al., 1999). Secondary prevention strategies were also emphasized. All patients, including CR drop-outs, were followed-up by telephone contact for 1 year post CR.

Quality of Life (QOL) was objectively measured using two self-report questionnaires, the SF-36 (v1) and the DASS21, and was assessed before and after the program.

The SF-36 (v1) Health Survey is a widely used generic questionnaire with standardized scores used to measure physical and social functioning, physical and emotional roles, bodily pain, vitality, mental health and general health perceptions (Ware and Sherbourne 1992). For this questionnaire, a higher score indicates a better level of physical and social functioning, vitality, mental health status and general health. Conversely, a higher score indicates a lower level of bodily pain. Cronbach's scales of the SF-36 (v1) exceed alpha 0.8, except for social functioning (a = 0.76). The questionnaire can be compared to previously published data describing QOL in the normal Australian population - Australian Bureau of Statistics (ABS), 1995.

The DASS21 is a 21 item self-report inventory that yields 3 factors: depression (DEP), anxiety (ANX) and stress (STR) (Lovibond S.H. & Lovibond P.F. 1995). The DASS21 is a set of three self-report scales (7 items per scale) designed to measure the negative emotional states of depression, anxiety and stress.

The Depression Scale assesses dysphoria, hopelessness, devaluation of life, self-deprecation, lack of interest/involvement, anhedonia, and inertia. The Anxiety Scale assesses autonomic arousal, skeletal muscle effects, situational anxiety, and subjective experience of anxious affect. The Stress Scale is sensitive to levels of chronic non-specific arousal. It assesses difficulty relaxing, nervous arousal, and being easily upset/agitated, irritable/over-reactive and impatient. In this questionnaire, the higher the score the higher the level of depression, anxiety and/or stress.

The DASS Anxiety Scale correlates 0.81 with the Beck Anxiety Inventory and the DASS depression scale correlates 0.74 with the Beck Depression Inventory in its original form, DASS42 (Lovibond P.F.and Lovibond S.H. 1995).

4. Results

In the study period, 161 patients with an ICD commenced the CR program on 178 occasions. Mean age ($\pm$ SD) was 61 $\pm$ 10 years, 85% of patients were male, and mean LVEF was 30 $\pm$ 10%.

Medical history included hyperlipidaemia 85%, hypertension 52%, previous myocardial infarction 48%, current smoking 29%, diabetes mellitus 26%, chronic obstructive airways disease 17%, previous cerebrovascular accident (CVA) 11% and depression 11%.

Cardioactive medications used were beta-blockers 85%, angiotensin converting enzyme inhibitors (ACEI) or angiotensin receptor blockers 72%, specific antiarrhythmic drugs 17%, nitrates 15% and digoxin 10%. Adherence to medication was emphasized, and regularly checked with both patients and carers.

Functional capacity testing was performed in all patients prior to CR commencement. Treadmill exercise tests (EST) were performed in 78%, 6 minute walk tests (6MWT) in 21% and timed up and go tests in 1%. Mean number of exercise sessions attended during the CR program was 9 $\pm$ 7. Program completion rate was 62%, with the drop-out rate for non-medical reasons being 14%. For those patients who completed CR, the same functional test was repeated at the end of the program.

There were no deaths or ventricular tachyarrhythmias in study patients while they were exercising or undergoing a functional capacity test. There were 4 deaths in the study group at 1 year follow-up (mortality 2%). Two of these patients died 6 months post CR program, and 2 others died while on the program. These latter 2 patients were admitted to hospital with heart failure which proved refractory to treatment.

Other admissions to hospital while patients were on the CR program were for the following reasons - acute heart failure 3%, displaced lead 1%, percutaneous interventions 1%, CVA 0.5%, ICD activations 0.5% and miscellaneous causes 2%.

Functional capacity increased significantly in patients completing the CR program. For those undertaking EST assessment, MET levels rose from 6.9 $\pm$ 2.2 pre CR to 9.6 $\pm$ 2.8 post CR, $p < 0.001$. For the 6MWT group, distance walked increased from 373 $\pm$ 114 metres pre CR to 430 $\pm$ 126 metres post CR, $p = 0.04$.

Resting heart rate at the initial functional assessment was 75 $\pm$ 14 beats/min, rising to 109 $\pm$ 21 beats/min at peak exercise ($p < 0.001$). Systolic BP rose from a baseline of 111 $\pm$ 18 mmHg to a peak of 131 $\pm$ 25 mmHg ($p < 0.001$) during the initial functional assessment.

For patients completing the CR program, QOL indicators also improved between pre and post CR assessments, with respect to most SF-36 domains, and also the DASS[21] Depression and Anxiety Scales (Table 1).

5. Discussion

The patients in this study had significant left ventricular dysfunction, as well as propensity for ventricular tachyarrhythmias, but were clinically well enough to commence a CR program and to participate in the exercise component which was a key core feature of CR at Westmead Hospital. The majority of participants completed the program, and all patients were accounted for at follow-up. Standard antifailure therapy was taken by a clear majority of patients, with over 80% being on beta blockers and over 70% on ACEI or angiotensin receptor blockers.

SF-36 Domains (n=77)	Pre Program	Post Program	p-value	ABS 1995 Mean (n >18,500)
General Health	62±20	66±21	0.09	72
Physical Functioning	54±23	74±21	<0.001	83
Role-Physical	26±37	55±40	0.049	80
Bodily Pain	65±24	82±22	<0.001	77
Vitality	54±22	69±19	<0.001	65
Social Functioning	64±28	82±21	<0.001	85
Role-Emotional	48±44	72±40	<0.001	83
Mental Health	72±20	77±18	0.21	76
Total	108±17	120±16	<0.001	
DASS21 (n=78)				
Depression	7.4±8.8	5.2±7.6	0.006	
Anxiety	6.9±6.8	5.2±6.1	0.005	
Stress	8.4±7.7	7.2±7.5	0.10	

Table 1. QOL assessments pre and post CR in ICD patients.

5.1 Safety of exercise

This study extended previous observations that exercise training as well as formal EST assessments are safe, and do not promote ICD activations.

There have been theoretical concerns that ventricular tachyarrhythmias can be provoked by adrenergic stimulation, such as occurs with exercise, but the present study and other studies of exercise testing or exercise training in patients with ICDs have now consistently shown that this concern is not warranted (Hussein & Thomas 2008). While this may in part be related to the high usage of beta blockers in the present study, there is data from both animal and clinical studies to suggest that exercise training might potentially reduce the incidence of ventricular tachyarrhythmias by shifting autonomic balance towards an increase in vagal tone, and by reducing the frequency of ischaemic episodes which may trigger arrhythmias (see reviews by Hussein & Thomas 2008; Lewin, et al., 2001).

5.2 Effects of exercise on functional capacity

Exercise prescription and training can also improve general physical fitness, and this in turn can decrease the likelihood of an early inappropriately fast sinus tachycardia with exercise, which could potentially lead to inappropriate ICD discharges if heart rate cut-offs for ICD shocks are exceeded. The heart rate response to exercise noted during the CR program can, in turn, help optimize the setting of heart rate cut-offs for ICD activation, so helping to reduce inappropriate ICD discharges.

Functional capacity improved substantially during the course of the 6 week CR program in this study, but MET levels achieved were still short of the 11-14 MET workloads achieved at the Westmead Hospital CR program in patients without ICDs (Kovoor, et al., 2006). The improvement in MET levels achieved in the Westmead ICD patients was 2-3 METS on average, which could potentially translate to a substantial reduction in mortality (up to 13% reduction for each increase in workload of 1 MET - Kokkinos et al., 2007), particularly if the improved functional capacity can be maintained after completion of the CR program.

Exercise training in patients with heart failure have demonstrated that most of the benefit appears to be the result of peripheral adaptations, although some improvements in cardiac function have also been documented (Briffa et al., 2009; Haykowsky et al., 2007). The present study did not re-evaluate LVEF at 1 yr post CR, and it is not known whether the low 1 year mortality observed was due to improvement in left ventricular function.

Demonstration to patients that they can safely exercise to relatively high workloads without setting off the ICD is an important way of building patient confidence and self esteem, as well as ensuring that they have improved endurance, reduced fatigue and increased muscular strength (Lampman & Knight 2000). This reinforces the desirability of continuing a regular exercise program after the CR program has been completed.

5.3 Effects on quality of life measures

Psychosocial problems of patients with ICDs include anxiety, depression, insomnia, fear of either shocks from the device or device malfunction, and reduced quality of life in general (Hussein & Thomas 2008; Sears et al., 2005; Sola & Bostwick 2005). As shown in Table 1, QOL in ICD patients in this study was poor when compared with the general Australian population, but did improve significantly over the course of the 6 week CR program. This study showed significant improvements in QOL indicators as assessed by both the SF-36 domains and $DASS^{21}$ scales.

The improvements in QOL documented in the present study were in the SF-36 domains of physical functioning, social functioning, physical and emotional roles, bodily pain and vitality. Anxiety and Depression DASS Scales also showed favourable outcomes during the course of the CR program. These major benefits probably derive from a combination of factors, including exercise training, and active educational and counselling sessions giving guidance on general health matters, secondary prevention, lifestyle change and psychosocial support. There may be a differential benefit for older and younger age groups (Crossmann et al., 2010) but this was not examined in the present study.

ICD patients are a heterogeneous group, both from the physical and psychological points of view. CR programs should have certain core components including exercise, education and psychological interventions. The individual needs of patients will have to be addressed by having sufficient flexibility of CR programs so as to tailor the individual programs to the needs of the patients.

6. Conclusion

This study shows that exercise testing and exercise training is safe in ICD patients who are clinically stable, and that exercise does not provoke ventricular tachyarrhythmias. The ICD patients also gain significant improvements in functional capacity and QOL outcomes.
Future studies will need to evaluate whether these benefits are maintained over time.

7. Acknowledgements

The contribution of the staff at the Cardiac Education and Assessment Program at Westmead Hospital, Sydney, is gratefully acknowledged.

8. References

Ades, P.A. Cardiac rehabilitation and secondary prevention of coronary heart disease (2001). *New Engl J Med* 345: 892-902.

Australian Bureau of Statistics (1995). *National Health Survey- SF-36 Population Norms – Australia.* ABS Catalogue No. 4399.0

Bellardinelli, R., Capestro, F., Misiani, A., Scipione, P. & Georgiou D. (2006). Moderate exercise training improves functional capacity, quality of life, and endothelium-dependent vasodilation in chronic heart failure patients with implantable cardioverter defibrillators and cardiac resynchronization therapy. *Eur J Cardiovasc Prev Rehabil* 13: 818-825.

Briffa, T.G., Kinsman, L., Maiorana, A.J., Zecchin, R., Redfern, J., Davidson, P.M., Paull, G., Nagle, A. & Denniss, A.R. (2009). An integrated and coordinated approach to preventing recurrent coronary heart disease events in Australia. Policy statement from the Australian Cardiovascular Health and Rehabilitation Association. *Med J Aust* 190: 683-686.

Chinnaiyan, K.M., Trivax, J., Franklin, B.A., Williamson, B. & Kahn, J.K. (2007). Stress testing in patients with implantable cardioverter-defibrillators: a preliminary report. *Prev Cardiol* 10: 92-95.

Crossmann, A., Schulz, S.M., Kuhlkamp, V., Ritter, O., Neuser, H., Schumacher, B., Bauer, W. & Pauli, P. (2010). A randomized controlled trial of secondary prevention of anxiety and distress in a German sample of patients with an implantable cardioverter-defibrillator. *Psychosomatic Medicine* 72: 434-441.

Dougherty, C.M., Glenny, R. & Kudenchuk, P.J. (2008). Aerobic exercise improves fitness and heart rate variability after an implantable cardioverter defibrillator. *J Cardiopulm Rehabil Prev* 28: 307-311.

Fan, S., Lyon, C.E., Savage, P.D., Ozonoff, A., Ades, P.A. & Balady, G.J. (2009). Outcomes and adverse events among patients with implantable cardiac defibrillators in cardiac rehabilitation. A case-controlled study. *J Cardiopulm Rehabil Prev* 29: 40-43.

Fitchet, A., Doherty, P.J., Bundy, C., Fitzpatrick, A.P. & Garratt, C.J. (2003). Comprehensive cardiac rehabilitation programme for implantable cardioverter-defibrillator patients: a randomized controlled trial. *Heart* 89: 155-160.

Haykowsky, M., Liang, Y., Pechter, D. & Jones, L. (2007). A meta-analysis of the effect of exercise training on left ventricular remodeling in heart failure patients: the benefit depends on the type of training performed. *J Am Coll Cardiol* 49: 2329-2336.

Hussein, N.A. & Thomas, M.A. (2008). Rehabilitation of patients with implantable cardioverter/defibrillator: a literature review. *Acta Cardiol* 63: 249-257.

Keteylan, S.J., Isaac, D., Thadani, U., Roy, B.A., Bensimhon, D.R., McKelvie, R., Russell, S.D., Hellkamp, M.S. & Krause, W.E. on behalf of the HF-ACTION Investigators (2009). Safety of symptom-limited cardiopulmonary exercise testing in patients with chronic heart failure due to severe left ventricular systolic dysfunction. *Am Heart J* 158: S72-S77.

Kokkinos, P., Myers, J., Kokkinos, J.P., Pittaras, A., Narayan, P., Manolis, A., Karasik, P., Greenberg, M., Papademetriou, V. & Singh, S. (2008). Exercise capacity and mortality in black and white men. *Circulation* 117: 614-622.

Kovoor, P., Lee, A.K., Carrozzi, F., Wiseman, V., Byth K., Zecchin, R., Dickson, C., King, M., Hall, J., Ross, D.L., Uther, J.B. & Denniss, A.R. (2006). Full return to normal activities including work at two weeks after acute myocardial infarction. *Am J Cardiol* 97: 952-958.

Lampman, R.M. & Knight B.P. (2000). Prescribing exercise training for patients with defibrillators. *Am J Phys Med Rehabil* 79:292-297.

Lewin, R.J., Frizelle, D.J. & Kaye, G.C. (2001). A rehabilitative approach to patients with internal cardioverter-defibrillators. *Heart* 85: 371-372.

Lovibond, S.H. & Lovibond, P.F. (1995). *Manual for the Depression Anxiety Stress Scales. (2nd. Ed.)* Psychology Foundation. ISBN 7334-1423-0. Sydney.

Lovibond, P.F. & Lovibond, S.H. (1995). The structure of negative emotional states: comparison of the Depression Anxiety Stress Scales (DASS) with the Beck Depression and Anxiety Inventories. *Behaviour Res and Therapy* 33: 335-343.

Sears, S.F., Lewis, T.S., Kuhl, E.A. & Conti, J.B. (2005). Predictors of quality of life in patients with implantable cardioverter defibrillators. *Psychosomatics* 46: 451-457.

Smart, N. & Marwick, T.H. (2004). Exercise training for heart failure patients: a systematic review of factors that improve patient mortality and morbidity. *Am J Med* 116: 673-706.

Sola, C. & Bostwick, M. (2005). Implantable cardioverter-defibrillators, induced anxiety, and quality of life. *Mayo Clin Proc* 80: 232-237.

Vanhees, L., Kornaat, M., Defoor, J., Aufdemkampe, G., Schepers, D., Stevens, A., van Exel, H., van den Beld, J., Heidbuchel, H. & Fagard, R. (2004). Effect of exercise training in patients with an implantable cardioverter-defibrillator. *Eur Heart J* 25: 1120-1126

Ware, J.E. & Sherbourne, C.D. (1992). The MOS 36-item short form health survey (SF-36). *Medical Care* 30: 473-481.

Wenger, N. (2008). Current status of cardiac rehabilitation. *J Am Coll Cardiol* 51: 1619-1631.

Zecchin, R.P., Chai, Y.Y., Roach, K.A., Speerin, R., Squire, J. & Denniss, A.R. (1999). Is nurse-supervised exercise stress testing safe practice? *Heart Lung* 28: 175-185.

16

ICDs and Risk Stratification in Magnetic Field Imaging

Dania Di Pietro Paolo[1], Tobias Toennis[2] and Sergio Nicola Erne[1]

[1]*BMDSys Production GmbH, Magdeburg*
[2]*Medizinische Abteilung Asklepios Klinik St. Georg, Hamburg*
Germany

1. Introduction

Sudden cardiac death (SCD) is the main cause of death in the USA with an annual incidence estimated between 184000 and 462000 (Goldberger et al., 2008). The typical therapy for preventing SCD is the use of Implantable Cardioverter Defibrillators (ICDs) in patients with low left ventricular ejection fraction (LVEF). Unfortunately the LVEF has limited sensitivity and specificity: The majority of SCDs occur in patients with preserved LVEF. Furthermore, SCD often occurs in active, outwardly healthy people with no known heart disease or other health problems: Most victims do have heart diseases such as Hypertrophic Cardiomyopathy, although they are unaware of this fact (Figure 1). ICDs are devices capable of terminating

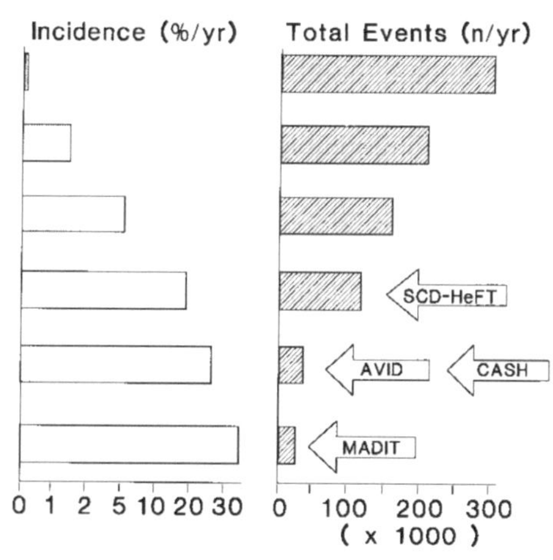

Fig. 1. Estimates of incidences and absolute numbers of SCD. Arrows indicate that trials such as MADIT, AVID and CASH have impact on a small population. SCD-HeFT probably affects a larger population at risk. Anyhow, these subgroups only represent a small part of the patients at highest risk of SCD (Myerburg et al., 1998).

malignant ventricular arrhythmias (Ventricular Tachycardia and/or Ventricular Fibrillation) that have recently been in the focus of large primary prevention studies yielding to an increase of implantation rates (i.e: the SCD-HeFT (Bardy et al., 2005) trial). The substantial number of

patients that fulfill the last trials criteria, in the face of economical constraints and the possible adverse effects, have prompted a research of additional arrhythmia risk markers to further identify patients at highest risk. In fact, the DINAMIT study (Hohnloser et al., 2004) shows that the use of ICDs can reduce the mortality due to arrhythmic events, but on the other hand, the overall mortality increases, due probably to the augmentation of heart failure deaths in the ICD group, presumably due to the ICD interventions. Because of this unprecedented expansion of ICD implantations, that only in few cases (between 21 to 35%) (Bardy et al., 2005) leads to an appropriate therapy (arrhythmic events followed by a shock), there is a continuous interest in a non-invasive predictor for risk-stratification (refer to section 2).
Within the last years, a new methodology is gaining interest in clinical use: Magnetic Field Imaging (MFI) / Magnetocardiography (MCG) (Yamada & Yamaguchi, 2005). Korhonen *et al.* (Korhonen et al., 2006) have performed a pioneer clinical study analyzing the intra QRS-fragmentation in averaged MCG/MFI data (for a mathematical description of the method refers to (Link et al., 1994) and (Mueller et al., 1999)), after attempts made using the high frequencies components of the QRS as marker of risk both in Electrocardiography (ECG) (Cain et al., 1990) and MCG (Leder et al., 2000). The results have showed the superiority of the method in comparison to ECG and, in all-cause mortality, an abnormal MFI score together with a LVEF <30% has shown a positive predictive accuracy (PPA) of 50% and a negative predictive accuracy (NPA) of 91% (Steinberg & Levitt, 2006). The population considered in this work was quite small (158 patients after myocardial infarction- MI) and therefore a bigger perspective clinical study is needed for validating the role of QRS-fragmentation as a risk stratificator.
In Germany one multi center study (MFI-RISTI) is ongoing to prove the utility of this parameter in patients prone to ventricular tachycardia (VT). Although pre-trial data in patients with cardiac dysfunction before implantation of ICDs has been presented, this kind of study is time consuming (in the order of years, if the follow-up phase is considered). An alternative approach is to perform retrospective studies on patients with already implanted ICDs (CORE-AIIM).

2. State of the art

In this section, an overview of the risk stratification methods developed till now is presented (Toennis & Kuck, 2009). These methods were developed in order to have a more precise indicator of Ventricular Fibrillation (VF) and /or Ventricular Tachycardia (VT), both in ischemic and non ischemic patients. The parameters that are used for risk stratification can be divided into different groups:

- conduction system
  - QRS-length
  - late potentials
- heterogeneous ventricular repolarization
  - QT-interval
  - QT-dispersion
  - T-wave alternans (TWA)
- imbalance of the autonomic tonus
  - heart rate variability (HRV)
  - heart rate turbulence (HRT)

  - baroreflex sensitivity (BS)
- left ventricular ejection fraction
- ventricular ectopy

2.1 Conduction system

2.1.1 QRS-length

The QRS-length is the easiest parameter to be determined, by measuring the length of the QRS complex on a 12-lead ECG. About 2% of the U.S. population has a QRS-length more than 120 ms and about 5% has either a right or left bundle-branch block (BBB). Among the patients with chronic congestive heart failure, the percentage of those with a QRS-prolongation increases up to 50%. If only those patients with left BBB (LBBB) are taken into consideration, it can be proved that LBBB may be considered an independent predictor of cardiovascular mortality due to SCD. The MADIT-II and the SCD-HeFT studies could not prove a dependence between QRS-prolongation and VT/VF events in patients with ICDs (Buxton et al., 2005).
QRS-length is not recommended, at this stage, for the risk stratification of SCD.

2.1.2 Late-potentials

Late potentials refer to low amplitude signals that occur after the end of the QRS, due to a delay of the conduction system. Low amplitude signals cannot be observed in patient with a BBB since they are hidden; furthermore those signals from regions of scar may also be obscured if the abnormal region is depolarized during the QRS. The validity of this method was proved in the CABG-Patch test. ICD implantation did not improve survivals, although arrhythmic deaths were reduced. Some studies pointed out that late potentials predicted death due to progressive heart failure rather than SCD (Yi et al., 1996).
The use of this parameter for SCD is not adequately supported at this time. Further studies are required to assess the utility of this test (Goldberger et al., 2008).

2.2 Heterogeneous ventricular repolarization

2.2.1 QT-interval

QT-interval is the summation of the ventricular action potentials duration. Since it varies with the heart variability, a corrected definition using the Bazett ' s formula is used. Although the reproducibility of the QT-interval is very high, the need for correction makes it difficult to compare values of this parameter for different patients. There are controversial studies where the QT-interval was related to higher mortality in patient with low EF, but with different results (Brendorp et al., 2001; Padmanabhan et al., 2003).
The use of this parameter for risk stratification is not supported.

2.2.2 QT-dispersion

QT-dispersion should reflect the dispersion of the myocardial recovery and should be associated with arrhythmia risk. There have been numerous studies that related the QT-dispersion to increased mortality, but no relation was found between QT-dispersion and outcome (Gang et al., 2003).
The use of this parameter for risk stratification is not supported.

2.2.3 T-wave alternans

T-wave alternans (TWA) is a reflection of repolarization alternans at level of the single cells. T-wave alternans is a rate-dependent phenomenon and tends to occur at lower heart rates in

patients prone to ventricular arrhythmias. In order to measure the TWA, a target heart rate with regular R-R (without ectopic beats present) has to be achieved. Because of this, a high percentage (from 12 to 41%) of patients that undergo the test, get an undetermined result. Different studies have been performed, but they have different results (Costantini et al., 2009; Gold et al., 2008).
Furthermore, it is worth to be remembered that TWA cannot be applied in patients with atrial fibrillation (AF- 9-30%) and in those who are not allowed to perform physical test (15%).
Finally, TWA cannot be suggested as parameter for risk stratification.

2.3 Imbalance of the autonomic tonus

2.3.1 Heart rate variability

The Heart rate variability (HRV) can be defined as the variation over time of the period between consecutive heartbeats. It is predominantly dependent on the extrinsic regulation of the heart rate (HR). It reflects the state of the autonomic nervous system that can be divided into two branches: the parasympathetic and the sympathetic nervous system. Normally cardiac arrhythmias occur in patients with enhanced sympathetic and diminished parasympathetic activity; furthermore the parasympathetic effects on the sinus node could predict mortality. The HRV can be calculated over a measurement that lasts between 3 and 8 minutes or using an Holter ECG. Atrial Fibrillation is an exclusion criterion for this method.

2.3.1.1 Short-term HRV

The short-term HRV is not reproducible, especially in patients with congestive heart failure. Moreover, there is a very strong interindividual variation in the relationship between short-term HRV and parasympathetic effect (Goldberger et al., 2001). For these reasons it cannot be used as parameter for the risk stratification of SCD.

2.3.1.2 Long-term HRV

In case the long-term HRV is used, the circadian rhythm has to be taken into account as well as the changes in HR according to the daily activity: This means that the power spectrum (PS) in the PS analysis is not stationary. In many studies it has been proved that there is an increase in mortality in those patients with a low HRV, but there is no evidence of a relation between low HRV and SCD (Gerritsen et al., 2001).
For this reason it cannot be used as parameter for risk stratification of SCD.

2.3.2 Heart rate turbulence

The term Heart Rate Turbulence (HRT) describes short-term fluctuations in sinus cycle length that follows spontaneous ventricular premature complexes (VPCs) (Schmidt et al., 1999). In normal subjects, it consists of a short initial acceleration followed by a deceleration of the heart rate compared with the pre-VPC rate. In order to use this method, at least 15 premature beats have to be analyzed in patients without AF. It was demonstrated that there is an increase in mortality in post-MI patients with low HRT.
HRT is a very attractive parameter for risk stratification, but a study involving the relation between low HRT and SCD has not been performed yet.

2.3.3 Baroreflex sensitivity

The baroreflex mechanism is a central part of the regulation of the cardiovascular system, particularly in the control of vagal and sympathetic outflow to the heart and the peripheral circulation. Baroreflex sensitivity (BRS) can be quantified by the analysis of the changes in

heart rate in response to changes in blood pressure. It has been demonstrated that there is a close link between reduced BRS and increased risk for serious ventricular tachyarrhythmias (Schwartz et al., 1992).
Although there are studies that suggest the utility of BRS as parameter for risk stratification of SCD in patients with CHD, further studies and a method to get a more reproducibility parameter are needed.

2.4 Left Ventricular ejection fraction

LFEF, that measures the left ventricular systolic function, is the most used parameter for the indication of implantation of an ICD. Reduced LVEF is considered a risk factor for overall mortality and SCD in the heart failure population. Although the LVEF has been demonstrated as the strongest independent predictor of SCD, its sensitivity and specificity are very low. In fact, if ,on the one hand, those persons with low EF have a higher probability to die from SCD, on the other hand, there is a considerable amount of people that die from SCD and have a preserved EF.

2.5 Ventricular ectopy and NSVT

Ventricular ectopic beats (VEBs) and non-sustained ventricular tachycardia (NSVT) are common arrhythmias that appear on the surface electrocardiogram (ECG) as a profound disturbance of normal cardiac rhythm (Campbell, 1993). In order to study them an Holter-ECG is necessary. Ectopy beyond 10 VPBs per hour does not affect the risk of mortality. The positive predictive value of VEBs after MI for predicting VT/VF or death is between 5% and 15% and the predictive value increases if it is combined with a low LVEF. Furthermore, patients with non ischemic cardiomyopathy are at increased risk of SCD and frequently have high grade ventricular ectopy and NSVT (Kron et al., 1988), but the relationship is not valid in case of ischemic cardiomyopathy. The method has low sensitivity (Toennis & Kuck, 2009).

3. Magnetic field imaging

3.1 Materials

Magnetic field imaging (MFI) is a new non-invasive modality that is able to combine the recording of external magnetic field (MF) generated by the electrical activity of the heart using a multi channel magnetic sensor array with its clinically applicable spatio-temporal visualization. Since heart MFs are very small when compared with the earth magnetic field (see Figure 2 for comparison), the acquisitions were in the past normally carried out in very heavy and expensive shielding rooms. With the advent of new technologies it is possible to redistribute the workload between hardware and software and this makes it possible the use of MFI in a daily clinical routine. Figure 3 shows an example of MFI acquisition system (Apollo CXS system). The sensor system is a 55-channels SQUID gradiometer system arranged in a hexagonal matrix, which covers an area of approximately 28 cm. The patients lie in a supine position during the recording. The sensor system is placed at approximately 1 cm distance from the anterior chest wall above the heart. For the details concerning the acquisition and the preprocessing please refer to (Di Pietro Paolo et al., 2011).
The here mentioned MFI recordings were carried out at the Asklepios Hospital St. Georg in Hamburg (Germany) using an Apollo CXS system (BMDSys Production GmbH, Germany).
Magnetic signals of 172 subjects were recorded: The control group consisted of 20 healthy volunteers and 44 subjects with normal coronary and normal LVEF, whereas the other group

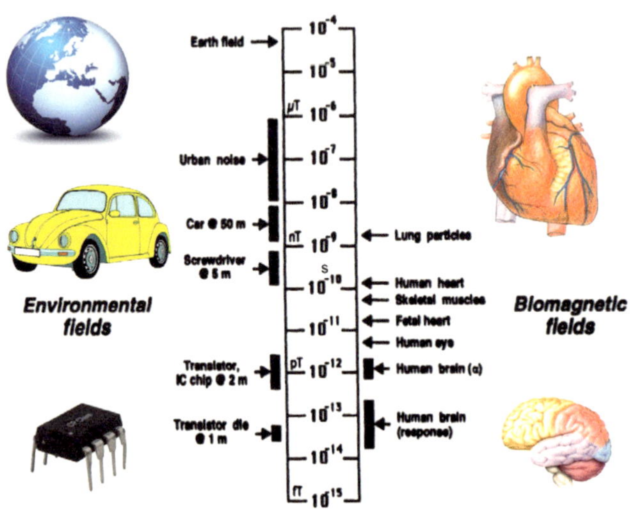

Fig. 2. Comparison of selected biomagnetic fields (heart, brain) and environment disturbances.

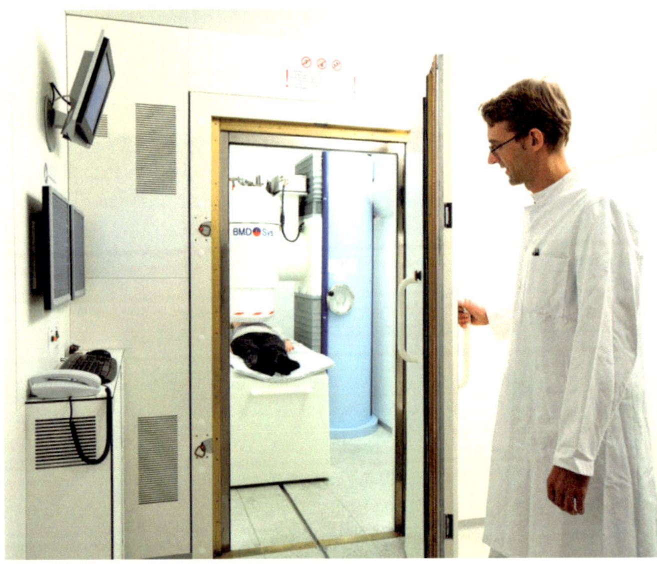

Fig. 3. Apollo CXS system: view from the preparation room into the acquisition room soon before the acquisition is carried out. The patient lies on the bed as close as possible under the dewar bottom.

consisted of 108 patients with primary prevention indication for ICD implantation, before the implantation.
The acquisition lasted about 5 minutes. All patients were followed up after implantation. The primary endpoint was the occurrence of ventricular arrhythmias.
Further information concerning the subjects characteristics can be found in the tables 1 and 2.

	ICD-group	volunteers	no CHD
N	108	20	44
Male	88(81%)	5(25%)	26(59%)
Female	20(19%)	15(75%)	18(41%)
Age	64 ± 12	39 ± 11	61 ± 11
Diabetes Mellitus	29(27%)	0	9(20%)
Hypertension	76(70%)	0	31(70%)
AF	35(32%)	0	7(16%)
LBBB	32(30%)	0	2(5%)
QRS	120 ± 33	90 ± 18	95 ± 18
LVEF	$27 \pm 7\%$	n.a.	$61 \pm 9\%$ [1]
β-Blockers	88(81%)	0	25(57%)
Amiodarone	25(23%)	0	2(5%)

Table 1. Subjects Characteristics: number of subjects, sex, medicaments, QRS-length, percentage of persons with Atrial Fibrillation (AF), Left Bundle Branch Block (LBBB) and Left Ventricular Ejection Fraction (LVEF).

	ICD-group
N	108
Isch. CM	74(69%)
DCM	31(29%)
Other (Brugada, Myocarditis,HOCM)	3(3%)
CABS	29(27%)
NYHA I	17(16%)
NYHA II	47(44%)
NYHA IIII	43(40%)
NYHA IV	1(1%)
ICD	100(93%)
VR	44(41%)
DR	25(23%)
CRT	31(29%)
no ICD	8(7%)

Table 2. ICD-Patients Characteristics: number of patients with Ischemic Cardiomyopathy (Isch. CM), Dilated Cardiomyopathy (DCM), Hyper-trophic obstructive cardiomyopathy (HOCM), Coronary artery bypass surgery (CABS), New York Heart Association (NYHA) Class I, II, III, and IV, ICDs in different typology (single chamber (VR), dual chamber (DR) and Cardiac Resynchronization Therapy (CRT)).

3.2 Methods-the Fragmentation Index (FI)

As aforementioned, QRS-fragmentation can be very useful for the risk stratification of SCD. A new parametrization of QRS- fragmentation has been introduced based on the findings of the past decades in order to make it possible to apply MFI using standardized equipments used in clinical environment and under clinical routine conditions. Until now, parameterization of

[1] data not available for all subjects

the fragmentation was based on the quantification suggested by (Endt et al., 1998) which in principle is a measure of the magnitude and number of extrema of the averaged and bandpass filtered QRS-complex signal. This direct approach has some intrinsic limitations:

- the weighting over the number of extrema makes the parameter very sensitive to the total noise.
- it only concentrates on one aspect of the fragmentation: the level difference.
- the score is clearly designed as a local quantity, since it refers to the signal of one channel

Furthermore, as already reported by (Mueller et al., 1999) the elementary parameters referring to a single channel have to be evaluated over all the available sensors with the goal to extract global values which are typical for the spatio-temporal evolution of the QRS-complex.
Here, the parameterization of the fragmentation without the weighting with the number of extrema has been proposed. Three parameters were calculated for each QRS interval in each channel:

1. The signal magnitude between the extrema: *step*

$$s_{step,i} = |y(t_{i+1}) - y(t_i)| \tag{1}$$

2. The sum over the slopes (derivative): *slope*

$$s_{slope,i} = \frac{|y(t_{i+1}) - y(t_i)|}{t_{i+1} - t_i} \tag{2}$$

3. The length of the linearized signal curve: *trace*

$$s_{trace,i} = \sqrt{(y(t_{i+1}) - y(t_i))^2 + (t_{i+1} - t_i)^2} \tag{3}$$

In Equation 1 and 2 the time intervals were normalized to an idealized QRS length of 80 ms. In this way a set of 3 indicators (step, slope and trace), each of them related to the sensor position was obtained. Mueller *et al.* (Mueller et al., 1999) pointed out that the availability of a large array of sensors is important because:

- only channels with high signal to noise ratio (> 40 % of the maximum QRS amplitude) are worth to be considered.
- channels "close" to the zero line in the dipolar pattern are more easily contaminated by breathing artifacts.

As a consequence, the maximum (*MAX*) and the root mean square (*RMS*) of the calculated parameters of all sensors satisfying the above mentioned conditions (signal amplitude > 40 % of the maximum QRS amplitude, sensor "far" from zero line) lead to 6 global parameters, 2 (*MAX* and *RMS*) for each of the 3 indicators (step, slope, and trace). The final goal was to obtain a unique scalar parameter. In order to perform the average of the 6 parameters defined above, a homogeneous metric had to be used. Therefore all parameters were normalized by the corresponding quadratic mean calculated averaging over a control group defined previously (eq. 4 and 5). Finally, all values were merged to one global, one dimensional scalar parameter: the Fragmentation Index (FI). In order to get the normalization parameters required before, the *RMS* was calculated for all six parameters ($\text{indicator}_{MAX,RMS}$) on the basis of the data of the control group:

$$RMS = \mu_{ind} = \sqrt{\frac{1}{N}\sum_{i=1}^{N} S_{ind}^{2}(i)} \tag{4}$$

where N is the number of subjects contributing to the normalization. That way, normalized parameters were obtained

$$S_{ind}^{*}(i) = \frac{S_{ind}(i)}{\mu_{ind}} \tag{5}$$

A set of 6 normalized parameters, showing the parameterization of the fragmentation, was defined using the signal averaged and band-pass filtered QRS-complex of the selected MFI channels. The Fragmentation Index was determined as the averaged value of the six above introduced parameters.

$$FI = \frac{1}{6}\sum S_{ind(MAX,RMS)}^{*} \tag{6}$$

Figure 4 shows a graphical view of the three parameters in a filtered QRS-complex. Figure 5 shows an example of channels that are used in the calculation of the global Fragmentation Index in a patient with low EF. The QRS-fragmentation Index was determined using the analysis software of Apollo CXS.

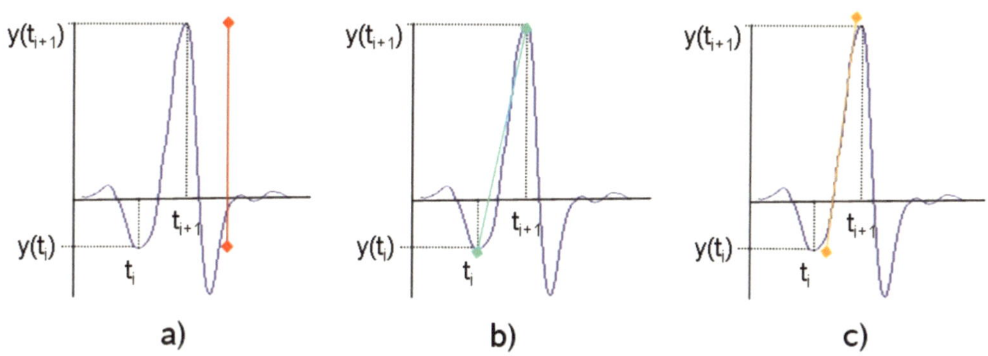

Fig. 4. Schematic explanation of the different fragmentation parameters: a) the difference between extrema: *step*, b) the length of the curve: *trace*, c) the derivative: *slope* (eq. 1, 2, and 3).

Figures 6 shows the QRS-fragmentation into two subjects: Figure 6a shows an example of QRS-fragmentation in a healthy volunteer whereas figure 6b in a patient with an ischemic cardiopathy.

4. Results

4.1 Results - MFI before ICD implantation

Preliminary results of the method have been presented in 2010 at the Herbsttagung und Jahrestagung of the German society of cardiology (Nuernberg) by Toennis et al (Toennis et al., 2010).

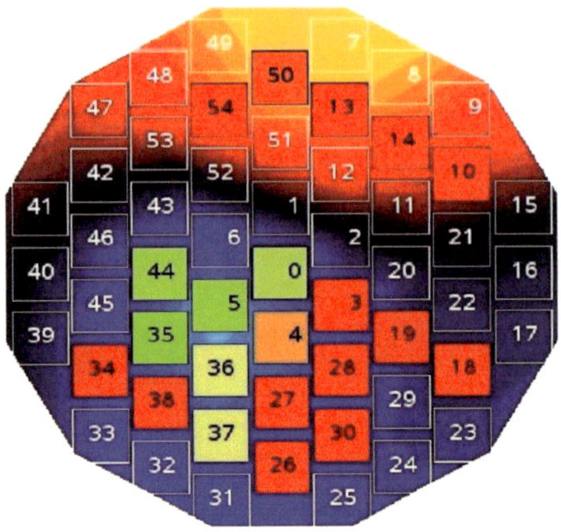

Fig. 5. Magnetic field map with channels position: The different colors of the channels correspond to different values of FI from green (low FI) to red (high FI): the transparent channels correspond to unused channels since too noisy (i.e 29) or too close to the 0 line (i.e: 1).

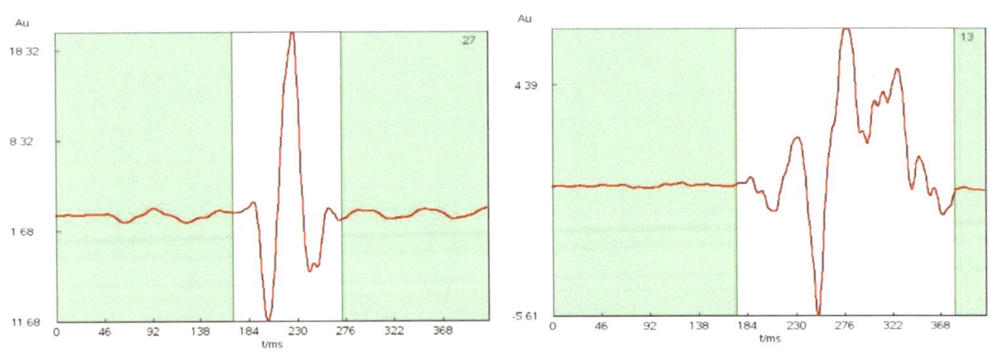

(a) (b)

Fig. 6. a) QRS-fragmentation of one healthy volunteer (FI=0.994), b) QRS-fragmentation in a patient with ischemic cardiomyopathy with EF=25% before ICD implantation (FI=2.10).

The QRS-fragmentation index was calculated in the 172 subjects and the 108 patients with primary prevention indication for ICD implantation had a follow-up of 6.6 months (median 10). There was no event (VT/VF) in the normal group and in those patients with a FI less than 1.25 (normal until light fragmentation). In the ICD group 2 patients died, one for an electrical storm and the other one for a progressive heart failure. Six patients had ventricular episodes (6%), 2 of them termined the episode by means of a DC-shock, 2 by using a anti-tachycardia pacing (ATP) therapy, 1 had one episode before the ICD was implanted (external shock) and the last one had nsVT that is without therapy. Five had an inadequate therapy (5%) caused in 4 out 5 cases by AF. An histogram of the results is in Figure 7.

This prospective study for validating the use of QRS-fragmentation as predictor for arrhythmic events needs time. A faster way for evaluating this method is doing retrospective studies on patients with already implanted ICDs.

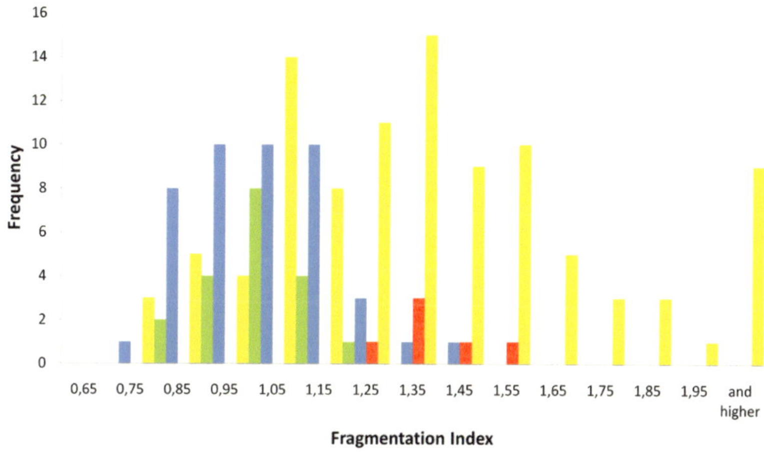

Fig. 7. QRS Fragmentation-Distribution according to the different groups: volunteers (green), Patients without coronary artery disease and normal EF (blue), patients with primary indication for ICD (yellow) and patient with ventricular arrhythmia episodes (red).

4.2 Results - MFI after ICD implantation

A preliminary study is presented using follow up data of 10 patients (10 males-0 females, age 54 ± 8) with already implanted ICD using a post-processing method based on Blind Source Separation (BSS) in order to extract the cardiac signals from biomagnetic signals that are disturbed by an ICD (Di Pietro Paolo et al., 2009). Until now, it has not been possible to perform biomagnetic measurements in patients with ICDs. In fact, the presence of this device in the thorax (normally located inside the chest on the left shoulder) of the patient leads to very strong interferences, that are orders of magnitude larger than the biomagnetic signal of the heart. For this reason, ICDs and pacemakers are among the exclusion criteria for studies concerning MFI. Di Pietro Paolo et al. (2009) extracted for the first time cardiac signals from measurements disturbed by an ICD, offering the possibility for a QRS-fragmentation analysis in such patients. Two out of the 10 patients had a ventricular arrhythmic event and both of them had a higher fragmentation level when compared to a patient that did not shock (Figure 8). On the basis of these results, a first retrospective study (MFI-COREAIIM), enrolling patients with already ICD implanted, has been started.

5. Discussion and conclusion

The gold standard to evaluate the risk to suffer from a VT/VF in future and for the implantation of an ICD is based on LVEF. LVEF does not directly measure arrhythmogenic substrate and statistics also show that only about 20% of those individuals, being evaluated to be at risk on the basis of LVEF, suffer from life threatening VT/VF within two years after diagnosis, respectively ICD implantation. On the other hand, looking at those persons that die from SCD there is consent that about 75% of them suffer from a preceding VT/VF episode before dying suddenly. This means that the LVEF has a small sensitivity and specificity: As already pointed out previously, the persons that die from SCD knowing to be suffering from a cardiac disease are only a small percentage when compared to the total number of persons dying from SCD every year (1/1000/y in the U.S).

There is, for this reason, still the need of non-invasive parameters for risk stratification of

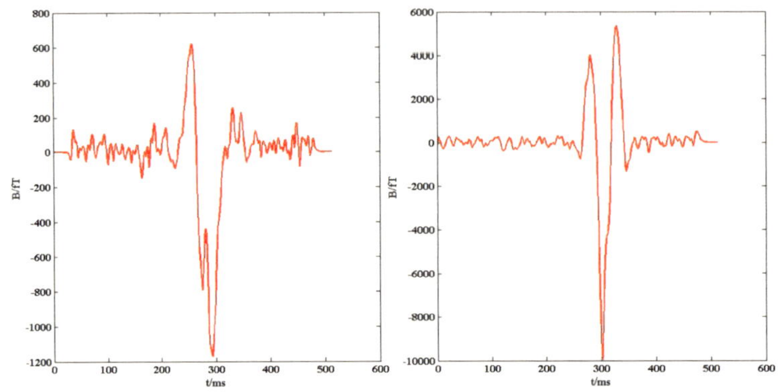

Fig. 8. Illustration of QRS-fragmentation recorded in two patients with implanted ICD, after post-processing: a) QRS fragmentation of a shocked patient, b) QRS-fragmentation of a patients that did not shock: Note the difference in the fragmentation level into the two cases.

patients at highest risk to die from SCD. In this chapter the main non invasive parameters introduced in the last period have been briefly described, but none of them was able to get better results when compared to LVEF. Another important point that should be consider is that most of the non-invasive parameters correlate with all cause of mortality, but the correlation with SCD is still unclear.

Magnetic Field Imaging can provide another parameter for SCD: the QRS-fragmentation. The easy application of a 5 minutes MFI examination and the lack of any risk or negative side-effects for the patient support the suggestion to use MFI as an efficient method to evaluate individuals risk. QRS fragmentation has already been shown to be a reasonable predictor for arrhythmic events and mortality in patients with cardiac dysfunction after myocardial infarction (Korhonen et al., 2006). The QRS-fragmentation was then parameterized to obtain a stable reproducible and operator-independent parameter: the Fragmentation Index. This method could complement the new risk stratification guidelines, as stability and reproducibility of the FI detected by means of non-invasive MFI have been shown. Based on these findings, two studies are ongoing: one is a prospective study (RISTI) that shows the correlation between high QRS-fragmentation (calculated before ICD implantation) and arrhythmic ventricular events whereas the other one is a retrospective study (CORE-AIIM) that investigates the relation between QRS-fragmentation and events in patients with an already ICD implanted.

Preliminary results of two ongoing studies have been referred, showing that high Fragmentation Index correlates (at this point of the trial) with an higher probability to suffer from a VT/VF.

6. References

Bardy, G. H., Lee, K. L., Mark, D. B., Poole, J. E., Packer, D. L., Boineau, R., Domanski, M., Troutman, C., Anderson, J., Johnson, G., McNulty, S. E., Clapp-Channing, N., Davidson-Ray, L. D., Fraulo, E. S., Fishbein, D. P., Luceri, R. M. & Ip, J. H. (2005). Amiodarone or an implantable cardioverter defibrillator for congestive heart failure, *New Engl J Med* 352(3): 225–237.

Brendorp, B., Elming, H., Jun, L., Koeber, L., Malik, M., Gorm-Boje, J. & Torp-Pedersen, C. (2001). QTc interval as a guide to select those patients with congestive heart failure and reduced left ventricular systolic function who will benefit from antiarrhythmic treatment with dofetilide, *Circulation* 103: 1422–1427.

Buxton, A., Sweeney, M., Wathen, M., Josephson, M., Otterness, M., Hogan-Miller, E., Stark, A. & Degroot, P. (2005). QRS duration does not predict occurrence of ventricular tachyarrhythmias in patients with implanted cardioverter-defibrillators, *J Am Coll Cardiol.* 46(2): 317–9.

Cain, M., Lindsay, B., Arthur, R., Markham, J. & Ambos, H. (1990). Noninvasive detection of patients prone to life-threatening ventricular arrhythmias by frequency analysis of electrocardiographic signals, *in* D. Zipes & J. Jalife (eds), *Cardiac. Electrophysiology. From Cell to Bedside*, WB Saunders, Philadelphia, PA, pp. 817–831.

Campbell, R. W. (1993). Ventricular ectopic beats and non-sustained ventricular tachycardia, *Lancet* 341: 1454–1458.

Costantini, O., Hohnloser, S. H., Kirk, M. M., Lerman, B. B., Baker, J. H. I., Sethuraman, B., Dettmer, M. M. & Rosenbaum, D. S. (2009). The ABCD (Alternans Before Cardioverter Defibrillator) Trial: Strategies using T-wave alternans to improve efficiency of sudden cardiac death prevention., *J. Am. Coll. Cardiol* 53: 471–479.

Di Pietro Paolo, D., Mueller, H.-P., Goernig, M., Haueisen, J. & Erne, S. (2009). Cardiac signal extraction in patients with implantable cardioverter defibrillators, *Med Eng Phys* 31(9): 1087 – 1094.

Di Pietro Paolo, D., Toennis, T. & Erne, S. (2011). Preprocessing in Magnetic Field Imaging data, *Proceedings of Biosig2011*, SciTePress, Rome, pp. 463–466.

Endt, P., Hahlbohm, H., Kreiseler, D., Oeff, M., Steinhoff, U. & Trahms, L. (1998). Fragmentation of band pass-filtered QRS-complex of patients prone to malignant arrhythmia, *Med Biol Eng Comput* 36: 723–728.

Gang, Y., Ono, T., Hnatkova, K., Hashimoto, K., Camm, A. J., Pitt, B., Poole-Wilson, A., P. & Malik, M. (2003). QT dispersion has no prognostic value in patients with symptomatic heart failure: An elite ii substudy, *PACE* 26(1p2): 394–400.

Gerritsen, J., Dekker, J. M., TenVoorde, B. J., Kostense, P. J., Heine, R. J., Bouter, L. M., Heethaar, R. M. & Stehouwer, C. D. (2001). Impaired autonomic function is associated with increased mortality, especially in subjects with diabetes, hypertension, or a history of cardiovascular disease, *Diabetes Care* 24(10): 1793–1798.

Gold, M., Ip, J., Costantini, O., Poole, J., McNulty, S., Mark, D., Lee, K. & Bardy, G. (2008). Role of microvolt T-wave alternans in assessment of arrhythmia vulnerability among patients with heart failure and systolic dysfunction: primary results from the T-wave alternans sudden cardiac death in heart failure trial substudy., *Circulation* 118(20): 2022–8.

Goldberger, J., Cain, M., Hohnloser, S., Kadish, A., Knight, B., Lauer, M., Maron, B., Page, R., Passman, R., Siscovick, D., Siscovick, D., Stevenson, W. & Zipes., D. (2008). American Heart Association/American College of Cardiology Foundation/Heart Rhythm Society scientific statement on noninvasive risk stratification techniques for identifying patients at risk for sudden cardiac death, *J. Am. Coll. Cardiol.* 52: 179–199.

Goldberger, J., Challapalli, S., Tung, R., Parker, M. & Kadish, A. (2001). Relationship of Heart Rate Variability to parasympathetic effect, *Circulation* 103: 1977.

Hohnloser, S. H., Kuck, K. H., Dorian, P., Roberts, R. S., Hampton, J. R., Hatala, R., Fain, E., Gent, M. & Connolly, S. J. (2004). Prophylactic use of an Implantable Cardioverter Defibrillator after acute myocardial infarction, *New Engl J Med* 351(24): 2481–2488.

Korhonen, P., Husa, T., Tierala, I., VääNänen, H., Mäkijärvi, M., Katila, T. & Toivonen, L. (2006). Increased intra-qrs fragmentation in magnetocardiography as a predictor of arrhythmic events and mortality in patients with cardiac dysfunction after myocardial infarction, *J Cardiovasc Electr* 17(4): 396–401.

Kron, J., Hart, M., Schual-Berke, S., Niles, N., Hosenpud, J. & McAnulty, J. (1988). Idiopathic dilated cardiomyopathy. role of programmed electrical stimulation and Holter monitoring in predicting those at risk of sudden death., *Chest* 93(1): 85–90.

Leder, U., Frankenstein, L., Haas, J., Baier, V., Haueisen, J., Nowak, H. & Figulla, H. (2000). Temporal proprieties of high frequency intra-qrs signals in myocardial infarction and healthy hearts, *Biomed. Technik* 45: 243–247.

Link, A., Trahms, L., Zimmermann, R. & Oeff, M. (1994). Complex binomial bandpass filters for analysis phase and envelope of high frequency components in cardiac signals, *Comput. Cardiol.* pp. 617–629.

Mueller, H.-P., Goedde, P., Czerski, K., Oeff, M., Agrawal, R., Endt, P., Kruse, W., Steinhoff, U. & Trahms, L. (1999). Magnetocardiographic analysis of the two-dimensional distribution of intra-qrs fractionated activation, *Phys. Med. Biol.* 44: 105–120.

Myerburg, R., Mitrani, R., Interian, A. & Castellanos, A. (1998). Interpretation of outcomes of antiarrhythmic clinical trials design features and population impact, *Circulation* 97: 1514 - 1521.

Padmanabhan, S., Silvet, H., Amin, J. & Pai, R. G. (2003). Prognostic value of QT interval and QT dispersion in patients with left ventricular systolic dysfunction: Results from a cohort of 2265 patients with an ejection fraction of <=40%, *Am Heart J* 145(1): 132 – 138.

Schmidt, G., Malik, M., Barthel, P., Schneider, R., Ulm, K., Rolnitzky, L., Camm, A., Bigger, J. J. & Schoemig, A. (1999). Heart-Rate Turbulence after ventricular premature beats as a predictor of mortality after acute myocardial infarction, *Lancet* 353(9162): 1390 1379.

Schwartz, P., La Rovere, M. & Vanoli, E. (1992). Autonomic nervous system and sudden cardiac death. experimental basis and clinical observations for post-myocardial infarction risk stratification., *Circulation* 85(1 Suppl.): 177–191.

Steinberg, J. S. & Levitt, H. (2006). Magnetocardiography throws its hat in the ring, *J Cardiovasc Electr* 17(3): 1–3.

Toennis, T. & Kuck, K.-H. (2009). Grenzen und Moeglichkeiten der nichtinvasiven Risikostratifikation fuer den ploetzlichen Herztod, *Herz* 34(7): 506–516.

Toennis, T., Ujeyl, A. & Kuck, K.-H. (2010). Magnetic Field Imaging zur Risikostratifizierung des ploetzlichen Herztodes bei Patienten mit primaerpraeventiver ICD Indikation, Herbsttagung, Nuernberg.

Yamada, S. & Yamaguchi, I. (2005). Magnetocardiograms in clinical medicine: unique information on cardiac ischemia, arrhythmias, and foetal diagnosis, *Intern. Med.* 44(1): 1–19.

Yi, G., Keeling, P., Goldman, J., Hnatkova, K., Malik, M. & McKenna, W. (1996). Comparison of time domain and spectral turbulence analysis of the signal-averaged electrocardiogram for the prediction of prognosis in idiopathic dilated cardiomyopathy, *Clin. Cardiol.* 19(10): 800–8.

17

Remote Monitoring of Implantable Cardioverter-Defibrillator Therapy

MJ Pekka Raatikainen and Ulla-Maija Koivisto[1]
Heart Center Tampere University Hospital, Tampere,
[1]Division of Cardiology, Oulu University Hospital, Oulu,
Finland

1. Introduction

With increasing awareness of the indications of implantable cardioverter defibrillator (ICD) therapy, the number of patients with ICDs has been growing rapidly. Patient with an ICD require high-quality care and intense follow-up to ensure safe and effective device performance. Given the expanding use and the complexity of these devices, there has been an urgent need to improve the safety and cost-effectiveness of ICD follow-up and to alleviate the burden of the pacemaker clinics. Remote monitoring is quickly becoming the standard of care for surveillance of patients with ICDs and other cardiovascular implantable electronic devices (CIED). Transtelephonic data transmission via analog phone lines has recently been replaced by sophisticated Internet-based, automatic monitoring systems, which enable transmission of ICD performance and therapy data via a mobile monitor located in the patient's home to a secure server. Within minutes, the data are available to the physician online via a secure Internet access 24/7.

Each company employs somewhat different technology and degree of automation in their systems. For several years Biotronik was the only company with fully automatic wireless data transmission, but recently also the other manufactures have developed GSM-based wireless systems. Currently remote monitoring systems are widely used for the surveillance of ICD patients in the USA and Europe and their use in the other parts of the world is increasing rapidly. We were the first to start using the Medtronic CareLink system in Europe in 2004. It has been estimated that at the moment more than 1 000 000 patients with CIEDs around the world are using remote monitoring systems. The technology is evolving toward fully automated wireless remote monitoring systems which allow instantaneous event transmission without any patient involvement and have the ability of rapidly bring to the physician attention all significant data. Recent trials have demonstrated that remote monitoring reduces clinic burden, and permits early detection of patient and device problems, enabling clinically appropriate intervention and an opportunity to enhance patient safety.

In this article, we describe the currently available remote monitoring systems (Table 1), review the available evidence in the literature regarding remote ICD follow-up and discuss some unresolved issues. In addition, we provide several examples that clarify the benefits of the remote ICD monitoring.

Manufacturer	Name of the system	ICD	CRT	PM	ILR
Biotronik	Home Monitoring	+	+	+	-
Boston Scientific	LATITUDE	+	+*	-	-
Medtronic	CareLink	+	+	+	+
St Jude Medical	Merlin.net	+	+	+	+

Table 1. Remote monitoring systems of the major CIED manufactures. ICD = implantable cardioverter defibrillator, CRT = cardiac resynchronization therapy with (CRT-D) or without defibrillator functions (CRT-D), PM = conventional pacemaker, ILR = implantable loop recorder. *The LATITUDE system is currently compatible only with CRT-D devices.

2. Overview of currently available remote monitoring systems

Since Biotronik pioneered the technology with FDA approval of their first system in 2001, remote monitoring systems have now been introduced by each of the major CIED manufacturers. Presently remote monitoring is primarily used for the surveillance of ICD systems, but the technology is also feasible for the follow-up of other CIEDs including pacemakers (PM), cardiac resynchronization devices (CRT), implantable loop recorders (ILR) and implantable cardiovascular monitors (ICM).
A remote monitoring system consists of an implanted device, a mobile patient monitor, a central database in a secure server, and a password-protected website, where clinicians can view and analyze the data saved in the memory of the patient's device (Figure 1). Systems differ regarding data transfer from the device to the patient monitor. In the early models data transfer required patient's active involvement as he/she had to interrogate the device manually with a specific wand. In the more recent systems data transmission is performed wirelessly from the implanted device to a patient monitor, but each company employs somewhat different technology and degree of automation in their systems.

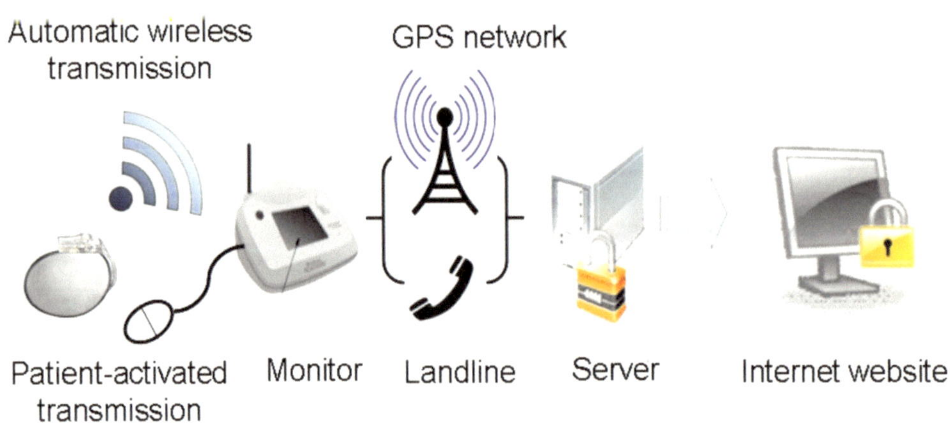

Fig. 1. Components of remote monitoring system. Systems differ regarding data transfer, which may require patient's active involvement or is performed wirelessly from the implanted device to a patient monitor. Data from the patient monitor is sent to a central database using either an analogue phone landline or via GSM network. The data are accessible to the clinical staff on a secure Internet site.

Patient initiated remote transmission requires that the patient manually interrogates and initiates the data transmission using a telemetry wand incorporated in the home transmitter. This encounter may be a scheduled follow-up interrogation or an unscheduled interrogation activated by a patient symptom (*e.g.* ICD shock) or detection of a device alert (audible tone or vibration). Wireless technology allows for automatic data transmission without any patient interaction. Automatic wireless interrogation requires that the implanted device is equipped with an integrated antenna for communication with the transmitter located close to the patient (Figure 2). Data transmission is initiated either at pre-scheduled time intervals or triggered immediately by programmed device alerts (*e.g.* abnormal lead impedance, delivery of ICD therapies, or changes in hemodynamic status).

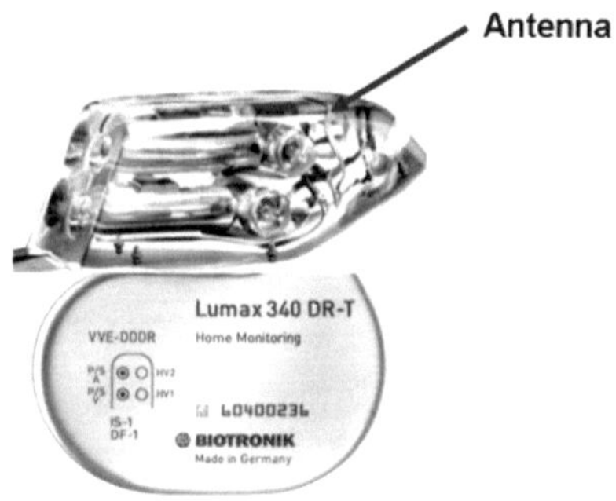

Fig. 2. An advanced ICD with an internal antenna for wireless data transmission to the patient monitor.

Data from the patient monitor is sent to a central database using either an analogue phone landline or via a GSM network. Within minutes from transmission, the processed data are accessible to the follow-up physician on a secure Internet webpage when and where he/she chooses. Available information includes all data within the device memory, which is comparable to the information provided during an in-clinic device follow-up visit. When a therapy-relevant event or device status change is detected, remote monitoring system also generates an event alert via email, SMS, or fax to the physician while simultaneously displaying the severity of alert on the internet website.

Devices with CRT-delivery have the capability to track the percentage of biventricular stimulation and several physiologically diagnostic parameters such as heart rate, heart rate variability, and patient activity. Some devices include also fluid status monitoring by assessing intrathoracic impedance. Fluid accumulation within the lungs leads to a decrease in impedance and provides an early indication of congestion. Remote monitoring system automatically generates wireless alert notification when the device detects a loss of CRT delivery or a change in hemodynamic status indicating risk for worsening heart failure.

3. Safety of remote ICD monitoring

Remote monitoring is easy to use and it provides a feasible alternative for long-term surveillance of patients with ICD. It allows the physician to view and analyze transmitted device data from any computer in a format similar to the information gathered during a typical in-clinic visit (Figure 3). In addition to the device parameters (*e.g.* battery voltage and longevity, lead impedance and trends, automatic capture thresholds) and the summary of stored ventricular and supraventricular arrhythmia episodes, the physician can also review the intracardiac electrograms of the arrhythmic events (Figure 4) and a real-time electrogram with the presenting rhythm. The information is automatically saved on the server for future comparison and analysis.

Clinical Status: Since Aug 09, 2006

Episodes		% Pacing	
VF	0	Sensed	98.4 %
FVT	4	Paced	1.6 %
VT	0		
SVT	0		
NST	45		

Observations (0)

- No observations based on currently interrogated data

ICD Status

Battery Voltage (ERI=2.62 V)	3.17 V	Dec 13, 2006
Last Full Energy Charge	7.49 sec	Oct 12, 2006
Last Capacitor Formation (Interval=Auto)		Oct 12, 2006

Lead Information

ICD	Medtronic	Marquis VR 7230	PKD610790S	May 20, 2005
RV/SVC	Medtronic	SPRINT FIDE	LFJ048743V	May 20, 2005

Lead Performance		Ventricular	
EGM Amplitude		10.3 mV	Dec 13, 2006
Pacing Impedance		408 ohms	Dec 13, 2006
Defibrillation Impedance		48 ohms	Dec 13, 2006
SVC (HVX) Impedance	63 ohms		Dec 13, 2006

Parameter Summary

Type	Detection		Rx1	Rx2	Rx3	Rx4	Rx5	Rx6
VF	On	188-500 bpm	30 J	30 J	30 J	30 J	30 J	30 J
FVT	via VF	188-250 bpm	Burst(1)	30 J	30 J	30 J	30 J	30 J
VT	On	150-188 bpm	Burst(3)	Ramp(3)	5 J	30 J	30 J	30 J

SVT Criteria On: Wavelet(Monitor)

Modes		Rates	
Mode	VVI	Lower	40 ppm

Lead Parameters	Ventricular
Amplitude	3 V
Pulse Width	0.4 ms
Sensitivity	0.3 mV

Fig. 3. Example of stored device data in the Medronic CareLink network. The patient had had 4 fast VT episodes.

Studies have shown a >90% successful transmission rate of automatically generated data collected by the device within several minutes and no direct safety issues with remote monitoring have been identified (Varma et al., 2005). It has been estimated that remote monitoring of ICD patients can potentially diagnose >99,5% of arrhythmia- and device-related problems (Heidbüchel et al., 2008). In our study physicians were satisfied with the performance of the system and found the data comparable to traditional device interrogation in the majority of the cases. In 2 of 137 cases, the physicians felt that an in-office visit would have provided more detailed information of the device function, because it was not possible to measure the pacing threshold remotely.

Remote monitoring systems do not allow remote programming of devices or manual determination of pacing thresholds. Although technically feasible, protecting patient safety is the primary concern not to enable remote programming yet. Meanwhile, most new devices have automatic features to measure pacing and sensing thresholds. The lack of possibility for remote programming appears also as an issue of minor relevance during the routine ICD follow-up. In a retrospectively analyzed data of 1739 ICD follow-up visits by Heidbüchel et al (2008), changes in device programming were made only in 4% of all scheduled follow-up visits. Likewise, problems with pacing threshold were detected only in 0,4% of the evaluations and typically in the early postoperative period. Due to the clustering of system-related complications in the early postoperative period, in-clinic visits are recommended for the post-implant and after 4-12 weeks follow-ups for patients with remote monitoring (Wilkoff et al., 2008).

4. Efficiency of remote ICD follow-up

According to the current HRS/EHRA expert consensus on the monitoring of CIEDs, patients with an ICD should be followed up in person after implantation and subsequently every 3-6 months (Wilkoff et al., 2008). More frequent monitoring may be required when the device approaches its elective replacement indicator. During the maintenance phase of follow-up and when the patient's medical condition is stable and no anticipated device programming is required, follow-ups can be accomplished remotely. It is also recommended that any patient with an ICD should be assessed in-clinic once a year.

Remote monitoring technology reduces the need for hospital visits and may facilitate, when needed, visits triggered by clinical event. It has been estimated that remote follow-up could be used to replace majority of scheduled in-clinic visits, as in only 10% of routine follow-ups does device interrogation lead to changes in medical treatment or device programming (Heidbüchel et al., 2008). Unscheduled clinic visits initiated by the patient due to perceived ICD shocks, other arrhythmic events or system related complications are actionable more often, in 40-90% of the cases. Thus, of the majority of the patient-initiated unscheduled clinic visits could be managed by remote monitoring with no need to visit the device clinic.

Our results showed that at least two out of three in-clinic visits can replaced by scheduled remote monitoring data transmission without compromising the safety of the patients (Raatikainen et al. 2008). The data from the TRUST trial demonstrated in the first prospective, randomized multicenter study that remote home monitoring with wireless automatic daily surveillance can safely and effectively replace conventional in-hospital ICD follow-up visits (Varma et al., 2010). The results showed that remote monitoring with only one scheduled annual in-clinic visit reduced the overall number of clinic visits by 45% without any negatively impact on quality of care or safety of the patients. Remote monitoring provided sufficient assessment in the majority of 3-monthly follow-ups, in 85,8% of the cases. In addition, the TRUST trial also demonstrated that automatic daily

surveillance provided early detection and notification of both symptomatic and asymptomatic arrhythmic events and device system anomalics allowing for earlier physician intervention than conventional in-hospital follow-ups. Detection was advanced by more than 30 days compared with conventional care.
According to our data the time needed by the patients for remote data transmission (6.9+3.7 min) was significantly shorter than the duration of an in-office visit, which took over six hours (391+282 min) when the travel time was included in the analysis. The average one-way distance and travel time to the hospital were 130+95 km (range 3–350) and 182+148 min (range 10–670 min), respectively. Most patients (90%) found the system convenient to use and classified the time needed for the remote data transmission for all follow-ups as very short (21%) or short (69%).

5. Workflow of the device clinic

It is obvious that remote monitoring reduces significantly the device clinic workload for routine cases by decreasing the number of non-actionable in-clinic visits. In addition, remote follow-up requires less physician and technician or nurse time than in-clinic follow-up. In an Italian study (Masella et al., 2008), remote follow-up with the CareLink system required on average 5 minutes per transmission compared with 15 minutes for in-clinic follow-up. In keeping with this, our data indicated that prescheduled data transmission significantly alleviated the time burden of the device clinic staff. In our study, two of four in-office visits were substituted by remote monitoring. As a result the physicians had at least 45 min and the nurses 90 min more time for other activities per patient during the 9-months study period, respectively (Raatikainen et al. 2008). New wireless remote monitoring systems allow automatic data transmission on a daily basis and instantaneous event transmission without any patient involvement. This permits physicians and clinic staff to focus on patients who urgently require a consultation for diagnostics or treatment.
Recently, remote monitoring with automatic data transmission has been shown to improve early detection of device malfunction and asymptomatic arrhythmias such as atrial fibrillation. On the other hand, it has been postulated that automatic transmission of all device- or therapy-related events via a fully automated wireless remote monitoring system may pose a challenge to workflow in ICD clinics. Transmitted data should be assessed in a regular timely fashion and responded to if events are observed. The remote monitoring system quickly and easily identifies patients who need immediate attention by automatically reviewing, filtering and communicating clinically relevant patient and device status data. Despite daily remote monitoring, the event alert notifications are triggered infrequently and most can be managed remotely. In the TRUST trial (Varma et al, 2010), about 90% of the alert notifications were managed remotely. Thus, replacement of routine in-clinic visits with remote monitoring only slightly raised the number of unscheduled in-clinic visits (0,7 vs. 0,5 per year). The commonest trigger for the transmission of event alert was the detection of atrial tachycardia or atrial fibrillation. In our study there were 18 unscheduled patient- or physician-initiated data transmissions during the study period. In accordance with the results of Varma et al. (2010), all of these were solved remotely and the patient did not need to come to the hospital for reassurance. An example of a symptom-initiated data transmission which was solved remotely is shown in Figure 2. Other events which have been commonly diagnosed and treated on the basis of symptom-initiated data transmissions include atrial fibrillation and "phantom" shocks.

In a study by Nielsen et al (2008), automatic wireless remote monitoring generated event notifications for 41% of ICD patients over a 10-month period. Most events caused by medical events such as arrhythmias and only about 3% of patients had technical events. Probability of any alert event after 1,5 years was 0.50. Less than one (mean of 0,86) event notifications was received per 100 patients per day. Ricci et al (2008) reported a mean time for remote data analysis of 59 min/week for the nurse and 12 min/week for the physician per 117 patient transmissions, when only 6% of events were forwarded to the physician for further evaluation. The time effort on the management of patients with remote monitoring is likely to reduce even more with the integrated automatic filtering functions.

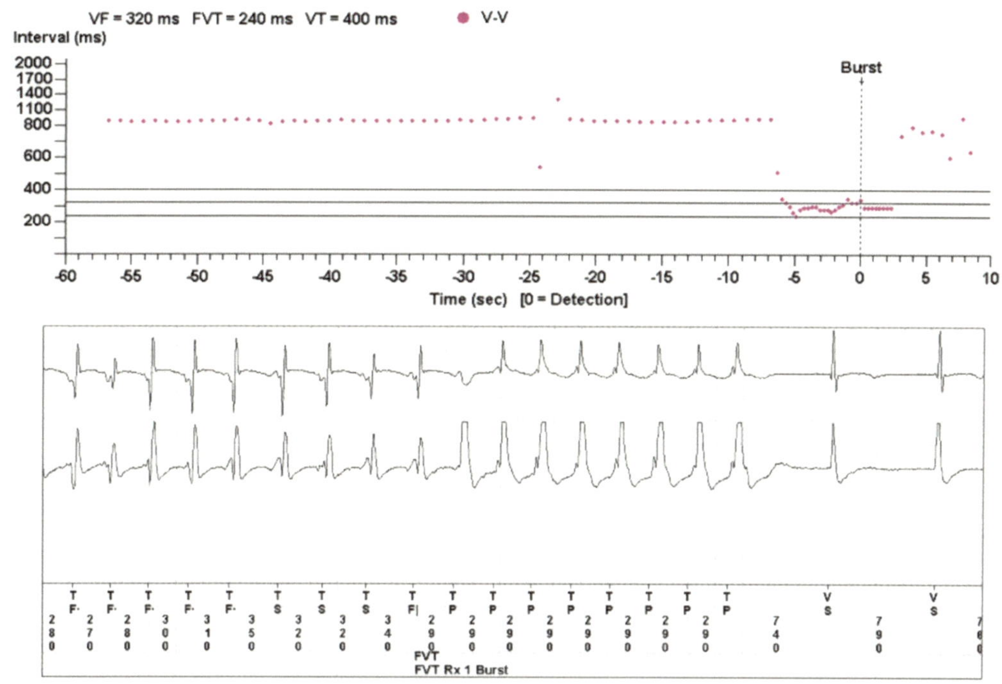

Fig. 4. Patient-initiated unscheduled data transmission. The patient had occasional palpitation about once a month. The remote data transmission revealed a fast VT episode that was appropriately treated by the device with single burst pace therapy and there were no need for an in-office visit. Shown are the interval (V–V) plot (A) and intracardiac ECG (B) obtained during the symptoms. In the more advanced systems the episode data would have been transmitted automatically.

6. Effect on patient care and safety

The information transmitted via the remote monitoring system is comparable to what is typically obtained during an in-clinic device follow-up. Hence, it provides the clinician with a comprehensive view of how the patient's heart and device are working. In addition, automatic remote monitoring early detects silent clinically relevant events and device system problems, allowing more timely treatment decisions and intervention. Earlier treatment intervention can ultimately result in improved clinical outcomes and reduce healthcare costs.

Lead failure is a long-term complication of ICD therapy. The annual rate of ICD leads requiring intervention increases with time and reaches 20% in 10-year-old leads (Kleemann et al., 2007). Inappropriate shocks due to noise oversensing are revealed as the most common presentation of lead failure. Studies have shown that early detection of lead failure by remote monitoring may reduce the risk of inappropriate ICD shocks (Hauck et al., 2009, Spencker et al., 2009). Spencker et al (2009) reported that fewer patients undergoing remote monitoring experienced ICD shocks for sensing failure prior to lead revision than those with standard in-clinic follow up. Inappropriate shocks occurred in 27,5% of the patients followed remotely compared with 46,5% of those followed up in-clinic. In 91% of all incidents, remote monitoring system transmitted an early alert message that enabled the correct diagnosis of lead failure. By accurately detecting lead failures, remote monitoring has also proven to be useful in the follow-up of ICD leads under advisory (Swerdlow et al., 2008, Theuns et al., 2009, Guédon-Moreau et al., 2010). An example of a lead problem which could actually have been detected by remote monitoring already a day before the inappropriate shock Figure 3.

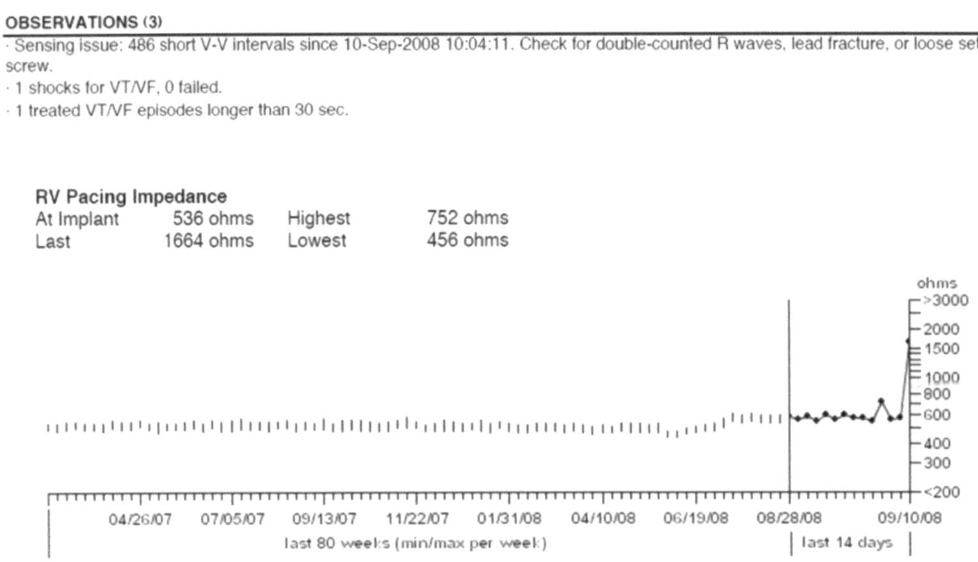

Fig. 3. Automatic data transmission showing high number of short V-V intervals suggesting double counting of R waves, lead fracture or loose set of screw. The impedance of the lead increased markedly on 09/10/08, *i.e.*, day before the patient had an inappropriate shock due to the lead fracture.

Recently the CONNECT trial for the first time showed that remote follow-up actually creates reliable outcome measures which improves care (Crossley et al., 2011). The study measured the time from an adverse event to a clinician's decision on how to handle it in patients with an ICD with or without CRT capabilities randomized to wireless remote monitoring with automatic clinician alerts versus standard in-clinic care. The results showed that remote monitoring significantly reduced the time from a clinically-actionable event to a clinical decision. The median time from a patient's clinical event (arrhythmias, cardiovascular disease progression, and device issues) to the physician's clinical decision was 22 days for those monitored in-clinic, versus 4.6 days for patients in the remote monitoring group. The data also showed that remote monitoring reduced average length of cardiovascular hospital stay by 18% (0,7 days). Due to the shorter length of stay, cardiovascular hospitalization costs were reduced by an estimated $1,793 per hospitalization. Furthermore, the data showed that replacement of routine in-clinic visits with remote monitoring did not significantly increase other healthcare utilization, such as emergency room visits, cardiovascular hospitalizations, and unscheduled clinic visits.

Type	ATP Seq	Shocks	Success	ID#	Date	Time hh:mm	Duration hh:mm:ss	Avg bpm V	Max bpm V	Activity at Onset
VF	0	35J	Yes	8	10-Sep-2008	22:22	:02:57	214	353	Active

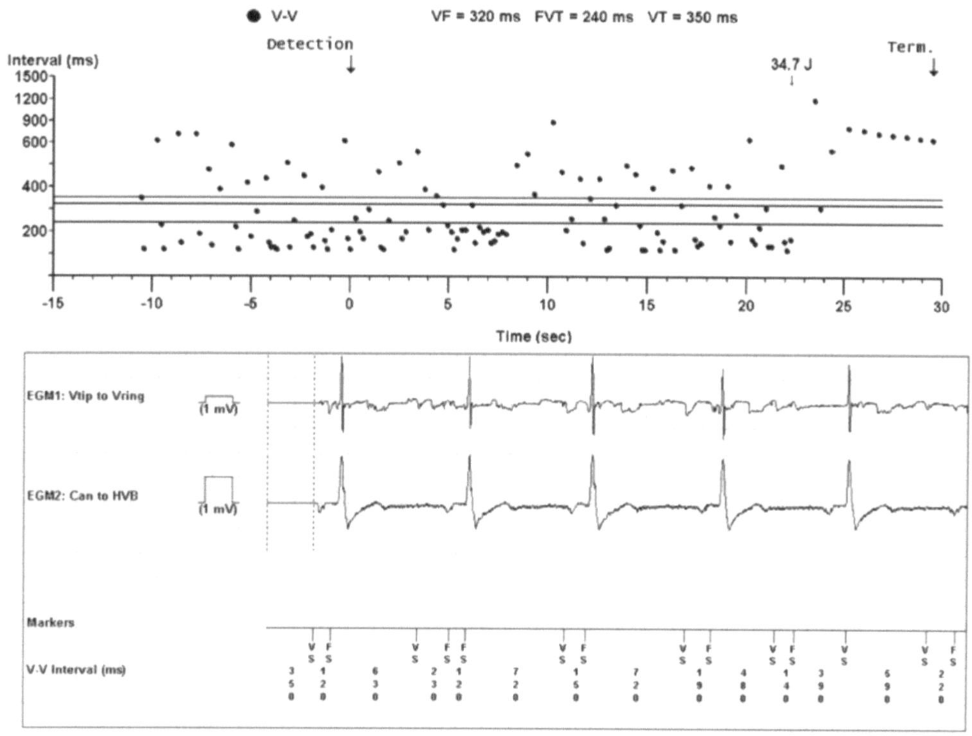

Fig. 4. Inappropriate shock due to lead fracture. Shown are the V-V interval plot and intracardiac ECG. It can be seen that the lead fracture resulted in oversensing of noise in the VT and fast VT zone which caused an inappropriate shock.

Inappropriate shocks are due to lead fracture (Figure 4.), misdiagnosis of sinus tachycardia (Figure 5.) or rapidly conducted AF/AT episodes are also a major concern among ICD recipients. Inappropriate shocks are painful for the patients and also potentially life-threatening. In a recent analysis (van Rees et al., 2011), the first inappropriate ICD shock increased the risk of death by 60%. Mortality risk increased with every subsequent shock. Detection of problems such as sinus tachycardia and T-wave oversensing through remote monitoring followed by prompt device reprogramming may prevent new episodes that could lead to inappropriate therapies (Sacher et al., 2009).

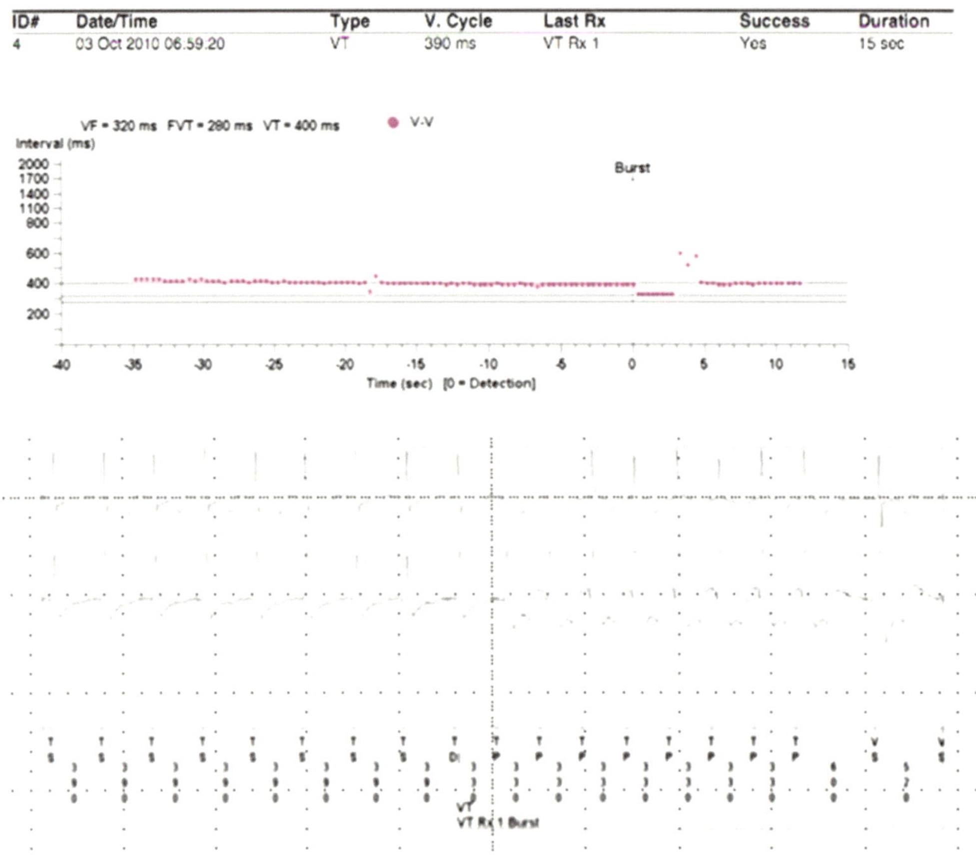

Fig. 5. Event notification via CareLink remote monitoring system. The V-V interval plot and the IEGM show inappropriate ATP-therapy delivery due sinus tachycardia. The patient was invited to device clinic for reprogramming of the device and adjustment of medication.

Several prospective randomized studies are presently underway on the clinical effectiveness of event-triggered active heart failure and AF management though remote monitoring in reducing cardiovascular related hospitalizations and mortality in patients with an ICD or a CRT-D device. In the ALTITUDE study (Saxon et al., 2010), analysis of a large manufacturer's database of ICD patients undergoing remote monitoring with LATITUDE system showed higher survival rates for patients followed remotely than those followed in-clinic only. Survival outcomes in ALTITUDE appeared also better than those observed previously in clinical trials, suggesting that closer management though remote monitoring allows to intervene more effectively with impact on survival.

An additional benefit is that remote monitoring provides convenient means to address the situation that the ICD or its leads can become subject to the an official safety advisory ("recall"). With remote monitoring, patients with advisory devices can be followed more closely, their issues addressed more promptly, and clinicians and device manufacturers get exquisitely detailed data on how the device is performing.

7. Patient preference

Several studies have shown a high degree of patient satisfaction with the convenience and ease of use of remote monitoring systems (Marzegalli et al., 2008, Masella et al., 2008, Raatikainen et al., 2008). From a patient's perspective, the biggest value of remote monitoring is convenience with fewer in-clinic visits and less time traveling to and from their clinics. Remote monitoring also leads to greater patient reassurance and improved patient follow-up adherence (Varma et al., 2010). Most patients prefer remote monitoring over in-clinic visits (Marzegalli et al., 2008, Masella et al., 2008). In TRUST trial, 98% of patients elected to retain remote monitoring as a follow-up mode on trial conclusion (Varma et al., 2010).

The current HRS/EHRA expert consensus states that remote monitoring of ICD devices is indicated when the patient's medical condition is stable and no anticipated device programming is needed (Wilkoff et al., 2008). The technology is not, however, intended to replace direct patient contacts completely. In-clinic visits are recommended for the post-implant follow-up, after 2-12 weeks and at least once a year. If the patient's cardiovascular status is unstable, in-clinic visit may be required to address the management of the underlying medical problem. The continuation of patient's clinical follow-up for the heart failure management should be ensured regardless of the place of care.

8. Cost effectiveness

As a result of expanding indication for use and complexity of the devices, the costs associated with ICD follow-up have risen sharply over the past several years. Remote monitoring may result in reduced overall costs to the healthcare system, although the cost-effectiveness will highly depend on differences in national healthcare systems. Potential cost savings of remote monitoring would include a reduced number of scheduled in-clinic visits and fewer hospitalizations due to early identification of problems followed by prompt intervention. It can be calculated that if remote monitoring were to be applied to all the patients with new ICDs, the annual saving for the healthcare system in Western Europe, would be 16–23 million Euros. In addition, remote monitoring gives physicians extra time to counsel patients with critical conditions, ensuring medical efficiency, and better overall patient management, which is expected to reduce the cost of the treatment even further.

The major indirect cost driver in the ICD follow-up is travelling to the hospital. Therefore, the greatest cost benefit is expected among patients who live far away from the device clinic and are still actively working (not retired). Several studies have evaluated the cost savings attributable to remote monitoring of ICD devices (Fauchier et al., 2005, Elsner et al., 2006, Raatikainen et al., 2008). The greatest benefit is seen among patients with long traveling distances to the device clinic. In a French study (Fauchier et al., 2005), remote monitoring appeared cost-effective for patients after a mean follow up of 33.5 months by saving on transportation costs. In our study (Raatikainen et al., 2008), replacing two scheduled routine in-clinic visits by remote monitoring reduced the total expenditure of ICD follow-up by 524€ per patient during the 9-month study period. In addition, an average of 100€ per patient was saved, because all unscheduled data transmissions during the study period were solved remotely and the patient did not need to come to the hospital for reassurance. Thus, depending on the number of unscheduled visits, it was calculated that the annual saving of remote monitoring was 524-749€ per patient (Table 2). Further prospective health economic studies are presently underway. They are aimed at assessing the economic impact of remote monitoring from the societal perspective and from the healthcare payer's perspective.

	In-clinic F-U	Remote F-U	Savings
Number of scheduled visits			
In-office visits*	164	82	
Remote data transmission**	0	82	
Direct cost			
In-office visit (210 € per visit)	34440.00 €	17220.00 €	17220.00 €
Remote monitoring (55 € per visit)	0.00 €	4510.00 €	-4510.00 €
Patient fee (22 € per in-office visit)	3608.00 €	1804.00 €	1804.00 €
Indirect cost			
Traveling (77.68 € per in-office visit)	12195.04 €	6097.52 €	6097.52 €
Accommodation (20.18 € / night)	40.36 €	20.18 €	20.18 €
Sickness allowance (44 € / day)	1672.00 €	836.00 €	880.00 €
Total costs	51955.40 €	30487.70 €	21467.70 €
Total costs per patient	1267.20 €	743.60 €	523.60 €

Table 2. Comparison between the cost of ICD follow-up according to the generally applied in-clinic follow-up scheme and remote monitoring. Adapted from Raatikainen et al. (2008).

9. Summary and future directions

In summary the major benefits of the currently available remote monitoring systems include:

- Improved quality of patient care
- Improved patient safety
- More efficient device clinic workflow
- Increased patient convenience
- Potential cost savings

The reality on the ground is that physicians should also have the ability to make adjustments to certain programmed ICD parameters remotely. As technology continues to evolve, a variety of new applications related to cardiac monitoring will emerge and an exponential growth in implementation of remote monitoring for the surveillance of a variety of devices including all new ICDs, pacemakers and other implantable disease monitors is likely to occur. Meanwhile, a wide range of medico-legal and reimbursement issues needs to be resolved before full implementation of the technology.

10. Conclusions

Remote monitoring has become the preferred method for ICD follow-up. It provides a tremendous convenience for the patients and reduces the burden of in-clinic follow-up on healthcare system. Continuous remote monitoring with fully automated wireless system also enables early detection of clinically relevant events and alerts physicians, allowing earlier medical intervention that increases the level of patient care. Despite 24/7 surveillance, the technology is not a substitute for an emergency system and should not create a false sense of complete security.

11. References

Crossley, GH., Boyle, A., Vitense, H., Chang, Y., Mead, RH. & CONNECT Investigators. The CONNECT (Clinical Evaluation of Remote Notification to Reduce Time to Clinical Decision) Trial: The Value of Wireless Remote Monitoring With Automatic Clinician Alerts. J Am Coll Cardiol 2011 57: 1181-1189.

Elsner, C., Sommer, P., Piorkowski, P., Taborsky, M., Neuser, H., Bytesnik, J., et al. A prospective multicenter comparison of Home Monitoring against regular follow-up in MADIT III patients: additional visits and cost impact. Comput Cardiol 2006;33:241-4.

Guédon-Moreau, L., Chevalier, P., Marquié, C., Kouakam, C., Klug, D., Lacroix, D., Brigadeau, F. & Kacet, S. Contributions of remote monitoring to the follow-up of implantable cardioverter–defibrillator leads under advisory. Eur Heart J (2010) 31(18): 2246-2252 .

Hauck, M., Bauer, A., Voss, F., Weretka, S., Katus, HA. & Becker, R. "Homemonitoring" for early detection of implantable cardioverter-defibrillator failure: a single-centre prospective observational study. Clin Res Cardiol. 2009 Jan;98(1):19-24. Epub 2008 Sep 5.

Heidbüchel, H., Lioen, P., Foulon, S., Huybrechts, W., Ector, J., Willems, R. & Ector, H. Potential role of remote monitoring for scheduled and unscheduled evaluations of patients with an implantable defibrillator. Europace (2008) 10(3): 351-357.

Kleemann, T., Becker, T., Doenges, K., Vater, M., Senges, J., Schneider, S., Saggau, W., Weisse, U. & Seidl, K. Annual rate of transvenous defibrillation lead defects in implan-table cardioverter-defibrillators over a period of .10 years. Circulation 2007;115: 2474 - 2480.

Marine, JE. Remote monitoring for prevention of inappropriate implantable cardioverter defibrillator shocks: is there no place like home? Europace (2009) 11(4): 409-411.

Marzegalli, M., Lunati, M., Landolina, M., Perego, GB., Ricci, RP., Guenzati, G., et al. Remote monitoring of CRT–ICD: the multicenter Italian CareLink evaluation—ease of use, acceptance, and organizational implications. Pacing Clin Electrophysiol 2008;31:1259-64.

Masella, C., Zanaboni, P., Di Stasi, F., Gilardi, S., Ponzi, P. & Valsecchi, S. Assessment of a remote monitoring system for implantable cardioverter defibrillators J Telemed Telecare 2008 14: 290-294.

Nielsen, JV., Kottkamp, H., Zabel, M., Aliot, E., Kreutzer, U., Bauer, A., Schuchert, A., Neuser, H., Schumacher, B., Schmidinger, H., Stix, G., Clémenty, J., Danilovic, D. & Hindricks, G. Automatic home monitoring of implantable cardioverter defibrillators. Europace (2008) 10(6): 729-735.

Raatikainen, MJP., Uusimaa, P., van Ginneken, MME, Janssen, JPG. & Linnaluoto, M. Remote monitoring of implantable cardioverter defibrillator patients: a safe, time-saving, and cost-effective means for follow-up. Europace (2008) 10(10): 1145-1151.

Ricci, RP., Morichelli, L. & Santini, M. Home monitoring remote control of pacemaker and implantable cardioverter defibrillator patients in clinical practice: impact on medical management and health-care resource utilization. Europace 2008;10:164–70.

Sacher, F., Probst, V., Bessouet, M., Wright, M., Maluski, A., Abbey, S., Bordachar, P., Deplagne, A., Ploux, S., Lande, G., Jaïs, P., Hocini, M., Haïssaguerre, M., Le Marec, H. & Clémenty, J. Remote implantable cardioverter defibrillator monitoring in a Brugada syndrome population. Europace (2009) 11(4): 489-494.

Saxon, LA., Hayes, DL., Gilliam, FR., Heidenreich, PA., Day, J., Seth, M., Meyer, TE., Jones, PW. & Boehmer, JP. Long-Term Outcome After ICD and CRT Implantation and Influence of Remote Device Follow-Up: The ALTITUDE Survival Study. Circulation 2010 122: 2359-2367.

Swerdlow, CD., Gunderson, BD., Ousdigian, KT., Abeyratne, A., Stadler, RW., Gillberg, JM., Patel, AS., et al. Downloadable algorithm to reduce inappropriate shocks caused by fractures of implantable cardioverter-defibrillator leads. Circulation 2008; 118:2122–2129.

Theuns, DA., Rivero-Ayerza, M., Knops, P., Res, JC. & Jordaens, L. Analysis of 57,148 transmissions by remote monitoring of implantable cardioverter defibrillators. Pacing Clin Electrophysiol 2009;32(Suppl. 1):S63 - S65.

van Rees JB., Borleffs, CJ., de Bie, MK., Stijnen, T., van Erven, L., Bax, JJ. & Schalij, MJ. Inappropriate Implantable Cardioverter-Defibrillator Shocks: Incidence, Predictors, and Impact on Mortality. J Am Coll Cardiol. 2011 Feb 1;57(5):556-62.

Varma, N., Epstein, AE., Irimpen, A., Schweikert, R., Love, C. and for the TRUST Investigators. Efficacy and Safety of Automatic Remote Monitoring for Implantable Cardioverter-Defibrillator Follow-Up: The Lumos-T Safely Reduces Routine Office Device Follow-Up (TRUST) Trial. Circulation 2010 122: 325-332.

Varma, N., Stambler, B. & Chun, S. Detection of atrial fibrillation by implanted devices with wireless data transmission capability. Pacing Clin Electrophysiol. 2005 Jan;28 Suppl 1:S133-6.

Wilkoff, BL,, Auricchio, A., Brugada, J., Cowie, M., Ellenbogen, KA., Gillis, AM., et al. HRS/EHRA expert consensus on the monitoring of cardiovascular implantable electronic devices (CIEDs). Europace 2008;10:707–25.